Updates in Pancreatic Endotherapy

Editors

DUVVUR NAGESHWAR REDDY
RUPJYOTI TALUKDAR

GASTROINTESTINAL ENDOSCOPY CLINICS OF NORTH AMERICA

www.giendo.theclinics.com

Consulting Editor
CHARLES J. LIGHTDALE

October 2023 • Volume 33 • Number 4

ELSEVIER

1600 John F. Kennedy Boulevard • Suite 1800 • Philadelphia, Pennsylvania, 19103-2899

http://www.theclinics.com

GASTROINTESTINAL ENDOSCOPY CLINICS OF NORTH AMERICA Volume 33, Number 4
October 2023 ISSN 1052-5157, ISBN-13: 978-0-443-18362-1

Editor: Kerry Holland
Developmental Editor: Isha Singh

Gastrointestinal Endoscopy Clinics of North America (ISSN 1052-5157) is published quarterly by Elsevier Inc., 360 Park Avenue South, New York, NY 10010-1710. Months of issue are January, April, July, and October. Business and Editorial Offices: 1600 John F. Kennedy Blvd., Suite 1800, Philadelphia, PA, 19103-2899. Periodicals postage paid at New York, NY and additional mailing offices. Subscription prices are $381.00 per year for US individuals, $703.00 per year for US institutions, $100.00 per year for US and Canadian students/residents, $419.00 per year for Canadian individuals, $830.00 per year for Canadian institutions, $501.00 per year for international individuals, $830.00 per year for international institutions, and $245.00 per year for international students/residents. To receive student/resident rate, orders must be accompanied by name of affiliated institution, date of term, and the *signature* of program/residency coordinator on institution letterhead. Orders will be billed at individual rate until proof of status is received. Foreign air speed delivery is included in all *Clinics* subscription prices. All prices are subject to change without notice. **POSTMASTER:** Send address change to *Gastrointestinal Endoscopy Clinics of North America*, Elsevier Health Sciences Division, Subscription Customer Service, 3251 Riverport Lane, Maryland Heights, MO 63043. **Customer Service: 1-800-654-2452 (US). From outside the United States, call 1-314-447-8871. Fax: 1-314-447-8029. E-mail: JournalsCustomerService-usa@elsevier.com (for print support) or JournalsOnlineSupport-usa@elsevier.com (for online support).**

Reprints. For copies of 100 or more, of articles in this publication, please contact the Commercial Reprints Department, Elsevier Inc., 360 Park Avenue South, New York, NY 10010-1710. Tel. 212-633-3874; Fax: 212-633-3820; E-mail: reprints@elsevier.com.

Gastrointestinal Endoscopy Clinics of North America is covered in *Excerpta Medica, MEDLINE/PubMed (Index Medicus), and MEDLINE/MEDLARS.*

Contributors

CONSULTING EDITOR

CHARLES J. LIGHTDALE, MD
Professor of Medicine, Division of Digestive and Liver Diseases, Columbia University Medical Center, New York, New York, USA

EDITORS

DUVVUR NAGESHWAR REDDY, MD, DM, DSc, AGAF, FRCP, FACG, MWGO, FAAAS
Chairman and Chief of Gastroenterology, Consultant Gastroenterologist, Asian Institute of Gastroenterology Hospitals, Hyderabad, Telangana, India

RUPJYOTI TALUKDAR, MD, FICP, AGAF, FISG, FRCP, FRSB
Director, Pancreatology, Clinician Scientist, Asian Institute of Gastroenterology Hospitals, Wellcome DBT India Alliance Labs, Translational Research Center, Head, Pancreas Research Group and Division of Gut Microbiome Research, Asian Healthcare Foundation, Hyderabad, Telangana, India

AUTHORS

VENKATA S. AKSHINTALA, MD
Division of Gastroenterology, Johns Hopkins Medical Institutions, Baltimore, Maryland, USA

TODD H. BARON, MD
Professor of Medicine, Division of Gastroenterology and Hepatology, The University of North Carolina at Chapel Hill, Chapel Hill, North Carolina, USA

JAHANGEER BASHA, MD, DM
Department of Gastroenterology, Asian Institute of Gastroenterology, AIG Hospitals, Hyderabad, Telangana, India

TORSTEN BEYNA, PD, Dr med
Chief of Department of Internal Medicine, Gastroenterology, Therapeutic Endoscopy, Medical Oncology, Pulmonology and Nephrology, Evangelisches Krankenhaus Duesseldorf, Duesseldorf, North Rhine-Westphalia, Germany

MARCO J. BRUNO, MD, PhD
Department of Gastroenterology and Hepatology, Erasmus University Medical Center, Rotterdam, the Netherlands

SUNG HYUN CHO, MD
Department of Gastroenterology, Asan Medical Center, University of Ulsan College of Medicine, Seoul, South Korea

GUIDO COSTAMAGNA, MD
Department of Translational Medicine and Surgery, Catholic University, Italy, Rome

GREGORY A. COTE, MD, MS
Professor of Medicine, Division of Gastroenterology, Oregon Health & Science University, Portland, Oregon, USA

YONGYAN CUI, MD
Department of Gastroenterology, Advanced Endoscopy Fellow, Virginia Mason Medical Center, Seattle, Washington

JACQUES DEVIÈRE, MD, PhD
Professor of Medicine, Department of Gastroenterology, Hepatopancreatology and Digestive Oncology, Erasme Hospital, Université Libre de Bruxelles, Brussels, Belgium

PRAMOD KUMAR GARG, MD, DM
Professor, Department of Gastroenterology, All India Institute of Medical Sciences, New Delhi, India

CHRISTIAN GERGES, Dr med
Chief of Department of Interventional Gastrointestinal Endoscopy, University Hospital Essen, Essen, North Rhine-Westphalia, Germany

ANDREW J. GILMAN, MD
Assistant Professor of Medicine, Division of Gastroenterology and Hepatology, The University of North Carolina at Chapel Hill, Chapel Hill, North Carolina, USA

MARC GIOVANNINI
Head of the Endoscopy Department, Paoli-Calmettes Institute, Marseille, France

SUMANT INAMDAR, MD, MPH
Associate Professor of Medicine, Division of Gastroenterology and Hepatology, Department of Medicine, University of Arkansas for Medical Sciences, Little Rock, Arkansas, USA

RICHARD A. KOZAREK, MD
Department of Gastroenterology, Emeritus Director of The Digestive Disease Institute at Virginia Mason Medical Center, Clinical Professor of Medicine, University of Washington, Seattle, Washington

SUNDEEP LAKHTAKIA, MD, DM
Department of Gastroenterology, Asian Institute of Gastroenterology, AIG Hospitals, Hyderabad, Telangana, India

SOUMYA JAGANNATH MAHAPATRA, MD, DM
Department of Gastroenterology, All India Institute of Medical Sciences, New Delhi, India

MARIOLA MARX
Unit of Hepato-Gastroenterology, CHUV, Lausanne, Switzerland

HORST NEUHAUS, Dr med
Professor Senior Consultant Gastroenterologist, RKM 740 Clinic, Duesseldorf, North Rhine-Westphalia, Germany

PARTHA PAL, MD, DNB, MRCP (UK)
Consultant Gastroenterologist, Department of Medical Gastroenterology, Asian Institute of Gastroenterology, Hyderabad, Telangana, India

MOHAN RAMCHANDANI, MD, DM
Department of Medical Gastroenterology, Asian Institute of Gastroenterology, Director, Interventional Endoscopy, AIG Hospitals, Hyderabad, Telangana, India

DUVVUR NAGESHWAR REDDY, MD, DM, DSc, AGAF, FRCP, FACG, MWGO, FAAAS
Chairman and Chief of Gastroenterology, Consultant Gastroenterologist, Asian Institute of Gastroenterology Hospitals, Hyderabad, Telangana, India

DONG-WAN SEO, MD, PhD
Department of Gastroenterology, Asan Medical Center, University of Ulsan College of Medicine, Seoul, South Korea

VIKESH K. SINGH, MD, MSc
Division of Gastroenterology, Johns Hopkins Medical Institutions, Baltimore, Maryland, USA

MANU TANDAN, MD, DM
Director, Asian Institute of Gastroenterology, Hyderabad, Telangana, India

SHYAM VARADARAJULU, MD
Center for Advanced Endoscopy, Research and Education, Orlando Health Digestive Health Institute, Orlando, Florida, USA

PHILIPPE WILLEMS, MD
Center for Advanced Endoscopy, Research and Education, Orlando Health Digestive Health Institute, Orlando, Florida, USA

DHIRAJ YADAV, MD, MPH
Professor of Medicine, Division of Gastroenterology, Hepatology and Nutrition, University of Pittsburg Medical Center, Pittsburgh, Pennsylvania, USA

Contents

In the last half century, endotherapy for pancreatic diseases has changed considerably. Although endoscopic retrograde cholangiopancreatography (ERCP) and endoscopic ultrasound (EUS) were introduced initially as diagnostic tools, they quickly evolved into therapeutic tools for preventing and managing complications of pancreatitis. More recently, therapeutic endoscopy has shown potential in palliation and cure of pancreatic neoplasms. This article discusses the changing landscape of pancreatic endotherapy as therapeutic ERCP and EUS were introduced and because they have evolved to treat different diseases.

The root cause for biliary pancreatitis is a transient impediment of the outflow of secretion from the pancreatic duct due to gallstones and sludge obstructing the ampulla of Vater. Based on meta-analyses and recent studies, clear recommendations can be formulated when and when not to perform an ERC in patients with biliary pancreatitis. ERC is indicated urgently in patients with biliary pancreatitis and concomitant cholangitis. Urgent ERC is not indicated in patients with predicted mild or severe biliary pancreatitis without cholangitis, even when stones or sludge are proven on EUS imaging.

 Video content accompanies this article at http://www.giendo. theclinics.com.

The management of walled-off necrosis has evolved substantially over the past 23 years since its first description. In this article, we review its history and the evidence supporting modern treatment, which is still subject to heterogeneity across centers and among endoscopists. This allows for creativity and customization of what can be an endoscopic marathon. Our typical practice is discussed with image and video guides aimed at improving procedure success.

Walled-off necrosis is a well-recognized complication of necrotizing pancreatitis that can cause sepsis, luminal or ductal obstruction, or persistent unwellness requiring multidisciplinary care. Recent data suggest that minimally invasive endoscopic treatment strategies are preferred over more invasive surgical approaches. Although endoscopic transmural drainage with or without necrosectomy is the primary approach for patients requiring an intervention, for collections not amenable to endoscopic approach, percutaneous drain placement followed by video-assisted retroperitoneal debridement or laparoscopic cystogastrostomy with internal debridement are other alternatives. More studies are required to optimize post-procedure care to shorten the length of stay and minimize resource utilization.

 Video content accompanies this article at http://www.giendo.theclinics.com.

Patients with acute pancreatitis might develop infected necrotic fluid collections which are associated with significant morbidity and mortality. Patients with infected necrotizing pancreatitis not responding to antibiotics require drainage and subsequent necrosectomy (Step-up approach). Percutaneous endoscopic necrosectomy (PEN) has evolved as a minimally invasive approach for necrosectomy through the percutaneous catheter route using a flexible endoscope and can be done under conscious sedation. It is best suited for predominantly laterally placed infected necrotic fluid collections and also can be performed at the bedside for sick patients admitted to an ICU. PEN has a clinical success rate of 80% with minimal adverse events.

Disconnected pancreatic duct (DPD) is common after acute necrotizing pancreatitis (ANP). Its clinical implications vary according to the course of disease. In the early phase of ANP, parenchymal necrosis along with disruption of pancreatic duct cause acute necrotic collection that evolves into walled-off necrosis (WON). In the later phase, DPD becomes evident as confirmed by magnetic resonance cholangiopancreatography. Clinical manifestations of DPD can vary from being asymptomatic, recurrent pain, recurrent pancreatic fluid collection (PFC), obstructive pancreatitis, or external pancreatic fistula (EPF). Few patients develop new-onset diabetes. Long-term indwelling plastic stents have been proposed to prevent the recurrent PFC.

effective, and should be regarded as an alternative endoscopic treatment of certain patients.

Endoscopic therapy is the first line of management for chronic pancreatitis (CP)-related benign biliary strictures. Multiple plastic stents (MPS) exchanged at regular intervals and temporary placement of fully covered self-expanding metal stents (FCSEMS) are preferred modalities of endotherapy. FCSEMS placement is non-inferior to MPS and requires fewer sessions of endoscopic retrograde cholangiopancreatography than MPS placement. The presence of head calcifications, severe CP, and length of stricture are predictors of failure or recurrence after endotherapy. Failure of endotherapy should be considered after 1 year when surgery should be considered.

Endoscopic ultrasound (EUS)-guided pancreatic duct drainage is one of the most challenging procedures in therapeutic endoscopy. Technical success is lower than for other therapeutic EUS procedures. However, when successful in a clear clinical indication, this procedure can offer a useful therapeutic alternative and improves the overall clinical success of the endoscopic approach. Current challenges include the standardization of clinical indications and of the techniques used for accessing the pancreatic duct, the strategy for mid-term and long-term management, and definition of the scope of the training that should be offered to a few highly experienced endoscopists.

Today, endoscopic ultrasound-guided radiofrequency ablation has become increasingly accepted for the treatment of different precancerous and neoplastic lesions of the pancreas, particularly in patients who are unfit for surgery. However, thermal ablation has long been suspected to induce pancreatitis or to injure adjacent structures. Published case reports and case series on this topic are of limited size and are often based on a heterogeneous study population, reporting on functional and nonfunctional pancreatic neuroendocrine tumors. Nevertheless, the overall results are promising, with high technical success and relatively low complication rates.

During the past two decades, there has been a significant evolution in endoscopic interventions in pancreatic cystic neoplasms (PCNs), ranging from diagnostic intervention (endoscopic ultrasound-guided through-the-needle biopsy [EUS-TTNB]) to therapeutic intervention (endoscopic ultrasound-guided pancreatic cystic ablation [EUS-PCA]). They have re-ceived attention as alternatives to conventional diagnostic and therapeutic modalities. EUS-TTNB can categorize PCN types accurately by providing histologic diagnoses that conventional diagnostic modalities cannot pro-vide. As pancreatectomy entails high morbidities, EUS-PCA can be per-formed safely to treat PCNs in patients who refuse surgery or have high surgical risks.

GASTROINTESTINAL ENDOSCOPY CLINICS OF NORTH AMERICA

SERIES OF RELATED INTEREST

Gastroenterology Clinics
(www.gastro.theclinics.com)
Clinics in Liver Disease
(www.liver.theclinics.com)

THE CLINICS ARE AVAILABLE ONLINE!
Access your subscription at:
www.theclinics.com

Foreword

Pancreatic Endotherapy: An Amazing Evolution

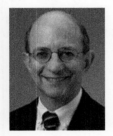

Charles J. Lightdale, MD
Consulting Editor

The stories are many of the progression of gastrointestinal endoscopy procedures from primarily diagnostic to therapeutic, but arguably the most exciting and disruptive story is that of pancreatic endotherapy. The story begins almost 50 years ago with the development of endoscopic retrograde cholangiopancreatography (ERCP), combining side-viewing duodenoscopes with x-ray fluoroscopy to visualize the biliary and pancreatic ductal systems. Some 10 years later came endoscopic ultrasonography (EUS), combining a side-viewing endoscope with a linear ultrasound transducer at the tip, producing an ultrasound beam parallel to the operating channel. EUS provided exquisitely detailed images of the entire pancreas and surrounding structures through the stomach and duodenum and allowed through-the-scope needles for tissue acquisition, and then guide wires, stents, and other devices for endotherapy.

The apocryphal advice to mid-twentieth century house staff fresh from medical school can be shortened to: "eat when you can, sleep when you can, and don't mess with the pancreas." The skilled and courageous interventional endoscopists who continue to develop pancreatic endotherapy using ERCP and EUS have brushed past this warning, replacing many more invasive surgical or interventional radiology procedures to the great benefit of patients. The Editors for this issue of the *Gastrointestinal Endoscopy Clinics of North America* are the world-famous Dr Nageshwar Reddy and Dr Rupjyoti Talukdar. They have assembled an over-the-top group of international expert authors detailing the amazing evolution of pancreatic endotherapy, the state-of-the-art, and visions of the future. This is an issue to be

Gastrointest Endoscopy Clin N Am 33 (2023) xiii–xiv
https://doi.org/10.1016/j.giec.2023.06.001
1052-5157/23/© 2023 Published by Elsevier Inc.

giendo.theclinics.com

treasured by all gastrointestinal endoscopists, especially by interventional endoscopists and those training in advanced endoscopy.

Charles J. Lightdale, MD
Department of Medicine
Columbia University Medical Center
161 Fort Washington Avenue
New York, NY 10032, USA

E-mail address:
CJL18@columbia.edu

Preface

Pancreatic Interventions: From the Quill to the Sonar

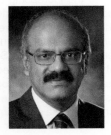
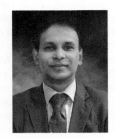

Duvvur Nageshwar Reddy, MD, DM, DSc   Rupjyoti Talukdar, MD, FRCP
Editors

Pancreatic ductal interventions have come a long way since the first canulation of a dog's pancreatic duct using the hollow quill of a goose feather by the Dutch medical student Reignier de Graff in 1663. Even though the initial endoscopic pancreatic ductal interventions were meant for diagnostic purposes, over the years these techniques have evolved with a therapeutic intent. Development of novel concepts has resulted in evolution of innovative techniques, aided by better imaging and instrumentation, and sustained by the courage of endoscopists. These factors have largely shifted the domain of pancreatic interventions from the surgeons to the endoscopists.

The evolution of instrumentation and pancreatic endoscopic intervention has been rapid. For instance, while it was in 1968 when McCune reported the first canulation of the ampulla with a fiberoptic duodenoscopy, 1974 saw the first endoscopic sphincterotomy with a side-viewing duodenoscope having a working channel and an elevator. Just 4 years later, in 1978, the first minor papilla sphincterotomy was conducted to treat pancreatitis in a patient with pancreas divisum. Eventually, pancreatic intervention progressed to endoscopic transmural drainage of pseudocysts in the mid-1970s, which was followed by direct endoscopic necrosectomy. Over time, pancreatic endotherapy was combined with extracorporeal shock wave lithotripsy, electrohydraulic lithotripsy, and laser lithotripsy in the treatment of pancreatic ductal stones.

Another development that has happened in parallel to the endoscopic techniques was the evolution of stent technology. The use of plastic stents appears to be rapidly superseded by metal stents in the management of pancreatic collections and biliary strictures related to pancreatic pathologies. Although a few stent designs could not pass the test of time, several others have shown promise and are on the path of evolution.

Gastrointest Endoscopy Clin N Am 33 (2023) xv–xvi
https://doi.org/10.1016/j.giec.2023.05.002
1052-5157/23/© 2023 Published by Elsevier Inc.

While endoscopic retrograde cholangiopancreatography (ERCP) has shifted from being a diagnostic modality to a therapeutic one, the advent of therapeutic endoscopic ultrasound (EUS) has revolutionized endotherapy for pancreatic diseases altogether. EUS has changed the approach to drainage of pancreatic collection alone or in combination with other modalities. EUS have also found indications in the palliative management of pancreatic neoplastic lesions. The other exciting area where EUS is being increasingly utilized is the access to the pancreatobiliary system in situations where conventional ERCP has failed. In view of the increasing utility, it won't be surprising if EUS-guided pancreatobiliary access becomes a primetime approach in the management of pancreatic diseases in the foreseeable future.

The rapid development and utilization of pancreatic endoscopic techniques and technologies do warrant a few concerns. Many of the recently developing EUS-based techniques require standardization and possibly do not have the best dedicated instrumentation. Added to this is the increasing number of gastroenterology and advanced endoscopy fellows who demonstrate keenness on practicing the newer techniques. These techniques demand a steep learning curve across a substantial volume of patients. These factors therefore naturally come with a concern for patient safety and requirement of regulations.

Based on the above premises, we felt the need for an updated discussion on the various aspects of pancreatic endotherapy from its evolution to the most recent developments. This culminated in the current issue of the *Gastrointestinal Endoscopy Clinics of North America*, wherein we attempted to bring together the best minds in the aforementioned subspecialties of pancreatic endotherapy to share the current evidence, their expertise, and vision.

Duvvur Nageshwar Reddy, MD, DM, DSc
Asian Institute of Gastroenterology Hospitals
Mindspace Road, Gachibowli
Hyderabad 500032, Telangana, India

Rupjyoti Talukdar, MD, FRCP
Pancreatology
Asian Institute of Gastroenterology Hospitals
Wellcome DBT India Alliance Labs
Translational Research Center
Division of Gut Microbiome Research
Asian Healthcare Foundation
Mindspace Road, Gachibowli
Hyderabad 500032, Telangana, India

E-mail addresses:
aigindia@yahoo.co.in (D.N. Reddy)
rup_talukdar@yahoo.com; rupppp@gmail.com (R. Talukdar)

Evolution of Pancreatic Endotherapy

YongYan Cui, MD, Richard A. Kozarek, MD*

KEYWORDS

- Pancreatic endotherapy
- Therapeutic endoscopic retrograde cholangiopancreatograhy
- Therapeutic endoscopic ultrasound • Pancreatic pseudocyst • Walled-off necrosis
- Pancreatic strictures • Pancreatic calculi

KEY POINTS

- Therapeutic endoscopic retrograde cholangiopancreatography (ERCP) and EUS are important tools for managing complications of pancreatitis and have significantly reduced the need for surgery.
- ERCP with transpapillary stenting remains key to managing pancreatic duct leaks. However, in more complex cases, therapeutic EUS or a multidisciplinary approach with interventional radiology can be helpful.
- EUS-guided antitumor therapy remains investigational, although shows potential in palliation and cure of pancreatic neoplasms.

INTRODUCTION

The pancreas was described circa 300 BC by the Greek physician Herophilus of Chalcedon during his decades of scientific dissections of human cadavers.[1,2] The organ was named circa 100 AD by Rufus of Ephesus from the Greek words *pan*, "all" and *kreas*, "flesh." It was not until the nineteenth century that physiologists began to recognize the pancreas' role in digestion and physicians began to describe pancreatic diseases. Microscopically verified cases of pancreatic adenocarcinoma were reported as early as 1858 and by the end of the nineteenth century, the signs and symptoms of cancer at the head of the pancreas were well known. In 1889, Mering and Minkowski found that extirpation of the pancreas in dogs caused glycosuria and diabetes. That same year, Fitz characterized the signs, symptoms, and complications of acute pancreatitis, thus establishing it as a disease entity.[1]

For more than a century, the treatment of pancreatic diseases fell almost exclusively within the purview of surgeons. In 1841, Wandesleben performed a pseudocyst drainage—the first documented pancreatic surgery. By 1867, Lucke reported the first

Department of Gastroenterology, Virginia Mason Medical Center
* Corresponding author. 1100 Ninth Avenue C3-Gas, Seattle, WA 98101.
E-mail address: Richard.kozarek@virginiamason.org

Gastrointest Endoscopy Clin N Am 33 (2023) 679–700
https://doi.org/10.1016/j.giec.2023.03.012
1052-5157/23/© 2023 Elsevier Inc. All rights reserved.

successful resection of a pancreatic cystic tumor. In the late nineteenth century, surgeons began debating the management of acute pancreatitis—whether conservative versus surgical treatment and furthermore whether early versus late surgery was favorable. Surgery prevailed as the treatment of choice until 1927 when the discovery of serum amylase revealed milder forms of pancreatitis that could respond to nonoperative therapy. This discovery, along with the recognition that surgical mortality rates were as high as 50% to 78%, shifted the treatment paradigm to a more conservative approach. In the 1960s, surgeons again began advocating for extensive pancreatic resections for patients with severe acute pancreatitis who had high mortality rates with medical treatment alone.[3,4] In recent decades, the pendulum swings of pancreatitis management have been less extreme.

As medical technology has expanded, so too have new treatments for pancreatic diseases. Although endoscopic retrograde cholangiopancreatography (ERCP) and endoscopic ultrasound (EUS) were introduced initially as diagnostic tools, they quickly evolved into therapeutic tools for treating pancreatic diseases. As such, in recent decades, gastroenterologists have had an increasingly important role in managing pancreatic diseases. The current article discusses the changing landscape of pancreatic endotherapy because therapeutic ERCP and EUS were introduced and because they have evolved to treat different diseases.

Endotherapy for Etiologies of Pancreatitis

In 1968, McCune reported the first endoscopic cannulation of the ampulla of Vater in living patients (**Table 1**). He used a fiberoptic duodenoscope and taped a small tube to the scope that allowed passage of a cannula that could be maneuvered into the ampulla. Citing a 25% cannulation rate and difficulty positioning the scope in the duodenum, McCune recognized the need for improved endoscopic instruments.[5] The following year, Oi helped develop a side-viewing duodenoscope that included a working channel with an elevator that improved manipulation of the cannula and presented the first ERCP at an international conference.[6] During the next few years, increased experience with ERCP led to higher cannulation rates, reported between 74% and 96%.[7] Finally in 1974, the first endoscopic sphincterotomy (ES) was performed, thus marking the beginning of therapeutic ERCP.[8]

Gallstone pancreatitis

Opie postulated in 1901 that gallstones that migrated and became impacted in the distal common bile duct (CBD) could impair pancreatic duct (PD) secretions, cause bile reflux into the PD, and lead to pancreatic inflammation.[9] However, it was not until the 1950s that biliary stone disease became widely recognized as a common cause of pancreatitis.[10] For decades, abdominal exploration with choledochotomy was the standard treatment of CBD stones.[11] After ERCP with ES was introduced, it was used in conjunction with nasobiliary catheters, biliary stents, balloons, and mechanical lithotripsy and became the procedure of choice for choledocholithiasis after cholecystectomy.[8]

Recurrent acute pancreatitis

With the widespread use of ERCP, anomalies of the PD were increasingly recognized as possible causes of recurrent acute pancreatitis (RAP). For the next 2 decades, an abundance of literature exploring the use of ES and endoprosthesis for management of these conditions emerged. These have been described below.

Pancreas divisum. Pancreas divisum is a common anatomic variant in which the pancreatic buds fail to fuse in utero, resulting in predominant drainage of pancreatic

Table 1
Timelines in pancreatic endotherapy

	Author, Year, and Reference
Pancreas divisum	
Minor papilla sphincterotomy to treat RAP in pancreas divisum	Cotton,[13] 1978
Minor papilla stents to treat RAP in pancreas divisum	McCarthy et al,[16] 1988
Choledocholcele	
Endoscopic snare removal of choledochocele	Deyhle et al,[19] 1974
Endoscopic sphincterotomy of choledochocele	Siegel,[20] 1981
Sphincter of Oddi disorder	
RCT demonstrating lack of efficacy of endoscopic sphincterotomy for type III SOD	Cotton et al,[24] 2014
Pancreatic pseudocyst	
Endoscopic transgastric needle aspiration of pseudocyst	Rogers,[31] 1975
Endoscopic cystoenterostomy via conventional transmural drainage	Kozarek et al,[33] 1985
Endoscopic cystoenterostomy with nasocystic drain left for irrigation	Sahel et al,[34] 1987
EUS-guided pseudocyst drainage	Wiersema,[40] 1996
Fully covered self-expanding stents used for pseudocyst drainage	Talreja et al,[42] 2008
Lumen-apposing metal stents invented	Binmoeller,[43] 2004
Cautery-enhanced lumen-apposing metal stents introduced	Teoh,[44] 2014
Walled-off necrosis	
Endoscopic drainage of walled-off necrosis	Baron et al,[47] 1996
Direct endoscopic necrosectomy	Seifert et al,[49] 2009
RCT demonstrating (1) low mortality rates with conservative management, (2) superiority of step-up therapy compared to surgical open necrosectomy for infected walled-off necrosis or peripancreatic necrosis	van Santvoort et al,[50] 2011
Dual-modality drainage	Ross et al,[52] 2014
Pancreatic duct leaks and disconnected duct syndrome	
Transpapillary drains or stents used to treat:	
Pancreatic duct leaks, some complicated by pancreatic fluid collections	Kozarek et al,[54] 1991
Pancreatic duct leaks complicated by ascites	Kozarek,[55] 1992
Pancreatic duct leaks complicated by pancreaticoenteric fistulae	Wolfsen et al,[56] 1992
Pancreatic duct leaks complicated by external pancreatic fistulae	Kozarek et al,[57] 1997
Disconnected duct syndrome managed with:	
Combination of transpapillary drainage, cystenterostomy, or nasocystic catheter	Deviere et al,[60] 1995
1. Outside-in technique 2. EUS-guided pancreaticobulbostomy	Arvanitakis et al,[61] 2007

(continued on next page)

Table 1
(*continued*)

	Author, Year, and Reference
1. Inside-out technique	Irani et al,[62] 2012
2. Reconnecting disconnected ducts	
Pancreatic calculi	
ERCP with basket stone retrieval	Inui et al,[63] 1983
ERCP with pancreatic sphincterotomy, stenting, pancreatoscopy with basket stone retrieval	Fuji et al,[64] 1985
Extracorporeal shock wave lithotripsy with ERCP	Sauerbruch et al,[66] 1987
ERCP with electrohydraulic lithotripsy	Howell et al,[72] 1999
Pancreatic duct strictures	
Retrospective study describing pancreatic stent placement associated with ductal changes, including stenoses	Kozarek,[39] 1990
Prospective study demonstrating efficacy of multi-stent placement for strictures refractory to single-stent placement	Costamagna,[76] 2006
EUS-guided pancreaticogastrostomy	Francois et al,[80] 2002
Celiac plexus block and neurolysis	
EUS-guided celiac plexus neurolysis	Wiersema & Wiersema,[83] 1996

fluid through the minor papilla.[12] Although most patients are asymptomatic, studies have shown that pancreas divisum is more prevalent in cases of unexplained RAP,[12,13] which may be due to increased intraductal pressures caused by minor papilla stenosis.[12] In 1978, Cotton performed the first minor papilla sphincterotomy to treat pancreatitis in patients with pancreas divisum.[13] Subsequent studies reported that patients with RAP who had pancreas divisum had fewer episodes of pancreatitis, fewer hospitalizations, and improvement in pain after minor papilla sphincterotomy.[14,15] In 1988, McCarthy and colleagues published the first experience of placing PD stents across the minor papilla in pancreas divisum with RAP and found that this was associated with fewer pancreatitis flares.[16] The efficacy of these interventions suggests that, at least in a subset of patients with pancreas divisum, endotherapy aimed at improving flow across the minor papilla is beneficial. However, randomized prospective trials aimed at delineating the effect of ES on pancreas divisum have been challenging to execute.[17] Thus, controversy remains about whether and which these patients benefit from pancreatic endotherapy with ES and stenting.

Choledochocele. In 1915, Wheeler first described a choledochocele after performing an exploratory laparotomy for workup of jaundice and discovering a small cyst at the orifice of the CBD.[18] Since that time, choledochoceles have been defined as cystic dilations of the intraduodenal portion of the distal CBD and have been distinguished from duodenal duplication cysts as having direct communication to the CBD, lack of fusion with the duodenal wall, and lack of a muscle layer beyond the muscularis mucosa.[18] Also known as type III choledochal cysts, choledochoceles have been associated with RAP.

Choledochoceles were previously treated surgically with excision or sphincteroplasty. However, the advent of ERCP has obviated surgery. Endoscopic removal of a choledochocele was documented as early as 1974, and the first use of ES for treatment was reported in 1981.[19,20] In 1992, a case series reported 7 patients with choledochoceles and RAP who underwent ES with complete resolution of symptoms.[21] Since that time, ES has remained primary treatment of choledochoceles.

Papillary stenosis and Sphincter of Oddi disorder. In 1887, Oddi described the anatomy of the muscle at the papilla of Vater and thereafter suggested that contraction of this muscle could lead to jaundice.[22] In the early 1900s, there was increasing recognition that Sphincter of Oddi (SO) abnormalities were associated with clinical presentations involving recurrent abdominal pain, elevated liver function tests, or even RAP.[1,22,23] With ERCP, sphincter of Oddi manometry (SOM) became a nonsurgical possibility and was reported as early as 1975.[24] The increasing use of SOM helped define parameters of normal transpapillary pressures and identify sphincter of Oddi disorders (SODs).

For the next few decades, ERCP was used to diagnose and treat SODs. In 2004, a review on SOD found that patients with papillary stenosis benefitted most consistently from ERCP with ES.[25,26] ERCP has been less beneficial in other SODs. In a landmark trial, Cotton and colleagues investigated patients with pancreaticobiliary-type pain after cholecystectomy who did not have significant laboratory or imaging findings. In this multicenter trial, patients were randomized to sphincterotomy versus sham. Patients in the sphincterotomy group with elevated pancreatic sphincter pressures were further randomized to biliary sphincterotomy alone or both biliary and pancreatic sphincterotomies. The results demonstrated that no clinical subgroups benefitted from sphincterotomy more than others and that sphincterotomy did not reduce disability related to pain.[27] This led to a change in the classification of SODs with the 2016 Rome IV criteria discarding "types I, II, and III SOD" and instead adopting "functional pancreatic (or biliary) sphincter disorder."[28]

Although ES remains the primary treatment of choice for papillary stenosis, it is not indicated for all patients with SOD. The use of SOM has also been greatly reduced, with its applicability limited to identifying hypertensive sphincters and assessing response to ES.[25,26]

Endotherapy for Complications of Pancreatitis

Pancreatic pseudocyst

Pancreatic pseudocysts (PP) are a common complication of pancreatitis that may require treatment if they become infected or symptomatic (see **Table 1**). For most of the 1900s, surgical cystoenterostomy was the primary method of PP drainage.[3,29] In the 1970s, ultrasound, computed tomography (CT), and fluoroscopic guided percutaneous drainage of PP were introduced as nonsurgical management alternatives.[30] Endoscopic drainage methods took longer to surface. In 1975, Rogers described the first transgastric needle aspiration of a PP through the biopsy channel of an endoscope.[31] However, it was not until 1984 that Hershfield and colleagues reported using ERCP to cannulate the minor papilla and incidentally found that it connected to a PP. During the procedure, he aspirated amylase-rich fluid and found that the PP had resolved on repeat imaging.[32]

In 1985, more intentional efforts of endoscopic PP drainage were reported in 4 patients who either failed surgery or were not surgical candidates. The procedure consisted of using a duodenoscope and diathermic needle-knife to create a fistulotomy between the PP and stomach or duodenum, whichever location appeared more amenable to drainage on earlier imaging. Two patients had complete PP resolution.[33] In 1987, Sahel and colleagues used a similar technique that relied on visualizing a bulge in the duodenal wall to identify the PP and then performing ERCP to determine the relationship between the PP and duodenum. After creating a cystoduodenostomy, a nasocystic drain was left in place for irrigation. They reported good results in 64% of patients.[34] This technique of relying on a visible bulge to create a cystoenterostomy became known as conventional transmural drainage (CTD).[29,35,36] In the late 1980s, experience with endoscopic PP drainage was growing. With the combination of CTD and nasocystic drains used for irrigation, PP drainage success rates were reported as greater than 96%.[29]

In the early 1990s, endoscopic drainage of PPs shifted in 3 manners. First, 2 case series reported successful use of plastic biliary stents to maintain the patency of the cystoenterostomy. This internal drainage method was as an improved alternative that would avoid discomfort of a nasal catheter and would result in the extinction of external nasocystic drainage.[37,38] Second, endoscopists began exploring the efficacy of ERCP with transpapillary PP drainage—with PD sphincterotomy and stent or drain placement into the duct. This method of drainage had high success rates, although it raised concerns of possible stent-related ductal changes (discussed later).[39] Finally, in the 1990s, the development of linear-array echoendoscopes with an accessory channel opened the doors to the possibility of EUS-guided therapeutic procedures.

In 1992, Grimm and colleagues demonstrated the utility of EUS in identifying an optimal puncture site for PP drainage close to the gastric or duodenal wall. In his report, a needle, guidewire, and catheter were advanced into the pseudocyst under EUS guidance before switching to a therapeutic duodenoscope for stent placement.[40] In 1996, Wiersema improved on this technique by using a new prototype linear-array echoendoscope with an elevator and a larger instrument channel that could create a cystoduodenostomy and place a stent without exchanging for a duodenoscope.[40] This was the first description of complete EUS-guided PP drainage, which would prove to have greater technical success than CTD and was a safe alternative for those without visible luminal compression[41] (**Fig. 1**).

Recognizing that many patients originally described as having pseudocysts actually had walled-off necrosis (WON). Over the years, new techniques were developed to optimize "PP" drainage including placing multiple stents and improving dilation of cystoenterostomies. In 2008, a larger shift was seen in the management of PPs. Although the use of self-expandable metal stents (SEMS) for PP drainage was first reported in 1994 in a patient with an infected pseudocyst, fully covered SEMS (FCSEMS) were not yet available, and the patient was left with a permanent uncovered SEMS. In 2008, a case series reported using FCSEMS to drain pancreatic fluid collections (PFCs) and demonstrated 78% clinical success with complete resolution of the PFCs.[42,43] Multiple subsequent studies used FCSEMS for drainage of PFCs but complications included stent migration, clogging, and exposed stent ends causing tissue trauma, bleeding, and perforation. In 2004, lumen-apposing metal stents (LAMS) were introduced as a solution to these complications. With bilateral double-walled flanges in a dumbbell shape, the tissue walls could be held in close apposition and minimize the risk of migration. Electrocautery-enhancement of the LAMS has further improved deployment of these stents to minimize leakage and maximize safety of PFC drainage.[43,44]

Management of PP has evolved during the last 50 years. EUS-guided cystgastrostomy has proven to be superior to surgical cystgastrostomy in reducing the length of stay, reducing cost, and improving quality of life for patients.[45] As such, EUS-guided drainage has remained the preferred management for symptomatic PP with LAMS demonstrating higher clinical success rates, lower adverse event rates, and reduced need for percutaneous drainage when compared with plastic stents.[46]

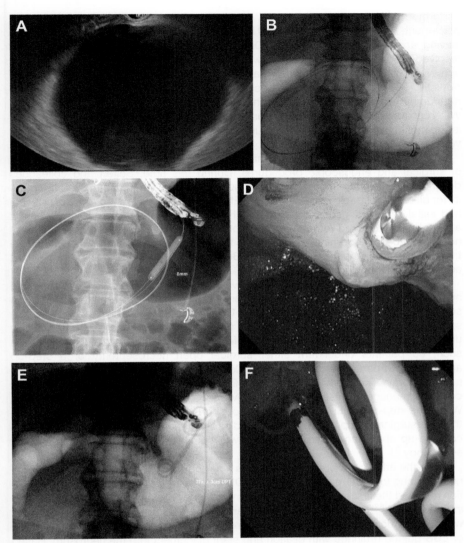

Fig. 1. EUS-guided drainage of a PP with double pigtail stents. (*A*) EUS view of PP before drainage. (*B*) After needle puncture, a dilating catheter is advanced over a guidewire into the PP. (*C, D*) The tract between the stomach lumen and guidewire is dilated, fluoroscopic and endoscopic views, respectively. (*E, F*) Two double pigtail stents are left in place, fluoroscopic and endoscopic views, respectively.

Walled-off necrosis

WON, a complication of acute necrotizing pancreatitis, can require drainage if infected or symptomatic.[45] Historically, surgical necrosectomy was considered the only management option.[47] However, because experience with endoscopic drainage of PP increased, similar techniques were applied to the management of WON. In 1996, Baron and colleagues published the first experience of endoscopic drainage of WON. The protocol used ERCP to assess the integrity of the PD then CTD was performed to create a tract into the WON collection, followed by dilation and stent placement. After 2 patients developed infection, the protocol was modified to include leaving a nasobiliary tube in the WON collection for irrigation until the collection resolved. Nine out of 10 patients whose collections were successfully entered achieved complete drainage, thus establishing the feasibility of endoscopic drainage of WON.[47] Endoscopists have since use this method as a prototype for entry into and debridement of WON collections with various endoscopic tools. Although CTD of WON can have high success rates, most endoscopists agree that EUS-guided access is superior in establishing a safe puncture site and minimizing risks of injury to adjacent vessels or organs.[41,48]

In the 2000s, natural orifice transluminal endoscopy emerged as a promising hybrid of surgical and endoscopic procedures. During this time, Seifert and colleagues described obtaining transgastric or transduodenal access into the retroperitoneal cavity for direct endoscopic necrosectomy (DEN). In long-term follow-up, 80% of patients had initial clinical success and 84% of these had sustained clinical improvement although 10% required retreatment. Complications included bleeding, perforation of necrosis into the abdominal cavity, fistula formation, air embolization, and pancreatitis. Furthermore, 7 patients died within 30 days and long-term follow-up included another 7 patients who died.[49]

With increasing treatment modalities available, including percutaneous drainage and video-assisted retroperitoneal debridement, the Dutch Pancreatitis Study Group sought to determine the optimal approach to managing WON. In this multicenter prospective trial, 639 patients with necrotizing pancreatitis were managed conservatively unless they had suspected or confirmed infected WON or peripancreatic necrosis. As such, 88 patients underwent either surgical open necrosectomy or a step-up approach with percutaneous drainage followed, if necessary, by minimally invasive necrosectomy. The study found that 62% of patients with necrotizing pancreatitis could be managed conservatively with low-mortality rates. For those with infected WON, the step-up group had lower rates of short-term and long-term complications than the surgical group.[50] Subsequent studies investigating endoscopic versus surgical step-up approaches demonstrated lower complication and mortality rates with endoscopy.[51]

Given the efficacy of both percutaneous and endoscopic drainage methods, it did not take long for dual-modality drainage (DMD) to be introduced. In 2014, our institution reported the first series of 117 patients who underwent DMD for symptomatic and infected WON.[52] These patients first underwent percutaneous drainage of the WON with interventional radiology (IR) and immediately afterward underwent either CTD or EUS-guided drainage with dilation and stent placement into the necrosum. Based on clinical course, some patients required irrigation through and upsizing of the percutaneous drain. With clinical improvement, the drains were capped and imaging was repeated to ensure that the collection did not recur before drain removal. At the time of publication, 103 patients completed treatment and had drains removed. Although this study demonstrated favorable clinical outcomes, this approach requires a collaborative relationship between gastroenterology and IR and reliable follow-up because the median duration of follow-up was 750 days.[52]

Although the initial WON drainage was performed with plastic stents, current guidelines recognize LAMS as superior in providing better egress of necrotic material[51] (**Fig. 2**). Furthermore, both endoscopic and percutaneous drainage are recommended as first-line nonsurgical approaches while DMD is reserved for more complicated WON. Notably, DEN is reserved for patients who do not respond to other nonsurgical approaches.[53]

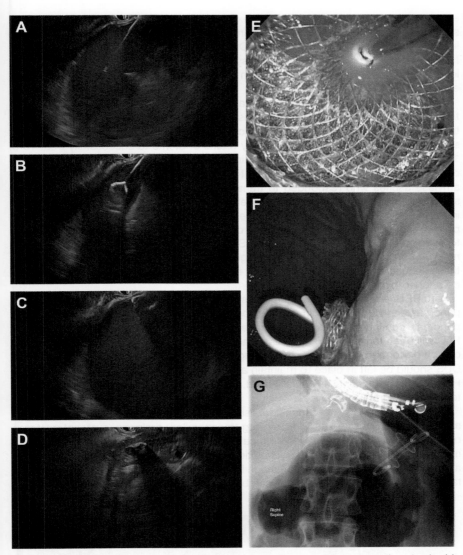

Fig. 2. EUS-guided drainage of WON with lumen apposing metal stent (LAMS) and a double pigtail stent within. *EUS views*: (*A*) Needle puncture through initial WON collection. (*B*) Distal flange of LAMS is deployed into collection. (*C*) Distal flange is retracted tightly against wall of WON. (*D*) Collection is notably smaller after more than 1L of fluid has drained. *Endoscopic views*: (*E*) Proximal flange of LAMS is deployed into the stomach lumen. (*F*) A double pigtail stent is placed within the LAMS. *Fluoroscopic view*: (*G*) Cystgastrostomy formed with LAMS and double pigtail stent within.

Pancreatic duct leaks and disconnected duct syndrome

PD leaks can develop as sequelae from pancreatitis, malignancy, abdominal trauma, or after abdominal surgery. Although minor leaks can resolve with conservative management, severe leaks often require interventions. Depending on the direction of location and flow, leaks can cause internal fistulae (including PP, WON, ascites, pleural effusion, pancreaticoenteric fistula) or external pancreatic fistulae (EPFs). Although some leaks may result from a partial disruption of the PD, complete disruptions can lead to disconnected duct syndrome (DDS) where the distal gland becomes isolated from the proximal gland—orphaned tail syndrome. Previously a surgical problem, PD leaks have been increasingly managed in a multidisciplinary fashion between gastro-enterology and IR.

As previously described, ERCP with transpapillary stenting has been used in isola-tion or in conjunction with other modalities for management of PP and WON. Our insti-tution has had a long history managing complications of PD leak with transpapillary stenting. In 1991, we used transpapillary drains or stents to successfully treat 16 of 18 patients with PD disruption, including 12 with PFCs[54] (**Fig. 3**). In 1992, we described the first endoscopic treatment of patients with PD leaks resulting in high-amylase ascites who responded to transpapillary stenting and paracentesis.[55] The same year, we demonstrated efficacy of endoscopic transpapillary stenting in manag-ing pancreaticoenteric fistulae that developed after patients with PFCs underwent percutaneous drainage.[56] In 1997, our group first reported using transpapillary stents for treating EPFs caused by PD leaks.[57] Since these initial descriptions, other studies have demonstrated transpapillary drainage as a safe and effective method for treating these sequelae of PD leaks with the best results obtained if the leak is partial and can be bridged by the stent.[48]

With DDS, endoscopic management is less straightforward because the upstream pancreas and duct are not in communication with the papilla. Because the isolated pancreas continues to secrete exocrine juices freely into the abdominal cavity, a PFC will often form. If a PFC is present and persistent, CTD or EUS-guided drainage can be performed. Contrary to the management of other PFCs, transmural stents for DDS should be left in place to maintain an outflow tract and prevent recurrence.[48,58] However, if metal stents are initially used, they should be exchanged for plastic stents to minimize complication rates.[59]

In 1995, Deviere and colleagues published the first experience of endoscopic man-agement of DDS and related PFCs using transpapillary drainage, cystoenterostomy, or nasocystic catheter drainage. Most patients required a combination of these treat-ments and 12 of 13 patients had resolution of PFCs.[60] Since this study, many hybrid approaches have been used to manage DDS and its complications. In 2007, Arvani-takis used transpapillary drainage combined with other techniques to treat EPF in

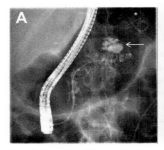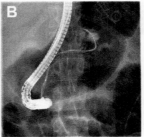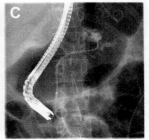

Fig. 3. Transpapillary stenting of PD leak complicated by new fluid collection. (*A*) Contrast injection of PD reveals dilated main duct with prominent side branches and a leak in the distal body of the pancreas (*arrow*), distinct from earlier WON collection that had been resolved with a lumen apposing metal stent and double pigtail stent within (*asterisk*). (*B*) Guidewire access is obtained into the new fluid collection. (*C*) A transpapillary stent is de-ployed to drain the PFC.

patients with DDS.[61] This included the first description of the outside-in technique where a needle and catheter were advanced over a guidewire that had been threaded through the EPF orifice (outside) to a site closely apposed to the stomach or duodenum wall (in). After a puncture was made, the needle, catheter, and guidewire were advanced into the duodenal or gastric lumen, where guidewire was retrieved by the scope, allowing endoscopic placement of a plastic stent from the lumen into the EPF tract. Another novel technique described was EUS-guided pancreaticobulbostomy, where EUS was used to access the dilated duct of the orphaned pancreas and a stent was placed from the duodenal bulb into the duct. Using these techniques along with PFC drainage, the EPF resolved in 15 of 16 patients.[61]

In 2012, our institution used the outside-in technique and described 2 other novel rendezvous techniques to treat EPF in DDS patients. First, the inside-out technique used EUS to find a site for a needle to advance from the stomach (inside) toward a preexisting drain placed within the EPF tract (out). After a guidewire was advanced through the needle into the EPF tract, the guidewire was secured externally. With access obtained, the newly created fistula was dilated before stents were placed between the stomach and EPF tract. The second technique of reconnecting the disconnected ducts was only possible in patients who were previously able to demonstrate both downstream (toward the head) and upstream (toward the tail) ducts on fistulograms. In this technique, IR injected contrast through a preexisting drain within the EPF tract, allowing full visualization of both duct segments. Then, a wire was passed from the cutaneous end of drain, past the duct disruption site, and through the ampulla. On the duodenal end, an endoscopist captured the wire and used it to guide a papillotome through the downstream duct and into the fistulous tract, which had been unsuccessful on earlier ERCPs. With visualization of the upstream duct, the wire could then be advanced toward the tail and facilitate balloon dilation and transpapillary stent placement. All patients had EPF closure without recurrence.[62]

Managing DDS and its complications is challenging. Although some groups have had success with transpapillary drainage alone, often a multimodality approach is required, and this may be in the form of transmural drainage, a rendezvous technique, or EUS-guided pancreaticoenterostomy. Current management is less streamlined and a multidisciplinary approach with surgery and IR is important.

Pancreatic calculi

Pancreatic calculi are sequelae of chronic pancreatitis that can obstruct PDs, lead to ductal hypertension, and cause pain (**Fig. 4**). In 1891, Pearce reported the first surgical stone removal.[10] In 1983, Inui and colleagues documented the first ERCP with stone extraction,[63] although Michel Cremer performed this earlier (*J. Deviere, personal communication*). In 1985, Fuji and colleagues described performing ERCP with ES in 10 patients with pancreatic calculi. In one patient, direct pancreatoscopy was used to facilitate basket retrieval of pancreatic calculi. In 3 patients, pancreatic stent placement was used to facilitate PD drainage. In total, 9 patients had improvement of pain.[64] This report was perhaps the first documented transpapillary pancreatic stent placement and validated the use of basket stone retrieval for pancreatic calculi. Shortly thereafter, balloon catheters were introduced as another method of extracting PD stones.[65]

In the following decade, endoscopists managed pancreatic calculi with ES, intraductal lavage, fragmentation with forceps, stone retrieval baskets, stone retrieval balloons, and dilating or stenting the main duct if strictures were present.[35] However, larger stones were not always amenable to these treatments. In 1987, Sauerbruch and colleagues demonstrated extracorporeal shock wave lithotripsy (ESWL) as an

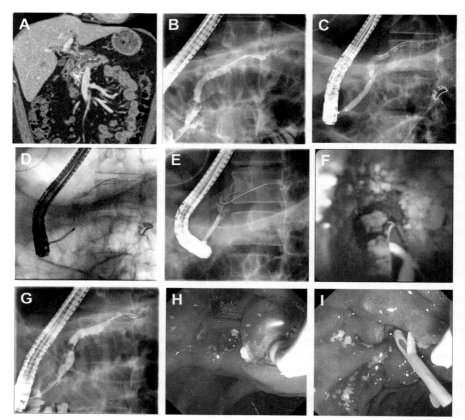

Fig. 4. Endoscopic management of a patient with chronic calcifying pancreatitis after undergoing ESWL. (*A*) CT scan before ESWL demonstrating multiple large stones in the head of the pancreas. (*B*) After ESWL, contrast injection demonstrates multiple filling defects and a stricture in the head of the pancreas. (*C*) After a pancreatic sphincterotomy is performed, the stricture in the head of the pancreas is dilated. (*D*) Basket stone retrieval is attempted but unable to advance past the stones. (*E*) A pancreatoscope is passed into the main PD. (*F*) Stones are visualized and EHL is performed, yielding stone fragments. (*G, H*) An extraction balloon is used to remove stone fragments, fluoroscopic and endoscopic views, respectively. (*I*) A stent is placed in the PD to facilitate further drainage.

effective method of breaking down biliary stones. The next year, the same group used ESWL to treat a patient with an obstructing PD stone who did not respond to earlier ERCP with ES.[66] Imaging after ESWL demonstrated successful disintegration of the stone, which was later removed with ERCP. Since this first experience, many studies have validated ESWL with ERCP as an effective strategy for managing larger pancreatic calculi, leading to long-term improvement in pain, reduced use of narcotics, and fewer hospitalizations.[67–69] Currently, the American Society for Gastrointestinal Endoscopy recommends ESWL as adjunctive therapy for symptomatic patients with pancreatic calculi refractory to standard endoscopic stone extraction techniques.[67]

Laser lithotripsy (LL) is another tool used for the fragmentation of large stones. In 1990, our institution reported using LL on a patient with chronic calcific pancreatitis (CCP) who failed surgical stone extraction and had an obstructive main duct calculus requiring surgical placement of a percutaneous pancreatostomy drainage catheter. Under endoscopic and fluoroscopic guidance, LL was applied directly to the stone and a transpapillary PD stent was left for drainage. The patient had complete resolution of pain, closure of the pancreaticocutaneous fistula, and no recurrent calculi.[70] Since this initial experience, a few case series have reported using pancreatoscopy-guided LL for pancreatic stone fragmentation with good results in patients who have failed ESWL but overall experience is still limited with LL.

Electrohydraulic lithotripsy (EHL) is another form of stone fragmentation that is less utilized than ESWL. EHL was first used to treat biliary stones in the mid-1970s. In 1992, the first experience of intraoperative EHL for pancreatic stones was reported in 2 patients with CCP who required lateral pancreaticojejunostomies.[71] During each operation, EHL allowed stone fragmentation under direct visualization, which facilitated subsequent stone extraction. In 1999, Howell and colleagues described using a 10F endoscope that could pass through the accessory channel of a therapeutic duodenoscope into the PD. Through the accessory channel of the 10F endoscope, an EHL probe was able to advance to the pancreatic stone, and EHL of the stone was performed under direct visualization. Five of 6 patients in this study had partial or complete PD clearance and relief of pain.[72] Similar success of pancreatoscopy with EHL has been seen with the Spyglass Direct Visualization System, a single-operator cholangiopancreatoscopy system.[73]

Management of PD calculi has evolved since the 1980s. In addition to standard ERCP techniques of balloon and basket stone extraction, ESWL, LL, and EHL have emerged as effective tools for stone fragmentation. Because data on intraductal lithotripsy are limited, ESWL is currently considered first-line in the management of larger stones.[67]

Pancreatic duct strictures

Benign PD strictures resulting from inflammation or fibrosis of the pancreas can cause upstream ductal hypertension, leading to pain or pancreatitis flares.[67] Endoscopic management of strictures has been documented as early as 1983 with ERCP with balloon dilation and 1986 with ES and pancreatic stent placement.[73,74] As previously described, pancreatic stents and drains were increasingly used in the late 1980s for indications including PD leaks and pancreas divisum. In 1990, our institution examined the long-term effects of PD stents that were placed for various diseases. Stents used were 5 to 7F and were exchanged at a mean of 4 months. We found that 36% of patients had ductal changes related to either stent occlusion, direct stent trauma, or side branch occlusion. These ductal changes included ductal dilation, irregular stenoses, and side branch ectasia—findings similar to those seen in chronic pancreatitis.[39] This study raised the concern that stent placement is not risk-free and highlighted the importance of determining the best protocols for PD stent placement.

For many years, standard treatment of PD strictures included dilation and insertion of a single plastic stent across a dominant stricture.[74,75] In 2006, a study challenged the paradigm of single-stent placement. Costamagna and colleagues reported a prospective study on patients with symptomatic PD strictures refractory to single-stent placement. Patients underwent balloon dilation followed by insertion of the maximum number of stents allowed by the stricture. The median number of stents placed through the major and/or minor papilla was 3. Although all patients developed temporary abdominal pain, they subsequently remained asymptomatic while the stents were in place. Of 19 patients, 84% had resolution of their strictures.[76] These results suggest that multiple plastic stenting can be effective and safe for refractory pancreatic strictures.

Many initial studies used stents of varying sizes between 5 F and 11.5 F. In 2009, a retrospective study reviewed patients who underwent PD stent placement for chronic pancreatitis and found that those with size 10 F stents had significantly fewer hospitalizations for abdominal pain when compared with those with size 8.5 F or smaller.[77] More recently, there has been growing interest in using FCSEMS to treat PD strictures. A meta-analysis including 19 studies with a total of 300 patients treated with FCSEMS reported a 91% pooled stricture resolution rate with a 6% recurrence rate. Although the results are promising, there was significant heterogeneity between the studies.[78] In a recent prospective study using soft FCSEMS to treat painful PD strictures, the technical success rate was high (97%) but the primary efficacy rate was low (26%) and there were high rates of stent migration (48%) and serious adverse events (31%). Further studies will be needed to determine the efficacy of FCSEMS.[79]

In patients with tight strictures that may preclude deep cannulation of the papilla, ERCP with transpapillary stenting may be challenging. In 2002, EUS-guided pancreaticogastrostomy was described as a technique for decompressing upstream-dilated PDs when ERCP was unsuccessful. In this procedure, an echoendoscope was used to guide a needle into the upstream-dilated PD. Under fluoroscopy, contrast injection demonstrated the duct, and a guidewire was then inserted to facilitate dilation of the tract and stent placement.[80] Since this initial description, other case series have described EUS-guided drainage of the PD. Studies with long-term data have reported complete or major pain relief in 70% to 90% of patients but the probability of remaining pain-free can drop over time.[81] Stent migration and occlusion rates have ranged between 20% and 55%.[81]

Over the years, the management of PD strictures has centered on dilation and stent placement. When single stents are placed, size 10F or larger are recommended. When strictures are refractory to single-stent placement, multistent placement can be considered.[67] Although studies have not been performed to assess duration of stent placement, some experts recommend planned exchanges every 6 months.[81] Of note, when encountering PD strictures, brushings for cytology should be considered to rule out underlying malignancy.[67,81]

Celiac plexus block and neurolysis

Despite endotherapy for pancreatic strictures and stones, pain management for chronic pancreatitis patients is often difficult. Since percutaneous transposterior celiac plexus block (CPB) was first described in 1914,[82] CPB has evolved with changing technology and has been performed under CT, fluoroscopic, and transcutaneous ultrasound guidance. In 1996, EUS-guided celiac plexus neurolysis (CPN) was first documented in patients with pain from pancreatic cancer or intra-abdominal metastases, with up to 88% experiencing pain improvement.[83] Although CPN and CPB differ in the injection solution, the technique is similar, and this initial experience demonstrated feasibility and safety of EUS-guided CPB.

Despite similarity in technique, CPN and CPB are not equally efficacious in treating pain for patients with pancreatic cancer and patients with chronic pancreatitis, respectively. Two meta-analyses reported that CPB provides temporary pain relief in 51% to 59% of chronic pancreatitis patients while CPN provides pain relief in 73% to 80% of patients with pancreatic cancer. Adverse events reported have included transient diarrhea, orthostasis, retroperitoneal abscess formation, and spinal cord infarction.[67,82,84] As such CPB should not be considered first-line treatment of chronic pancreatitis pain and should only be considered in patients with severe pain affecting quality of life or recurrent hospitalizations. However, CPN is generally accepted as a relatively effective method of pain control for patients with pancreatic cancer and has been suggested to have greater benefit when used earlier as opposed to as salvage therapy.[85]

Endotherapy for Pancreatic Neoplasms

In the last 2 decades, EUS has expanded its application and played an active role in the management of pancreatic neoplasms (**Table 2**). The following section discusses EUS-guided radiotherapy, tissue ablation, and antitumor injections. Although some of these techniques are promising, they remain experimental and require further studies to delineate their utility.

Endoscopic ultrasound-guided radiotherapy

Stereotactic radiotherapy is a treatment that delivers external radiation into tumors by using real-time image guidance.[86] Fiducials are radiographic markers that serve as reference points for stereotactic radiotherapy and were initially placed surgically or percutaneously.[87] In 2006, EUS guidance was successfully used to place fiducials in patients with mediastinal and abdominal lesions.[86] Since this experience, many centers have reported EUS-guided placement of fiducials into pancreatic neoplasms. Although generally safe, migration can occur with tumor treatment and inflammation, and there is a 1% risk of minor bleeding.[87]

Although fiducials facilitate external radiotherapy, brachytherapy exposes tumors to internal radiotherapy. In EUS-guided brachytherapy, radioactive seeds are implanted into or adjacent to tumor and release radiation that induces tissue injury and tumor ablation.[87,88] In 2006, EUS-guided implantation of iodine-125 seeds was reported in 15 patients with unresectable pancreatic adenocarcinoma. Seven patients had partial or minor response and complications occurred in 20% of patients, including 3 who developed pancreatitis.[89] Although there have been a few other studies on EUS-guided brachytherapy, these have been limited by a small number of subjects and lack of a control group.[87]

Endoscopic ultrasound-guided radiofrequency ablation

Radiofrequency ablation (RFA) is a minimally invasive technique that generates localized heat to induce thermal necrosis of targeted tissue.[87] Experience with RFA began in animal models and later was used intraoperatively in humans. In 2015, EUS-RFA was successfully used in 6 patients with pancreatic cystic neoplasm (PCN). Two patients had complete resolution of the cysts and 3 had 48% reduction in size.[90] In a

Table 2
Investigational endotherapy for pancreatic neoplasms

Endotherapy	Year of Initial Experience (Reference Number)	Potential Pancreatic Disease Applications
EUS-guided fiducial placement	Pishvaian et al,[86] 2006	Unresectable pancreatic cancer
EUS-guided brachytherapy	Sun et al,[89] 2006	Unresectable pancreatic cancer
EUS-guided radiofrequency ablation	Pai et al,[90] 2015	PCNs, PNETs, unresectable pancreatic cancer
EUS-guided ethanol ablation	Gan et al,[95] 2005	PCNs, PNETs
EUS-guided immunotherapy injection	Chang et al,[99] 2000	Unresectable pancreatic cancer
EUS-guided chemotherapy injection	Levy et al,[100] 2016	Unresectable pancreatic cancer

Abbreviations: PCN, pancreatic cystic neoplasm; PNET, pancreatic neuroendocrine tumor.

subsequent larger series of 17 PCNs, 11 had complete disappearance, and one had a diameter reduced by greater than 50% 1 year after treatment; all 12 had complete resolutions of mural nodules.[91]

EUS-RFA has also had favorable results with pancreatic neuroendocrine tumors (PNETs). In the larger series cited above, 12 of 16 PNETs disappeared 1 year after treatment. These results were validated in a meta-analysis of 12 studies that included 61 patients, reporting a 96% efficacy rate without differences noted between functional and nonfunctional PNETs (NF-PNETs).[92]

Although EUS-RFA is associated with 10% risk of abdominal pain,[93] it has overall proved promising for treating pancreatic neoplasms. Few studies have demonstrated safety and feasibility of using EUS-RFA for unresectable pancreatic cancer; however, these have yet to demonstrate an impact on disease progression and survival.[93]

Endoscopic ultrasound-guided ethanol ablation

Ethanol is an ablative agent that causes cell death by inducing cell membrane lysis, protein denaturation, and vascular occlusion.[94] In 2002, EUS-guided ethanol ablation was first used to treat liver metastases.[87] By 2005, EUS-guided ethanol ablation was reported in 23 patients with PCNs with 35% achieving complete resolution within 12 months; the ethanol concentration ranged between 5% and 80%.[95] Later studies used 80% to 100% ethanol and reported PCN resolution rates widely ranging between 9% and 85% with inconsistent results regarding whether cyst type or size affect clinical response.[96]

EUS-guided ethanol ablation has also been used to treat PNETs. In 2006, EUS-guided ethanol ablation of a symptomatic insulinoma led to the resolution of hypoglycemic episodes and of the PNET on imaging. Other limited case reports using EUS-guided ethanol ablation for symptomatic insulinomas have reported similar favorable responses.[97] Additionally, in a study that included 10 NF-PNETs, EUS-guided ethanol ablation was able to achieve complete response in 6 and incomplete response in 3.[98]

Although EUS-guided ethanol ablation has shown promise in treating pancreatic neoplasms, it is currently reserved for patients who are not surgical candidates or for those who refuse surgery. Further studies are needed to determine its efficacy on different types of PCNs and to standardize treatment protocols (ie, ethanol concentration, number of treatments).

Endoscopic ultrasound-guided antitumor injections

Although the previously discussed EUS-guided treatments have focused on PCNs and PNETs, EUS-guided antitumor injections have been directed at treating pancreatic cancer. In 2000, the first EUS-guided immunotherapy was performed in 8 patients with advanced unresectable pancreatic cancer. These cancers were injected with a lymphocytic culture that could theoretically produce cytokines and activate antitumor effector cells. Only 2 patients had partial tumor response.[99] Other EUS-guided immunotherapy injections have been performed with dendritic cells and TNFerade (a recombinant agent that delivers tumor necrosis factor alpha [TNF-α] to cancer cells). Neither has been shown to have significant benefit.[87]

EUS-guided chemotherapy injection has shown more promise in treating pancreatic neoplasms. Initial experience with chemotherapy injection was with either gemcitabine or paclitaxel and was performed as an adjunct to EUS-guided ethanol ablation for PCNs. These studies suggested a higher rate of complete resolution of PCNs with chemotherapy injection as compared with ethanol injection alone.[96] In 2016, EUS-guided injection of gemcitabine was performed in patients with inoperable locally advanced pancreatic cancer who were receiving conventional chemoradiation. In this study, 20% of patients with unresectable stage III disease were downstaged and underwent R0 resection.[100] Further studies are needed to assess safety and efficacy of EUS-guided antitumor injections.

SUMMARY

In the last half century, endotherapy for pancreatic diseases has evolved considerably. With more accessory tools available, both ERCP and EUS have grown in their therapeutic capabilities in managing pancreatic disease and have reduced the need for surgery. Although the management of pancreatitis and its complications has been stagnant in the last 2 decades, endotherapy for pancreatic neoplasms is only in the early stages of development and has shown potential for both palliation and cure.

CLINICS CARE POINTS

- Symptomatic or infected PFCs can be safely drained with EUS-guided cystoenterostomy.
- WON should be managed conservatively. However, if the WON becomes infected or symptomatic, endoscopic and percutaneous step-up therapies have been showed to have lower complication and mortality rates when compared with surgical approaches. Furthermore, DMD has favorable clinical outcomes but requires collaboration with IR and reliable patient follow-up.
- Complications of PD leaks can be treated with endoscopic transpapillary stenting or drainage. However, the management of DDS often requires the addition of therapeutic EUS techniques or a multidisciplinary approach with IR.
- When large pancreatic calculi cannot be managed with traditional endoscopic extraction methods, stone fragmentation with ESWL, LL, and EHL can be considered.
- Although endoscopic transpapillary stenting is used to treat PD strictures, long-term observations suggest that PD stenting can induce changes including ductal dilation, stenoses, and side branch ectasias.
- EUS-guided CPB and neurolysis differ in the injection solution used but have been used to treat pain for chronic pancreatitis and patients with pancreatic cancer, respectively. However, CPB should not be considered first-line treatment of chronic pancreatitis pain.
- EUS-guided antitumor therapy remains investigational, although shows potential in palliation and cure of pancreatic neoplasms.

DISCLOSURES

Y. Cui: no financial disclosures. R. Kozarek: no financial disclosures.

REFERENCES

1. Busnardo AC, DiDio LJ, Tidrick RT, et al. History of the pancreas. American journal of surgery 1983;146(5):539–50.
2. Wiltse LL, Pait TG. Herophilus of Alexandria (325-255 B. C.). The father of anatomy. Spine (Phila Pa 1976) 1998;23(17):1904–14.
3. Navarro S. The art of pancreatic surgery. Past, present and future. The history of pancreatic surgery. Gastroenterol Hepatol 2017;40(9):648 e1–e648, e11. El arte de la cirugia pancreatica. Pasado, presente y futuro. doi:.
4. O'Reilly DA, Kingsnorth AN. A brief history of pancreatitis. J R Soc Med 2001; 94(3):130–2.

5. McCune WS, Shorb PE, Moscovitz H. Endoscopic cannulation of the ampulla of vater: a preliminary report. Ann Surg 1968;167(5):752–6.
6. Wallace MB, Fockens P, Sung JJY. Gastroenterological endoscopy. Thieme 2018;xix:418.
7. Cotton PB. Cannulation of the papilla of Vater by endoscopy and retrograde cholangiopancreatography (ERCP). Gut 1972;13(12):1014–25.
8. Buscaglia JM, Kalloo AN. Pancreatic sphincterotomy: technique, indications, and complications. World J Gastroenterol 2007;13(30):4064–71.
9. Behrns KE, Ashley SW, Hunter JG, et al. Early ERCP for gallstone pancreatitis: for whom and when? J Gastrointest Surg 2008;12(4):629–33.
10. Andersen DK, Frey CF. The evolution of the surgical treatment of chronic pancreatitis. Ann Surg 2010;251(1):18–32.
11. Sherman S, Hawes RH, Lehman GA. Management of bile duct stones. Semin Liver Dis 1990;10(3):205–21.
12. Guo A, Poneros JM. The Role of Endotherapy in Recurrent Acute Pancreatitis. Gastrointest Endosc Clin N Am 2018;28(4):455–76.
13. Cotton PB. Congenital anomaly of pancreas divisum as cause of obstructive pain and pancreatitis. Gut 1980;21(2):105–14.
14. Lehman GA, Sherman S, Nisi R, et al. Pancreas divisum: results of minor papilla sphincterotomy. Gastrointestinal endoscopy 1993;39(1):1–8.
15. Kozarek RA, Ball TJ, Patterson DJ, et al, Brandabur JJ, Raltz SL. Endoscopic approach to pancreas divisum. Digestive diseases and sciences 1995;40(9): 1974–81.
16. McCarthy J, Geenen JE, Hogan WJ. Preliminary experience with endoscopic stent placement in benign pancreatic diseases. Gastrointest Endosc 1988; 34(1):16–8.
17. Cote GA, Durkalski-Mauldin V, Williams A, et al. Design and execution of sham-controlled endoscopic trials in acute pancreatitis: Lessons learned from the SHARP trial. Pancreatology 2022. https://doi.org/10.1016/j.pan.2022.12.011.
18. Law R, Topazian M. Diagnosis and treatment of choledochoceles. Clin Gastroenterol Hepatol 2014;12(2):196–203.
19. Deyhle P, Schnaars P, Meyer HJ, et al. [Electrosurgical removal of a choledochocele through an endoscope introduced by mouth (author's transl)]. Dtsch Med Wochenschr 1974;99(3):71–2. Perorale endoskopisch-elektrochirurgische Abtragung einer Choledochocele.
20. Siegel JH, Harding GT, Chateau F. Endoscopic incision of choledochal cysts (choledochocele). Endoscopy 1981;13(5):200–2.
21. Martin RF, Biber BP, Bosco JJ, et al. Symptomatic choledochoceles in adults. Endoscopic retrograde cholangiopancreatography recognition and management. Arch Surg 1992;127(5):536–8, discussion 538-9.
22. Guelrud M. Papillary stenosis. Endoscopy 1988;20(Suppl 1):193–202.
23. Toouli J. What is sphincter of Oddi dysfunction? Gut 1989;30(6):753–61.
24. Gregg JA, Carr-Locke DL. Endoscopic pancreatic and biliary manometry in pancreatic, biliary, and papillary disease, and after endoscopic sphincterotomy and surgical sphincteroplasty. Gut 1984;25(11):1247–54.
25. Petersen BT. An evidence-based review of sphincter of Oddi dysfunction: part I, presentations with "objective" biliary findings (types I and II). Gastrointestinal endoscopy 2004;59(4):525–34.
26. Petersen BT. Sphincter of Oddi dysfunction, part 2: Evidence-based review of the presentations, with "objective" pancreatic findings (types I and II) and of presumptive type III. Gastrointest Endosc 2004;59(6):670–87.

27. Cotton PB, Durkalski V, Romagnuolo J, et al. Effect of endoscopic sphincterotomy for suspected sphincter of Oddi dysfunction on pain-related disability following cholecystectomy: the EPISOD randomized clinical trial. JAMA 2014; 311(20):2101–9.

28. Cotton PB, Elta GH, Carter CR, et al. Rome IV. Gallbladder and Sphincter of Oddi Disorders. Gastroenterology 2016. https://doi.org/10.1053/j.gastro.2016. 02.033.

29. Cremer M, Deviere J, Engelholm L. Endoscopic management of cysts and pseudocysts in chronic pancreatitis: long-term follow-up after 7 years of experience. Gastrointest Endosc 1989;35(1):1–9.

30. Barkin JS, Smith FR, Pereiras R Jr, et al. Therapeutic percutaneous aspiration of pancreatic pseudocysts. Dig Dis Sci 1981;26(7):585–6.

31. Rogers BH, Cicurel NJ, Seed RW. Transgastric needle aspiration of pancreatic pseudocyst through an endoscope. Gastrointestinal endoscopy 1975;21(3): 133–4.

32. Hershfield NB. Drainage of a pancreatic pseudocyst at ERCP. Gastrointestinal endoscopy 1984;30(4):269–70.

33. Kozarek RA, Brayko CM, Harlan J, et al. Endoscopic drainage of pancreatic pseudocysts. Gastrointest Endosc 1985;31(5):322–7.

34. Sahel J, Bastid C, Pellat B, et al. Endoscopic cystoduodenostomy of cysts of chronic calcifying pancreatitis: a report of 20 cases. Pancreas 1987;2(4): 447–53.

35. Huibregtse K, Schneider B, Vrij AA, et al. Endoscopic pancreatic drainage in chronic pancreatitis. Gastrointest Endosc 1988;34(1):9–15.

36. Kozarek RA, Patterson DJ, Ball TJ, et al. Endoscopic placement of pancreatic stents and drains in the management of pancreatitis. Ann Surg 1989;209(3): 261–6.

37. Binmoeller KF, Seifert H, Walter A, et al. Transpapillary and transmural drainage of pancreatic pseudocysts. Gastrointestinal endoscopy 1995;42(3):219–24.

38. Smits ME, Rauws EA, Tytgat GN, et al. The efficacy of endoscopic treatment of pancreatic pseudocysts. Gastrointestinal endoscopy 1995;42(3):202–7.

39. Kozarek RA. Pancreatic stents can induce ductal changes consistent with chronic pancreatitis. Gastrointestinal Endoscopy 1990;36(2):93–5.

40. Wiersema MJ. Endosonography-guided cystoduodenostomy with a therapeutic ultrasound endoscope. Gastrointestinal endoscopy 1996;44(5):614–7.

41. Adler JM, Sethi A. Interventional Endoscopic Ultrasonography in the Pancreas. Gastrointest Endosc Clin N Am 2018;28(4):569–78.

42. Talreja JP, Shami VM, Ku J, et al. Transenteric drainage of pancreatic-fluid collections with fully covered self-expanding metallic stents (with video). Gastrointest Endosc 2008;68(6):1199–203.

43. Binmoeller KF, Nett A. The Evolution of Endoscopic Cystgastrostomy. Gastrointest Endosc Clin N Am 2018;28(2):143–56.

44. Teoh AY, Binmoeller KF, Lau JY. Single-step EUS-guided puncture and delivery of a lumen-apposing stent for gallbladder drainage using a novel cautery-tipped stent delivery system. Gastrointest Endosc 2014;80(6):1171.

45. Fisher JM, Gardner TB. Endoscopic therapy of necrotizing pancreatitis and pseudocysts. Gastrointest Endosc Clin N Am 2013;23(4):787–802.

46. Yang J, Chen YI, Friedland S, et al. Correction: Lumen-apposing stents versus plastic stents in the management of pancreatic pseudocysts: a large, comparative, international, multicenter study. Endoscopy 2019;51(11):C5.

47. Baron TH, Thaggard WG, Morgan DE, et al. Endoscopic therapy for organized pancreatic necrosis. Gastroenterology 1996;111(3):755–64.
48. Varadarajulu S, Rana SS, Bhasin DK. Endoscopic therapy for pancreatic duct leaks and disruptions. Gastrointest Endosc Clin N Am 2013;23(4):863–92.
49. Seifert H, Biermer M, Schmitt W, et al. Transluminal endoscopic necrosectomy after acute pancreatitis: a multicentre study with long-term follow-up (the GE-PARD Study). Gut 2009;58(9):1260–6.
50. van Santvoort HC, Bakker OJ, Bollen TL, et al. A conservative and minimally invasive approach to necrotizing pancreatitis improves outcome. Gastroenterology 2011;141(4):1254–63.
51. Yasuda I, Takahashi K. Endoscopic management of walled-off pancreatic necrosis. Dig Endosc. Mar 2021;33(3):335–41.
52. Ross AS, Irani S, Gan SI, et al. Dual-modality drainage of infected and symptomatic walled-off pancreatic necrosis: long-term clinical outcomes. Gastrointest Endosc 2014;79(6):929–35.
53. Baron TH, DiMaio CJ, Wang AY, et al. American Gastroenterological Association Clinical Practice Update: Management of Pancreatic Necrosis. Gastroenterology 2020;158(1):67–75 e1.
54. Kozarek RA, Ball TJ, Patterson DJ, et al. Endoscopic transpapillary therapy for disrupted pancreatic duct and peripancreatic fluid collections. Gastroenterology 1991;100(5 Pt 1):1362–70.
55. Kozarek RA, Jiranek GC, Traverso LW. Endoscopic treatment of pancreatic ascites. American Journal Of Surgery 1994;168(3):223–6.
56. Wolfsen HC, Kozarek RA, Ball TJ, et al. Pancreaticoenteric fistula: no longer a surgical disease? J Clin Gastroenterol 1992;14(2):117–21.
57. Kozarek RA, Ball TJ, Patterson DJ, et al. Transpapillary stenting for pancreaticocutaneous fistulas. J Gastrointest Surg 1997;1(4):357–61.
58. Larsen M, Kozarek R. Management of pancreatic ductal leaks and fistulae. J Gastroenterol Hepatol 2014;29(7):1360–70.
59. Verma S, Rana SS. Disconnected pancreatic duct syndrome: Updated review on clinical implications and management. Pancreatology 2020;20(6):1035–44.
60. Deviere J, Bueso H, Baize M, et al. Complete disruption of the main pancreatic duct: endoscopic management. Gastrointestinal endoscopy 1995;42(5):445–51.
61. Arvanitakis M, Delhaye M, Bali MA, et al. Endoscopic treatment of external pancreatic fistulas: when draining the main pancreatic duct is not enough. American Journal of Gastroenterology 2007;102(3):516–24.
62. Irani S, Gluck M, Ross A, et al. Resolving external pancreatic fistulas in patients with disconnected pancreatic duct syndrome: using rendezvous techniques to avoid surgery (with video). Gastroenterol Endosc 2012;76(3):586–93, e1-3.
63. Inui K, Nakae Y, Nakamura J, et al. A case of non-calcified pancreatolithiasis which was removed by endoscopic sphincterotomy of the pancreatic duct. Gastroenterol Endosc 1983;25(8):1246–53.
64. Fuji T, Amano H, Harima K, et al. Pancreatic sphincterotomy and pancreatic endoprosthesis. Endoscopy 1985;17(2):69–72.
65. Ponsky JL, Duppler DW. Endoscopic sphincterotomy and removal of pancreatic duct stones. Am Surg 1987;53(10):613–6.
66. Sauerbruch T, Holl J, Sackmann M, et al. Disintegration of a pancreatic duct stone with extracorporeal shock waves in a patient with chronic pancreatitis. Endoscopy 1987;19(5):207–8.

67. ASoP Committee, Chandrasekhara V, Chathadi KV, et al. The role of endoscopy in benign pancreatic disease. Gastrointest Endosc 2015;82(2):203–14.

68. Rosch T, Daniel S, Scholz M, et al. Endoscopic treatment of chronic pancreatitis: a multicenter study of 1000 patients with long-term follow-up. Endoscopy 2002; 34(10):765–71.

69. Kozarek RA, Brandabur JJ, Ball TJ, et al. Clinical outcomes in patients who undergo extracorporeal shock wave lithotripsy for chronic calcific pancreatitis. Gastrointest Endosc 2002;56(4):496–500.

70. Feldman RK, Freeny PC, Kozarek RA. Pancreatic and biliary calculi: percutaneous treatment with tunable dye laser lithotripsy. Radiology 1990;174(3 Pt 1): 793–5.

71. Tanaka M, Yokohata K, Kimura H, et al. Intraoperative endoscopic electrohydraulic lithotripsy of pancreatic stones. Int J Pancreatol 1992;12(3):227–31.

72. Howell DA, Dy RM, Hanson BL, et al. Endoscopic treatment of pancreatic duct stones using a 10F pancreatoscope and electrohydraulic lithotripsy. Gastrointest Endosc 1999;50(6):829–33.

73. van der Wiel SE, Stassen PMC, Poley JW, et al. Pancreatoscopy-guided electrohydraulic lithotripsy for the treatment of obstructive pancreatic duct stones: a prospective consecutive case series. Gastrointest Endosc 2022;95(5): 905–914 e2.

74. Nguyen-Tang T, Dumonceau JM. Endoscopic treatment in chronic pancreatitis, timing, duration and type of intervention. Best Pract Res Clin Gastroenterol 2010;24(3):281–98.

75. Talukdar R, Reddy DN. Pancreatic Endotherapy for Chronic Pancreatitis. Gastrointest Endosc Clin N Am 2015;25(4):765–77.

76. Costamagna G, Bulajic M, Tringali A, et al. Multiple stenting of refractory pancreatic duct strictures in severe chronic pancreatitis: long-term results. Endoscopy 2006;38(3):254–9.

77. Sauer BG, Gurka MJ, Ellen K, et al. Effect of pancreatic duct stent diameter on hospitalization in chronic pancreatitis: does size matter? Pancreas 2009;38(7): 728–31.

78. Tringali A, Costa D, Rota M, et al. Covered self-expandable metal stents for pancreatic duct stricture: a systematic review and meta-analysis. Endosc Int Open 2022;10(9):E1311–21.

79. Sherman S, Kozarek RA, Costamagna G, et al. Soft self-expanding metal stent to treat painful pancreatic duct strictures secondary to chronic pancreatitis: a prospective multicenter trial. Gastrointest Endosc 2022. https://doi.org/10. 1016/j.gie.2022.09.021.

80. Francois E, Kahaleh M, Giovannini M, et al. EUS-guided pancreaticogastrostomy. Gastrointestinal endoscopy 2002;56(1):128–33.

81. Dumonceau JM, Delhaye M, Tringali A, et al. Endoscopic treatment of chronic pancreatitis: European Society of Gastrointestinal Endoscopy (ESGE) Guideline - Updated August 2018. Endoscopy 2019;51(2):179–93.

82. Kaufman M, Singh G, Das S, et al. Efficacy of endoscopic ultrasound-guided celiac plexus block and celiac plexus neurolysis for managing abdominal pain associated with chronic pancreatitis and pancreatic cancer. J Clin Gastroenterol 2010;44(2):127–34.

83. Wiersema MJ, Wiersema LM. Endosonography-guided celiac plexus neurolysis. Gastrointestinal endoscopy 1996;44(6):656–62.

84. Puli SR, Reddy JB, Bechtold ML, et al. EUS-guided celiac plexus neurolysis for pain due to chronic pancreatitis or pancreatic cancer pain: a meta-analysis and systematic review. Digestive diseases and sciences 2009;54(11):2330–7.

85. Wyse JM, Chen YI, Sahai AV. Celiac plexus neurolysis in the management of unresectable pancreatic cancer: when and how? World journal of gastroenterology 2014;20(9):2186–92.

86. Pishvaian AC, Collins B, Gagnon G, et al. EUS-guided fiducial placement for CyberKnife radiotherapy of mediastinal and abdominal malignancies. Gastrointestinal endoscopy 2006;64(3):412–7.

87. Mukewar S, Muthusamy VR. Recent Advances in Therapeutic Endosonography for Cancer Treatment. Gastrointest Endosc Clin N Am 2017;27(4):657–80.

88. Bratanic A, Bozic D, Mestrovic A, et al. Role of endoscopic ultrasound in anticancer therapy: Current evidence and future perspectives. World J Gastrointest Oncol 2021;13(12):1863–79.

89. Sun S, Xu H, Xin J, et al. Endoscopic ultrasound-guided interstitial brachytherapy of unresectable pancreatic cancer: results of a pilot trial. Endoscopy 2006;38(4):399–403.

90. Pai M, Habib N, Senturk H, et al. Endoscopic ultrasound guided radiofrequency ablation, for pancreatic cystic neoplasms and neuroendocrine tumors. World J Gastrointest Surg 2015;7(4):52–9.

91. Barthet M, Giovannini M, Lesavre N, et al. Endoscopic ultrasound-guided radiofrequency ablation for pancreatic neuroendocrine tumors and pancreatic cystic neoplasms: a prospective multicenter study. Endoscopy 2019;51(9):836–42.

92. Imperatore N, de Nucci G, Mandelli ED, et al. Endoscopic ultrasound-guided radiofrequency ablation of pancreatic neuroendocrine tumors: a systematic review of the literature. Endosc Int Open 2020;8(12):E1759–64.

93. Dhaliwal A, Kolli S, Dhindsa BS, et al. Efficacy of EUS-RFA in pancreatic tumors: Is it ready for prime time? A systematic review and meta-analysis. Endosc Int Open 2020;8(10):E1243–51.

94. Zhang WY, Li ZS, Jin ZD. Endoscopic ultrasound-guided ethanol ablation therapy for tumors. World J Gastroenterol 2013;19(22):3397–403.

95. Gan SI, Thompson CC, Lauwers GY, et al. Ethanol lavage of pancreatic cystic lesions: initial pilot study. Gastrointest Endosc 2005;61(6):746–52.

96. Du C, Chai NL, Linghu EQ, et al. Endoscopic ultrasound-guided injective ablative treatment of pancreatic cystic neoplasms. World J Gastroenterol 2020; 26(23):3213–24.

97. Qin SY, Lu XP, Jiang HX. EUS-guided ethanol ablation of insulinomas: case series and literature review. Medicine (Baltimore) 2014;93(14):e85.

98. Park DH, Choi JH, Oh D, et al. Endoscopic ultrasonography-guided ethanol ablation for small pancreatic neuroendocrine tumors: results of a pilot study. Clin Endosc 2015;48(2):158–64.

99. Chang KJ, Nguyen PT, Thompson JA, et al. Phase I clinical trial of allogeneic mixed lymphocyte culture (cytoimplant) delivered by endoscopic ultrasound-guided fine-needle injection in patients with advanced pancreatic carcinoma. Cancer 2000;88(6):1325–35.

100. Levy MJ, Alberts SR, Bamlet WR, et al. EUS-guided fine-needle injection of gemcitabine for locally advanced and metastatic pancreatic cancer. Gastrointest Endosc 2017;86(1):161–9.

Endoscopy in Gallstone Pancreatitis

Marco J. Bruno, MD, PhD

KEYWORDS

- Biliary pancreatitis • Choledocholithiasis • ERCP • Gallstone pancreatitis

KEY POINTS

- In patients with biliary pancreatitis and concomitant cholangitis, ERC is indicated urgently.
- In patients with predicted mild biliary pancreatitis without cholangitis, urgent ERC is not indicated.
- In patients with predicted severe biliary pancreatitis without cholangitis, urgent ERC does not ameliorate the disease course, even when stones or sludge are proven on endoscopic ultrasonography imaging.
- To prevent recurrent biliary events after biliary pancreatitis, a cholecystectomy is the option of choice with endoscopic sphincterotomy to be considered in patients unfit for surgery.

INTRODUCTION

The most common gastrointestinal indication for acute hospital admissions in the United States is acute pancreatitis of which a biliary etiology accounts for 45% of the cases.[1,2] Most of the patients suffering from an acute pancreatitis attack, including those with a biliary origin, recover quickly after a few days of hospital observation while receiving adequate pain control. About 20% of patients, however, develop local and systemic complications including systemic inflammatory response syndrome, infected necrosis, and multi-organ failure. Despite aggressive treatment, the mortality rate in these patients ranges between 20% and 40%. For decades, gastroenterologists and endoscopists have sought to halt the disease progression in patients suffering from an acute biliary pancreatitis attack by means of early endoscopic retrograde cholangiography (ERC) for removing biliary stones and/or sludge with the aim to decompress the biliary tree and ampulla and improve pancreatic ductal outflow.

NATURE OF THE PROBLEM

A transient impediment of the flow of secretion from the pancreatic duct caused by gallstones and sludge obstructing the ampulla of Vater has been postulated as the

Department of Gastroenterology & Hepatology, Erasmus University Medical Center, Doctor Molewaterplein 40, Rotterdam 3015 GD, the Netherlands
E-mail address: m.bruno@erasmusmc.nl

Gastrointest Endoscopy Clin N Am 33 (2023) 701–707
https://doi.org/10.1016/j.giec.2023.04.003
1052-5157/23/© 2023 Elsevier Inc. All rights reserved.

giendo.theclinics.com

root cause for the development of acute biliary pancreatitis.[3,4] Interestingly, the duration of the pancreatic duct obstruction seems related to the severity of inflammation of the pancreas.[5] These observations led to the hypothesis that early ERC aimed at removing biliary stones and/or sludge with decompression of the ampulla of Vater and improvement of pancreatic ducal outflow would beneficially influence the disease course preventing the pancreatitis attack to become severe.

Before even contemplating to perform an intervention like an ERC, the first consideration is to accurately diagnose a biliary cause as being responsible for the acute pancreatitis attack. Whereas diagnosing acute pancreatitis usually is not difficult, demonstrating a biliary cause often proves more challenging. Moreover, even when an acute pancreatitis episode is biliary in origin, spontaneous stone passage is known to occur. Earlier studies have shown that spontaneous passage of biliary stones is estimated to occur in 21% to 33% of cases within 4 to 6 weeks, with smaller size stones (<8 mm), which are particularly associated with biliary pancreatitis, passing more often spontaneously.[6,7] More recent prospective studies show that in patients suspected of acute biliary pancreatitis, in 50% to 60% of cases no stones or sludge are found on endoscopic ultrasonography (EUS) or ERC.[8,9]

The question to perform an ERC in acute biliary pancreatitis therefore is multifaceted and based on the following considerations: (1) to establish a biliary etiology, (2) to take into account the possibility of spontaneous stone passage, (3) the likelihood that (early) ERC with sphincterotomy is expected to alter the disease course for better, and (4) the possibility that ERC may cause harm and aggravates the disease course.

DIAGNOSIS

Traditionally, a biliary cause for an episode of acute pancreatitis is considered when stones in the common bile duct (CBD) are visualized on imaging or in case of dilation of the CBD or an abnormal liver panel.[10] Earlier studies on the outcome of ERC in patients with acute biliary pancreatitis relied on (the combination) of the latter two criteria which should be regarded circumstantial evidence for a diagnosis of biliary pancreatitis with varying degrees of probability depending on which cutoff values are used.

Symptoms and blood tests are unreliable to diagnose a biliary cause for an acute pancreatitis attack, particularly early in the course of the disease.[11] However, elevations in the concentrations of bilirubin, alkaline phosphatase, gamma-glutamyl transferase, alanine aminotransferase (ALT) and aspartate aminotransferase (AST) may be indicative for a biliary etiology with a positive predictive value exceeding 80% when ALT is equal or greater than two times the upper limit of normal within 48 hour of hospital admission[8] or equal or greater than three times the upper limit of normal regardless of timing.[12,13]

Although abdominal ultrasound is a highly sensitive investigation for the detection of cholecystolithiasis, it lacks sensitivity to diagnose choledocholithiasis in acute pancreatitis (20%), mainly because of the inability to visualize the CBD in its entirety due to overlying bowel loops.[11,14] Computed tomography for the detection of CBD stones has a sensitivity of 40%.[12] Magnetic resonance cholangiopancreatography (MRCP) has a high overall sensitivity for the detection of choledocholithiasis in patients with acute pancreatitis of 90%, but stones smaller than 5 mm can be easily missed by MRCP.[15] This potentially bears clinical significance. Small stones in particular are thought to be associated with biliary pancreatitis.[16,17] The most sensitive modality to diagnose CBD stones or sludge is EUS with a near perfect specificity and a reported sensitivity between 89% and 96%.[12,18,19] Because of its close approximation to the luminal tract, visualization of the biliary tree, in particular the CBD, is excellent. ERC may never be used as the principle diagnostic tool to look for biliary stones because of its associated complications such as aggravation of the ongoing pancreatitis, perforation, and bleeding.[12,20]

PROCEDURAL APPROACH

ERC in patients with suspected acute biliary pancreatitis in essence is not any different than in regular stone cases. The disease severity and condition of the patient dictate how much support is required from an anesthesiologist and which type of sedation can be used: conscious sedation, propofol sedation, or general anesthesia with intubation. Coagulation must be checked and found within limits, or corrective actions should be taken. In critical patients suffering from associated cholangitis and not fit to undergo an urgent ERC, one should opt for immediate percutaneous drainage.

Management and Outcomes

As gallstones or biliary sludge are thought to initiate but also aggravate pancreatitis in the case of an ongoing obstruction, many researchers have explored the utility and benefit of urgent biliary decompression by ERC.

According to guidelines, urgent ERC with endoscopic sphincterotomy (ES) is warranted in patients with acute biliary pancreatitis and concomitant cholangitis and not recommended in patients with acute biliary pancreatitis with a predicted mild disease course. Limited guidance and evidence, however, are available on the indication of urgent ERC with ES in patients with acute biliary pancreatitis and a predicted severe disease course.[10,21,22]

Several clinical trials have been published in recent decades on the indication of urgent ERC with ES in patients with acute biliary pancreatitis and a predicted severe disease course. Most studies have certain shortcomings that prohibit making a balanced and science-based judgment. First, patient inclusion was not always according to the defined in- and exclusion criteria. Multiple studies wrongly included patients with concomitant cholangitis, patients with a predicted mild disease course, and even patients with a non-gallstone aetiology.[23–27] Second, in most trials, ERC was performed between 24 to 72 hours after admission.[23–25,28] Presumably, for biliary decompression to be effective in preventing complications, ERC needs to be done as early as possible after the onset of symptoms. Apart from the fact that early de-obstruction of biliary and pancreatic outflow may be related to a better outcome, successful biliary cannulation may also be hampered by progressive mucosal and papillary edema later in the disease course. Third, in most RCTs, a biliary sphincterotomy was not performed routinely.[23–25,29] These limitations potentially bear important relevance as smaller-sized stones and microlithiasis can be easily missed on cholangiogram during ERC. Forth, the study population sizes of the RCTs and subsequent meta-analyses were too small to detect an effect of ERC in the group of patients with gallstone pancreatitis with a predicted severe disease course, with and without cholestasis, but without cholangitis.

Recently, a randomized controlled trial (acute biliary pancreatitis: urgent ERCP with sphincterotomy versus conservative treatment [APEC] study) was published in which urgent biliary decompression using ERC with ES was compared with a conservative strategy in patients with predicted severe acute biliary pancreatitis without cholangitis.[8] In the protocol preparation and study execution, extensive efforts were made to avoid shortcomings of previous studies. The timing "urgent" was defined as performing an ERC with sphincterotomy within 24 hours after hospital presentation and within 72 hours after symptom onset. If biliary cannulation was successful, a sphincterotomy was always performed regardless of whether stones were visualized on the cholangiogram. The outcome of this study was that urgent biliary decompression with ERC with ES did not reduce the composite endpoint of major complications, or mortality, as compared with conservative treatment.

The probability for a biliary origin and hence the indication for performing an ERC with sphincterotomy in the APEC study was based on CBD dilation, an increase in ALT, or sludge or stones on imaging (located in the gallbladder or CBD). As already indicated, elevated liver enzymes and radiological signs of CBD stones correlate poorly with the actual presence of CBD stones or sludge during ERC.[8,30] In the APEC trial, for example, in 55% of the patients in the urgent ERC group, no stones or sludge were found during ERC. With hindsight, ERC with ES for biliary decompression in these patients may have been not (longer) indicated and even harmful (eg, aggravation of pancreatitis, hemorrhage, perforation).[31,32]

The most sensitive modality for diagnosing CBD stones or sludge, and hence to determine the indication for ERC with ES, is EUS.[16,33] With this in mind, the prospective multicenter APEC-2 cohort study was designed and carried out in which ERC with ES was only carried out in case of EUS-proven biliary stones or sludge.[9] In the APEC-2 study, CBD stones or sludge were found in 58% of patients during urgent EUS within 24 hours after presentation at the emergency department and within 72 hours of start of symptoms. Immediate ERC with ES following a positive EUS was performed successfully in 90% of cases with a low complication rate (2%). The study outcome was revealing and humbling. Urgent EUS-guided ERC with ES did not reduce the composite endpoint of major complications or mortality as compared with the conservative arm of the APEC randomized trial, despite the most timely and optimal selection of patients.[31]

Based on the current literature, meta-analyses and the results of the APEC and the APEC-2 study (see above), there is no indication to perform an urgent ERC in patients with acute biliary pancreatitis, regardless of predicted severity. The only indication for urgent ERC is (suspected) cholangitis. In the case of clinical signs of persistent CBD stones, ERC with ES for stone removal should be scheduled at a later stage, preferably when the acute attack has subsided. As many (smaller) biliary stones pass spontaneously, it is our routine practice also in these cases to (re)confirm the indication for ERC with EUS in the same session.

The role and timing of cholecystectomy in acute biliary pancreatitis
After an initial attack of biliary pancreatitis, patients run the risk of developing a recurrent episode of biliary pancreatitis or other biliary events, including acute cholecystitis and cholangitis.[32,34]

A prospective study including 233 patients with acute biliary pancreatitis reported a 31-fold chance of recurrence in patients in whom the gallbladder was left in situ with severity and mortality rates of the recurrent episodes similar to those of the primary attack.[35] International guidelines therefore advise performing a cholecystectomy after a biliary pancreatitis or consider an ES in patients unfit for surgery.[36,37] In patients with mild pancreatitis, cholecystectomy is advised directly after recovery or in the first 2 to 4 weeks after discharge for mild biliary pancreatitis.[20,21,34] A recent RCT showed that compared with interval cholecystectomy 25 to 30 days after recovery, same-admission cholecystectomy within 72 hours after recovery of a first episode of mild biliary pancreatitis reduced the rate of recurrent gallstone-related complications in patients with mild gallstone pancreatitis with a very low risk of cholecystectomy-related complications.[38] There is limited scientific evidence to guide the optimal timing to perform a safe cholecystectomy in patients with clinically severe pancreatitis having local complications such as pancreatic necrosis. Usually, cholecystectomy is delayed until local complications have resolved.[9] In a recent *post hoc* analysis of a multicenter prospective cohort, the optimal timing of cholecystectomy after necrotizing biliary pancreatitis, in the absence of peripancreatic collections, was found to be within 8 weeks after discharge.[37]

CLINICS CARE POINTS

- If a patient presents with a (suspected) biliary pancreatitis endoscopic retrograde cholangiopancreaticography (ERCP), do not perform an urgent ERC in an attempt to ameliorate the disease course, regardless of predicted severity, unless the patient has concomitant cholangitis.
- If a patient has retained stones in the biliary tree, schedule an elective ERCP for stone removal once the acute pancreatitis episode has subsided.
- Make sure that every patient who suffered from a biliary pancreatitis episode is scheduled for an elective cholecystectomy to prevent further complication, which in case of a mild episode this should preferably be scheduled during the same admission.

DISCLOSURE

The author declares to act as a paid consultant and lecturer for Boston Scientific, Cook medical, and Pentax Medical, and to have received funds for investigator initiated and industry sponsored studies from Boston Scientific, Cook Medical, United States, Pentax Medical, InterScope, Mylan, United States.

REFERENCES

1. Iannuzzi JP, King JA, Leong JH, et al. Global incidence of acute pancreatitis is increasing over time: a systematic review and meta-analysis. Gastroenterology 2022;162:122–34.
2. Roberts SE, Morrison-Rees S, John A, et al. The incidence and aetiology of acute pancreatitis across Europe. Pancreatology 2017;17:155–65.
3. Lerch MM, Saluja AK, Runzi M, et al. Pancreatic duct obstruction triggers acute necrotizing pancreatitis in the opossum. Gastroenterology 1993;104:853–61.
4. Opie EL. The aetiology of acute haemorrhagic pancreatitis. Bull Johns Hopkins Hosp 1901;xii:182–8.
5. Acosta JM, Rubio Galli OM, Rossi R, et al. Effect of duration of ampullary gallstone obstruction on severity of lesions of acute pancreatitis. J Am Coll Surg 1997;184:499–505.
6. Collins C, Maguire D, Ireland A, et al. A prospective study of common bile duct calculi in patients undergoing laparoscopic cholecystectomy: natural history of choledocholithiasis revisited. Ann Surg 2004;239:28–33.
7. Frossard JL, Hadengue A, Amouyal G, et al. Choledocholithiasis: a prospective study of spontaneous common bile duct stone migration. Gastrointest Endosc 2000;51:175–9.
8. Schepers NJ, Hallensleben NDL, Besselink MG, et al, Dutch Pancreatitis Study Group. Urgent endoscopic retrograde cholangiopancreatography with sphincterotomy versus conservative treatment in predicted severe acute gallstone pancreatitis (APEC): a multicentre randomised controlled trial. Lancet 2020;396:167–76.

9. Hallensleben ND, for the Dutch Pancreatitis Study Group. Urgent endoscopic ultrasound-guided ERC in predicted severe acute biliary pancreatitis (APEC-2): a multicenter prospective study. United Eur Gastroenterol 2021;9(S8):101–2. OP131.

10. Working Group IAP/APA Acute Pancreatitis Guidelines. IAP/APA evidence-based guidelines for the management of acute pancreatitis. Pancreatology 2013;13: e1–15.

11. van Santvoort HC, Bakker OJ, Besselink MG, et al, Dutch Pancreatitis Study Group. Prediction of common bile duct stones in the earliest stages of acute biliary pancreatitis. Endoscopy 2011;43:8–13.

12. Liu CL, Fan ST, Lo CM, et al. Clinico-biochemical prediction of biliary cause of acute pancreatitis in the era of endoscopic ultrasonography. Aliment Pharmacol Ther 2005;22:423–31.

13. Tenner S, Dubner H, Steinberg W. Predicting gallstone pancreatitis with laboratory parameters: a meta-analysis. Am J Gastroenterol 1994;89:1863–6.

14. Moon JH, Cho YD, Cha SW, et al. The detection of bile duct stones in suspected biliary pancreatitis: comparison of MRCP, ERCP, and intraductal US. Am J Gastroenterol 2005;100:1051–7.

15. Kondo S, Isayama H, Akahane M, et al. Detection of common bile duct stones: comparison between endoscopic ultrasonography, magnetic resonance cholangiography, and helical-computed-tomographic cholangiography. Eur J Radiol 2005;54:271–5.

16. Diehl AK, Holleman DR Jr, Chapman JB, et al. Gallstone size and risk of pancreatitis. Arch Intern Med 1997;157(15):1674–8.

17. Venneman NG, Buskens E, Besselink MG, et al. Small gallstones are associated with increased risk of acute pancreatitis: potential benefits of prophylactic cholecystectomy? Am J Gastroenterol 2005;100:2540–50.

18. Stabuc B, Drobne D, Ferkolj I, et al. Acute biliary pancreatitiss: detection of common bile duct stones with endoscopic ultrasound. Eur J Gastroenterol Hepatol 2008;20:1171–5.

19. De Lisi S, Leandro G, Buscarini E. Endoscopic ultrasonography versus endoscopic retrograde cholangiopancreatography in acute biliary pancreatitis: a systematic review. Eur J Gastroenterol Hepatol 2011;23:367–74.

20. Cotton PB, Garrow DA, Gallagher J, et al. Risk factors for complications after ERCP: a multivariate analysis of 11,497 procedures over 12 years. Gastrointest Endosc 2009;70:80–8.

21. Tenner S, Baillie J, DeWitt J, et al. American College of Gastroenterology guideline: management of acute pancreatitis. Am J Gastroenterol 2013;108:1400–15.

22. Crockett SD, Wani S, Gardner TB, et al, American Gastroenterological Association Institute Clinical Guidelines C. American gastroenterological association institute guideline on initial management of acute pancreatitis. Gastroenterology 2018;154:1096–101.

23. Chen P, Hu B, Wang C, et al. Pilot study of urgent endoscopic intervention without fluoroscopy on patients with severe acute biliary pancreatitis in the intensive care unit. Pancreas 2010;39:398–402.

24. Fan ST, Lai EC, Mok FP, et al. Early treatment of acute biliary pancreatitis by endoscopic papillotomy. N Engl J Med 1993;328:228–32.

25. Neoptolemos JP, Carr-Locke DL, London NJ, et al. Controlled trial of urgent endoscopic retrograde cholangiopancreatography and endosc opic sphincterotomy versus conservative treatment for acute pancreatitis due to gallstones. Lancet 1988;2:979–83.

26. Zhou MQ, Li NP, Lu RD. Duodenoscopy in treatment of acute gallstone pancreatitis. Hepatobiliary Pancreat Dis Int 2002;1:608–10.
27. Folsch UR, Nitsche R, Ludtke R, et al. Early ERCP and papillotomy compared with conservative treatment for acute biliary pancreatitis. The German Study Group on Acute Biliary Pancreatitis. N Engl J Med 1997;336:237–42.
28. Oria A, Cimmino D, Ocampo C, et al. Early endoscopic intervention versus early conservative management in patients with acute gallstone pancreatitis and biliopancreatic obstruction: a randomized clinical trial. Ann Surg 2007;245:10–7.
29. Acosta JM, Katkhouda N, Debian KA, et al. Early ductal decompression versus conservative management for gallstone pancreatitis with ampullary obstruction: a prospective randomized clinical trial. Ann Surg 2006;243:33–40.
30. Anderloni A, Galeazzi M, Ballare M, et al. Early endoscopic ultrasonography in acute biliary pancreatitis: A prospective pilot study. World J Gastroenterol 2015;21:10427–34.
31. Hallensleben ND, Stassen PMC, Schepers NJ, et al. for the Dutch Pancreatitis Study Group. Urgent endoscopic ultrasound-guided endoscopic retrograde cholangiopancreatography in predicted severe acute biliary pancreatitis (APEC-2): a multicentre prospective study, Gut, 2023, doi: 10.1136/gutjnl-2022-328258. Online ahead of print.
32. Forsmark CE, Baillie J. AGA institute technical review on acute pancreatitis. Gastroenterology 2007;132:2022–44.
33. Giljaca V, Gurusamy KS, Takwoingi Y, et al. Endoscopic ultrasound versus magnetic resonance cholangiopancreatography for common bile duct stones. Cochrane Database Syst Rev 2015;2:CD011549.
34. Banks PA, Freeman ML. Practice guidelines in acute pancreatitis. Am J Gastroenterol 2006;101:2379–400.
35. Hernandez V, Pascual I, Almela P, et al. Recurrence of acute gallstone pancreatitis and relationship with cholecystectomy or endoscopic sphincterotomy. Am J Gastroenterol 2004;99:2417–23.
36. Uhl W, Warshaw A, Imrie C, et al. International Association of Pancreatology: IAP guidelines for the surgical management of acute pancreatitis. Pancreatology 2002;2:565–73.
37. Hallensleben ND, Timmerhuis HC, Hollemans RA, et al. Dutch Pancreatitis Study Group. Optimal timing of cholecystectomy after necrotising biliary pancreatitis. Gut 2022;71:974–82.
38. da Costa DW, Bouwense SA, Schepers NJ, et al, Dutch Pancreatitis Study Group. Same-admission versus interval cholecystectomy for mild gallstone pancreatitis (PONCHO): a multicentre randomised controlled trial. Lancet 2015;386(10000): 1261–8.

Endoscopic Necrosectomy

Andrew J. Gilman, MD, Todd H. Baron, MD*

KEYWORDS

- Direct endoscopy necrosectomy • Pancreatic necrosis • Pancreatitis • Endoscopy

KEY POINTS

- Direct endoscopic necrosectomy (DEN) is best performed by endoscopists in a tertiary center.
- A combination of chemical and mechanical debridement can be used to perform DEN.
- Paracolic gutter extension often portends the need for percutaneous access.
- The use of plastic stents across lumen apposing metal stents, between DEN sessions, can reduce adverse event rates.
- A variety of devices, some emerging and some familiar, are available for DEN and will be discussed.

 Video content accompanies this article at http://www.giendo.theclinics.com.

INTRODUCTION

Endoscopic drainage of pancreatic necrosis was first described in 1996, 27 years ago, with subsequent direct endoscopic necrosectomy (DEN) first described in 2000.[1,2] Since then both have undergone significant advances. Treatment of pancreatic necrosis was once exclusively surgical but has transitioned to a multimodal approach with endoscopy as the backbone.[3–7] Initial transmural treatment of walled-off necrosis (WON) involved only endoscopic identification of extrinsic compression with transmural drainage using plastic stent placement, now uniformly performed with endoscopic ultrasound (EUS) guidance and lumen apposing metal stents (LAMS).[8–10] Creation of access points into WON is discussed elsewhere in this issue. This article focuses on management of WON after access has been obtained but has been shown to be insufficient in leading to resolution.

Division of Gastroenterology & Hepatology, University of North Carolina, 130 Mason Farm Road, Bioinformatics Building CB# 7080, Chapel Hill, NC 27599-7080, USA
* Corresponding author.
E-mail address: todd_baron@med.unc.edu
Twitter: @a_gilman (A.J.G.); @EndoTx (T.H.B.)

Gastrointest Endoscopy Clin N Am 33 (2023) 709–724
https://doi.org/10.1016/j.giec.2023.04.010
1052-5157/23/© 2023 Elsevier Inc. All rights reserved.

giendo.theclinics.com

NATURE OF THE PROBLEM

Endoscopic treatment of WON involves numerous nuances and flavors. There is no clear-cut optimal workflow with guidelines focusing on platitudes of treatment, opening the door for further study and customization of DEN to the endoscopist's experience and the patient's response.[11,12]

Chemical Debridement

Before physical debridement of DEN became part of routine care, drainage was often augmented by chemical debridement. Discontinuation of gastric acid suppression after drainage allows gastric acid to breakdown solid debris. In one retrospective multicenter study, no proton pump inhibitor (PPI) use was found to be associated with less DEN sessions without a difference in bleeding or infection rates.[13] However, no PPI use was also associated with a higher rate of LAMS stent occlusion, suggesting that gastric acid dissolves and mobilizes necrosis. This risk may be mitigated by concurrent use of plastic stents across LAMS. Therefore, it is recommended to discontinue PPI after transmural drainage assuming there is not an acute indication for its use.

Additional chemical agents have been used variably in the treatment of WON. Aggressive irrigation was initially described using endoscopic placement of a nasocystic tube. This practice has generally fallen out of favor given the unclear additive benefits when LAMS are placed and the relative lack of patient acceptance. Hydrogen peroxide instillation has been used despite uncertain benefits from retrospective studies.[14,15] It has also been used as an irrigant infused through percutaneously placed necrosectomy catheters.[16] Instillation of antibiotics has also been described, also with uncertain clinical benefits.[17,18] Although significant increases in adverse events (AEs) associated with use of either of these have not been reported, the lack of clear benefit combined with the theoretical risk of aspiration (for hydrogen peroxide) precludes our group's routine use of them.

Streptokinase irrigation has also been reported with the aim of dissolution and mobilization of solid debris.[19] Although one study showed that streptokinase use was associated with a lower rate of surgical intervention and mortality, robust data are lacking.

Management of WON is ever evolving and with the introduction of LAMS and DEN we have found limited clinical benefit to chemical debridement. Outside of stopping PPI when able they are not part of our practice.

Mechanical Debridement (Direct Endoscopic Necrosectomy) and Indications

As changes in management shifted toward incorporating physical debridement, an initial question posed was whether endoscopic drainage with irrigation alone was sufficient or if the augmentation of DEN produced clinically meaningful benefits. Although a subset of patients can achieve WON resolution without DEN, it clearly has a role in improving endoscopic outcomes (higher resolution rate with lower need for surgery or percutaneous drains, lower recurrence) yet with similar AEs.[20] In practice, DEN is recommended and often pursued in the presence of substantial solid debris identified either by endosonographic images or after subsequent cross-sectional imaging reveals a large amount of solid necrosis or the collection has failed to resolve, even when only small volume.[11,12]

Pre-drainage imaging studies can predict treatment response, which can be important in managing both patient and health care providers' expectations. The composition of a collection and its percentage of solid versus liquid content can influence outcome since mostly liquid collections often resolve with LAMS placement alone.[21] Similarly, pre-drainage CT characteristics including size of the collection, its location, the presence of hemorrhage, and concern for pancreatic duct disconnection can allow one to predict the number of DEN sessions needed for resolution.[22] However, difficulty with prediction of degree of underlying solid composition prior to evacuation of the liquid component limits the utility of CT.[23–25] Similarly, EUS is limited by poor interobserver agreement for percentage solid component, though good agreement for procedural planning.[26] MRI can provide reasonable estimates of composition though sacrifices spatial resolution, which may be beneficial for procedural planning.[24] Most patients undergo initial drainage followed by repeat CT imaging to assess remaining solid material and, if present, proceed with DEN as clinically indicated.

In one recent retrospective study, this so-called "step-up therapy" was required in slightly >50% of patients who underwent drainage with LAMS placement, demonstrating that DEN plays a frequent role in management.[27] Step-up therapy is utilized for both endoscopic and surgical approaches. Endoscopic step-up begins with endoscopic transmural drainage and proceeds to DEN if there is a lack of clinical improvement/resolution by imaging. Surgical step-up begins with percutaneous drainage and proceeds to minimally invasive debridement (typically video-assisted retroperitoneal debridement [VARD]) as needed. Endoscopic step-up appears to have similar complication rates and mortality compared to surgical step-up with the advantage of a decrease in rate of external fistulae and shorter hospital stays, leading to its prioritization when available.[28] In our practice, we have found that most patients do not progress past percutaneous drainage in the surgical step-up pathway, but this is contingent on the use of aggressive DEN.

Severity of illness of patients with WON can be compelling and the pressure to act is high. These patients are best managed through multidisciplinary collaboration involving experienced gastroenterology, diagnostic and interventional radiology, critical care, and surgical teams.[11,12] One recent study found that an annual volume of 15 EUS-guided drainages of pancreatic fluid collections was associated with the lowest risk of AEs.[29]

ANATOMY
Paracolic Extension

The variety of shapes and distribution of WON underlines the need to tailor approaches to an individual patient while remaining within the experience and ability of the endoscopist. This especially holds true when progress on resolution of WON with DEN alone stalls, as is frequently the case in the presence of paracolic gutter extension and greatly increases the need to incorporate surgical step-up, beginning with percutaneous drainage.[30]

Although some patients will have a single ovoid central pancreatic collection, multilobulated or multiple discrete collections with thin communications are frequently encountered and often found with paracolic extension. A transgastric approach targeting the most anterior and superior aspect of WON establishes a gradient that can be problematic for large collections. Even with the most aggressive multi-gate drainage and DEN, the deepest depths of these pockets have an uphill battle against gravity to pass contents into the stomach or duodenum.

To combat this, our group has explored aggressive reduction in resistance to flow within the cavity to lower the pressure gradient needed to yield egress of debris as close to the stomach or duodenum as possible. Overcoming the barrier to passage from the deep recesses of the cavity can facilitate resolution. To this end we have used fully covered self-expandable metal stents (FC-SEMS) deployed entirely within the WON cavity, particularly at the site of thin communications between larger collections. **Figs. 1–5** illustrate a case where this technique successfully augmented drainage of a deep paracolic extension. A less aggressive, yet similar in theory, method has been the use of very long double pigtail plastic stents (DPPS) (**Figs. 6 and 7**). Cutting a nasobiliary drain to create a custom length single pigtail plastic stent may also be possible for very deep paracolic extension. Transcolonic drainage could potentially serve a similar role.

Surgical step-up enters the algorithm when the above approaches fail, and necrotic debris cannot be cleared from the paracolic gutters. In the spirit of ownership of WON as a gastroenterological problem, some centers have explored percutaneous necrosectomy as an endoscopic procedure. Similar to transluminal drainage, FC-SEMS can be placed across percutaneous drain tracts to allow endoscopic entry into WON followed by DEN as is done transluminally.[31–33] The principle is the same as when comparing simple EUS transluminal drainage to DEN–solid debris needs large conduits and mechanical removal, and often limited bore plastic catheters are not sufficient. One concern with augmenting percutaneous tracts is the creation of an eventual pancreaticocutaneous fistula, the risk of which is unknown with percutaneous FC-SEMS. This may be mitigated by a stepwise removal of entry sites into WON, with transluminal being the last.

EQUIPMENT AND MATERIALS

As with esophageal food impactions, a variety of devices are available to assist with DEN, often a lengthy and arduous procedure. Our most commonly used item is the "spiral" snare (SnareMaster, Olympus America, Center Valley, PA, USA). Its unique wire properties allow for more secure entrapment of debris while preventing inadvertent cutting, though an experienced endoscopy tech is still essential. By anchoring the

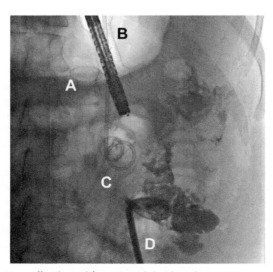

Fig. 1. Paracolic gutter collection with contrast injection via percutaneous drain to delineate dimensions. (*A*) LAMS at site of gastroenterostomy. (*B*) FC-SEMS and DPPS at cystgastrostomy. (*C*) Percutaneous jejunostomy tube. (*D*) Percutaneous drain into paracolic portion of collection.

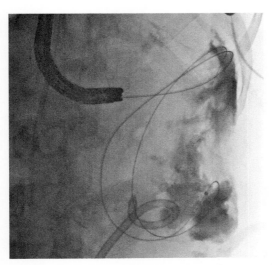

Fig. 2. Passage of catheter and wire into deep recesses of collection, adjacent to percutaneous drain.

tip against the wall of the cavity and laying the snare down, as though preparing for polypectomy, large pieces can be securely grasped and pulled through an LAMS, even when liquid obscures direct visualization of solid material (Videos 1–3). Some groups have also described using cautery to create grooves in solid debris to further enhance grip.[34]

Numerous other devices can also be used, with options only limited by creativity and availability. Common through-the-scope devices also include the Rescue Grasper and RescueNet (Boston Scientific, Marlborough, MA, USA) and Talon Grasper (Steris

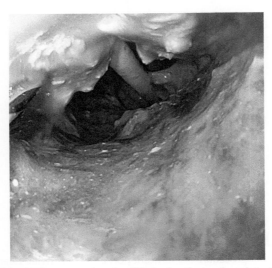

Fig. 3. Traversal of the endoscope using the "finder" catheter deep into the collection, with direct visualization of the percutaneous drain.

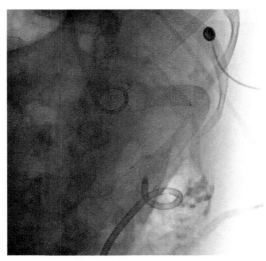

Fig. 4. Placement of FC-SEMS fully within the cavity bridging between transgastric and percutaneous entry points.

Healthcare, Mentor, OH, USA) (Video 4). Their use can also be combined with a distal attachment cap that can improve the efficacy of "grasping" with suction without clogging the working channel.[35] Novel over-the-scope graspers have also been developed to allow safe and efficient DEN (Xcavator, Ovesco Endoscopy AG, Tübingen, Germany).[36] An intriguing high pressure water jet device similar to a pressure washer has also undergone preclinical testing and was effective and rapidly reducing the size of solid debris.[37]

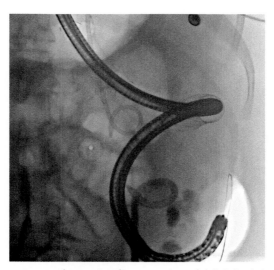

Fig. 5. On a subsequent procedure a significant portion of debris had cleared through the 2 FC-SEMS to the stomach. The endoscope was able to traverse deeply within to complete DEN in this portion.

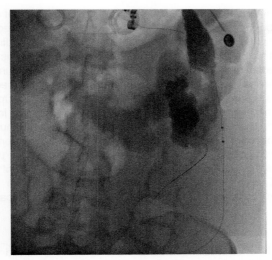

Fig. 6. Catheter and wire delineating deep recesses of paracolic gutter extension.

Even endoscopic submucosal dissection (ESD) techniques and tools have made their way into DEN. One group described tunnel creation through tracing a plastic stent placed solely with fluoroscopic visualization, followed by balloon dilation along the course of the stent to improve visualization and tissue evacuation.[38] ESD knives can also provide fine-tuned, rotatable grasping.[39] Necessity is the mother of invention, and the laborious nature of DEN has and will continue to spawn creative solutions.

Endoscopic morcellators have gained recent attention (EndoRotor, Interscope, Inc, Northbridge, MA, USA).[40] A through-the-scope catheter with a controllable rotating cutting edge, when combined with suction, can potentially lead to rapid clearance

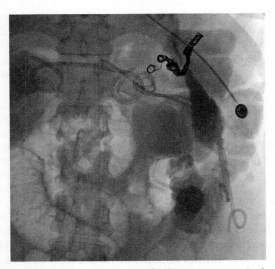

Fig. 7. Long DPPS placed into the collection to facilitate transgastric drainage.

of debris. Concerns about a rotating knife within a cavity and risk of damaging major vasculature have been partially alleviated by the lack of device-related AEs in a recent prospective multicenter trial of 30 patients.[41] Gastrointestinal bleeding occurred in 2 patients, believed to be procedure and not device related. In this study, patients only required a median of 1.5 DEN sessions but with a mean procedure time of 117 minutes and mean device time of 71 minutes. These durations do not seem to be shorter than typical DEN sessions, so the time benefit is unclear. One group highlighted the controlled nature and improved visualization that may lead to less inadvertent injury to major vessels.[42] The device has also been used via percutaneous tracks, further blurring the lines between surgical (VARD) and endoscopic management.[43]

Although morcellators and other devices show the promise for use during DEN, more data are needed regarding their safety and improvement of outcomes. The ongoing lack of Current Procedural Terminology (CPT) codes for DEN is also an impediment to introduction and adaptation of devices that require capital purchases.

ADVERSE EVENTS

AEs following DEN offer a few additional risks to those incurred with initial EUS drainage of WON. Principle concerns are perforation (in the form of dislodgement/disconnection of the FC-SEMS or LAMS maintaining access to the WON as well as perforation of the wall not in contact with the transmural site), intracavitary bleeding, infection, stent occlusion, pneumoperitoneum, fistula formation, and fatal air embolism.[11,44–47] Most high-quality externally validated data regarding AE rates focus on EUS drainage rather than DEN itself.

The potential for severe bleeding underlines the recommendation of pursuing DEN in centers with interventional radiology and surgical backup. One study reported a bleeding rate of 5.2% per procedure or 11.9% per patient which was similar to previous reports.[48] In this study, direct endoscopic visualization of a vessel, cirrhosis, and thrombocytopenia conferred a significantly increased risk of bleeding. Given the multiple major vessels that can course nearby, severe bleeding can result from DEN as from arterial pseudoaneurysms. Often endoscopic management of intraprocedural bleeding can be limited by visualization and obscurement of the source. Traditional endoscopic hemostasis devices can be used, including clips, cautery (grasper or probe based), epinephrine, and even argon plasma coagulation.[49] Spray-based hemostatic powders (Hemospray, Cook Medical, Bloomington, IN, USA) may be helpful as a rescue device. Its use would be contingent on a relatively dry cavity with an identifiable bleeding source, which may not be possible within WON cavities.

Double Pigtail Plastic Stent Use

DPPS placement through an LAMS has often been suggested as a means of reducing AE rates. The WON cavity is dynamic and changes between the time of LAMS placement and removal. As the cavity decreases in size, the back wall or an egressing piece of solid necrosis may lead to occlusion of the LAMS lumen. The flanges of the stent may also abrade the back wall leading to bleeding–one of the rationales for removal of LAMS prior to 60 days (as the cavity significantly collapses down). The role of DPPS then is to serve as a tent pole for the stent.

This theoretical benefit of DPPS has been variably observed. One retrospective study of 46 patients who underwent LAMS placement for pseudocyst drainage found a non-significant trend toward decreased infection with placement of DPPS.[50] A separate retrospective study of 41 patients found DPPS use significantly lowered global AE rate, despite the higher patient ASA score; bleeding was the most frequently occurring event (though not statistically significantly different).[51] A recent, randomized controlled trial included 67 patients and found DPPS resulted in significantly lower global AE rate and stent occlusion, but did not significantly alter bleeding.[52] Infection rates after LAMS placement (with or without DPPS) were not reported.

Given the lack of clear and convincing evidence supporting the advantages of DPPS with LAMS, their use is not mandatory. Although no studies have shown an increase in risk in their use, the need to remove and replace them with each DEN session will certainly add time and cost for an already lengthy procedure without a dedicated CPT code. However, more convincing data may become available as more patients have them utilized–each of the above studies may not be powered to detect differences in outcomes. A yet explored potential benefit may also be the mitigation of risks of LAMS which dwell for longer than the dwell time based upon LAMS manufacturer labeling (eg, 60 days for WON using the AXIOS device). Our group routinely uses DPPS with all LAMS for WON.

PREPROCEDURE PLANNING

- Prior to initiating drainage of WON with potential future DEN, consider transfer of the patient to a facility with interventional radiology and surgical backup, if none are available locally.
- Personally review all available pertinent cross-sectional imaging.
- Obtain contrast-enhanced CT if not recently done. Repeat imaging after initial drainage but before considering DEN.
- If the WON has not responded to drainage (symptoms with any remaining size or large amount of remaining cavity size/contents), consider DEN.
- Prior to initiating DEN, personally commit to the likely need for multiple repeated sessions.
  - Given the theoretical need for LAMS removal at 60 days, it is advised to make significant headways against WON volume reduction prior to this time.
- Informed consent and discussion with the patient with emphasis on multiple sessions and potential for slow resolution/recovery.
- Ensure there are no barriers to completing another DEN session prior to starting:
  - Adequate time slot–we suggest at least 1 hour for each DEN session.
  - Preferred equipment available–some of the devices routinely used in DEN are not otherwise used. Low or no stock of an item may not be discovered until after it is requested during the procedure. This can be particularly critical for hemostasis devices.
- Consider stopping PPI if there are no strong indications for continuing, as discussed under *Chemical Debridement*.

PREP AND PATIENT POSITIONING

- Endoscope choice
  - A gastroscope with a therapeutic channel should be used, at minimum. The lessened likelihood of clogging of the channel can lead to a smoother and more efficient experience. This will be required if 10 French DPPS are intended to be used at the end of the DEN session, or if a dislodged LAMS needs replacement.
  - For WON that might respond to suction and lavage alone, consider a gastroscope with an extra-large working channel, such as the GIF-XTQ160 (Olympus America, Center Valley, PA, USA). If the solid pieces are small enough, or made small enough during the procedure, this endoscope can facilitate a quick DEN.
  - Significant disadvantages are the reduced agility and large outer diameter which can make WON entry impossible depending on the position of the LAMS.

- Strongly consider intubation:
  - Although not mandatory for procedural completion, there are a number of potential aspiration risks from DEN including the removal of solid debris through the mouth rather than depositing in the gastric antrum, presence of fluid within the cavity, and use of irrigation during the procedure, especially when using hydrogen peroxide as mentioned above in *Chemical Debridement.*
  - Potential disadvantages:
    - Procedural duration (though as above it can be crucial to success to ensure ample time is available).
    - Inability to extubate (critically ill but not currently intubated patients may be difficult to extubate postprocedure).
- Consider fluoroscopy:
  - Particularly if the WON cavity is large or contains percutaneous drain. Although not essential, fluoroscopy can aid navigation into deep recesses of the collection. This can be particularly helpful when attempting to augment paracolic drainage toward the stomach. Its use becomes more important if entry into the WON is maintained without LAMS, as the cystgastrostomy tract can become quite narrow even after only short periods of time.
  - Potential disadvantages:
    - Higher (though not definite) need for intubation.
    - Not needed for DPPS placement post-DEN if LAMS is present.
    - Physical burden on endoscopy team (protective lead use can make an already lengthy procedure seem much longer).
- Use of CO_2 insufflation rather than air *is essential* to reduce the risk of fatal air embolization.

PROCEDURAL APPROACH

- Predetermine goals for the session:
  - Because most patients often require more than one DEN session, it can be helpful to set goals/stopping points for each session. We typically assign a loose time constraint of one hour. This often can coincide with specific milestones: clearance of the entryway, clearance of the main cavity, access to distant subcavities (such as in paracolic gutter extension), and clearance of those cavities. Although an individual patient may have each of the above steps take more or less time, they can all easily take an hour. Having a goal in mind can reduce the burden of performing this cumbersome procedure.
- Access to the cavity depends on initial drainage modality
  - LAMS:
    - Remove any indwelling plastic stents
    - Although reusing the same plastic stents after DEN may be possible, this could risk dislodgment of the LAMS. It can also be helpful to use progressively longer DPPS that mirror your progress through clearance to facilitate egress of deeper portions of the cavity (**Fig. 8**).
    - We place DPPS across the LAMS at the end of every DEN session, as discussed above under section "Adverse events."
  - DPPS:
    - Remove stents either before or after wire cannulation.
    - Balloon dilate the cystgastrostomy tract to 20 mm.
    - Place new stents across the tract at the end of the DEN session.

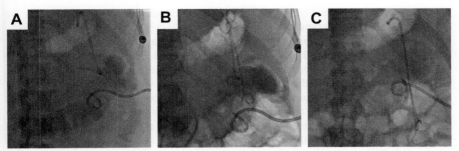

Fig. 8. Progressively longer DPPS (*A–C*) tracking the progress of DEN and facilitating egress between procedures.

- Clearance of the entryway
  - During the first DEN session, we often encounter necrotic debris impacted within and occluding LAMS. Clearance can be challenging given the frequent acute angulation required to enter the stent. Short throw devices can be helpful here (such as grasping forceps), though care needs to be taken to not grasp the LAMS. Suction can also be helpful though may lead to frequent endoscope clogging.
- Clearance of the main cavity
  - We almost exclusively use the spiral snare at this stage. Achieving efficiency with it can prove to be an unexpectedly steep learning curve. Anchoring the snare tip against the cavity wall followed by directing the sheath to the opposite wall to "lay down" the snare perpendicular to the axis of the endoscope can maximize debris entrapment, even with poor visualization (see Videos 1–3). This is a similar maneuver to colonic polypectomy when the target is straight in front and cannot be rotated to 6 o'clock.
  - Care should be taken to avoid injury to vessels within the cavity. Pink walls with oozing blood upon irritation are to be expected and should resolve spontaneously without intervention (Video 5).
  - If significant bleeding occurs and is not responsive to traditional hemostatic techniques, discussed above in AEs, there should be a low threshold for escalation of care and involvement of interventional radiology for embolization. Bleeding in these scenarios can become massive and fatal if not promptly identified and remedied.
- Access to distant subcavities
  - Fluoroscopy and recent cross-sectional imaging can be particularly helpful in this phase. If a percutaneous drain has been placed, a "finder" wire can be passed to probe a route toward it. If needed, balloon dilation can then facilitate endoscope entry into these subcavities, which are often connected to the main cavity through thin passageways.
  - Placement of stents from the gastric lumen all the way down to subcavities at this stage can augment egress toward the stomach and maintain progress achieved in this stage. We often use DPPS, though have used fully intracavitary FC-SEMS in the past (see **Figs. 1–5**).
- Clearance of subcavities
  - This is the final stage of DEN. Robust access into these areas achieved previously can lead to a trail of breadcrumbs of egressing debris. If access cannot be achieved percutaneous debridement may be beneficial, as discussed in section *"Paracolic extension"*.

- Attempt to complete DEN sessions prior to 60 days so that LAMS can be removed within this time.
  - Current FDA indications for use labeling states that LAMS are intended for implantation of up to 60 days. However, in common clinical practice an informal goal of 4 weeks of implantation time is often targeted.
  - As above there is a theoretical risk of increased AEs, particularly bleeding, if LAMS remain in place for longer periods. We expect this risk to be mitigated by concurrent DPPS use though this has not been scientifically confirmed.
  - If additional DEN sessions are needed, it would be reasonable to keep LAMS in place slightly longer than 2 months or to convert access into the WON cavity via DPPS alone, as was done prior to LAMS availability.
- When possible, we delay removal of transgastric or transduodenal access until after all percutaneous access has been removed. This is done to reduce the rate of pancreaticocutaneous fistula formation.

MANAGEMENT, OUTCOMES, AND RECOVERY

- It is reasonable to perform DEN as an outpatient procedure. The need for additional DEN sessions should not be a factor preventing discharge of a patient.
- Each patient may have some pain after each session, which is normal. This should resolve within 1 day and be replaced with a better tolerance of oral intake with less nausea and vomiting.
- Expectation setting for patients can be critical. We often advise that it can take months to a year or more for a patient to fully recover from necrotizing pancreatitis that requires DEN.
- These patients may develop new-onset (or worsening) pancreatic insufficiency, both exocrine and endocrine. Monitoring for this, starting pancreatic enzyme replacement therapy, and ensuring a patient has a primary care physician can improve outcomes in this recovery phase. For these reasons, it is advised to have clinic follow-up with patients for at least one visit after completion of DEN.
- Monitoring WON response to treatment with cross-sectional imaging is crucial. We obtain contrast-enhanced CT prior to the first and suspected last DEN sessions. After LAMS removal, we repeat imaging again to ensure a fluid collection (pseudocyst) has not developed. If this occurs, consider if there is disconnected pancreatic duct, discussed elsewhere in this issue.
- Consider internal monitoring of success and AE rates for quality control.

SUMMARY

The management of WON has evolved substantially over the past 23 years since it was first described. In this article, we reviewed its history and the evidence supporting modern practice, which is still subject to heterogeneity across centers and based on many factors, including endoscopist experience. This allows for creativity and customization of what can be an endoscopic marathon. Our typical practice was discussed with image and video guides aimed at improving procedure success.

CLINICS CARE POINTS

- DEN is best performed at centers with experience in the techniques involved and with both interventional radiology and surgical backup.

- Some patients may respond to drainage alone. A lack of improvement in symptoms and a large residual cavity after drainage are indications for DEN. This process has been coined "endoscopic step-up".
- A combination of chemical and mechanical debridement can be used. Stopping PPI use can be effective and safe. Hydrogen peroxide use is under ongoing investigation and appears to be safe but with questionable benefit.
- Paracolic gutter extension often portends the need for percutaneous access and introduction of "surgical step-up". There have been recent forays into endoscopic approaches, but involvement of teams outside of gastroenterology is critical in this scenario.
- The use of plastic stents across LAMS, between DEN sessions, can reduce AE rates.
- A variety of devices, some emerging and some familiar, are discussed. Some of these may play an integral role in DEN of the future as additional evidence becomes available.

DISCLOSURE

A.J. Gilman has nothing to disclose. T. H. Baron is a consultant and speaker for Ambu, Boston Scientific, Cook Endoscopy, Medtronic, Olympus America, and W.L. Gore.

SUPPLEMENTARY DATA

Supplementary data related to this article can be found online at https://doi.org/10.1016/j.giec.2023.04.010.

REFERENCES

1. Baron TH, Thaggard WG, Morgan DE, et al. Endoscopic therapy for organized pancreatic necrosis. Gastroenterology 1996;111:755–64.
2. Seifert H, Wehrmann T, Schmitt T, et al. Retroperitoneal endoscopic debridement for infected peripancreatic necrosis. Lancet 2000;356:653–5.
3. van Brunschot S, Hollemans RA, Bakker OJ, et al. Minimally invasive and endoscopic versus open necrosectomy for necrotising pancreatitis: a pooled analysis of individual data for 1980 patients. Gut 2018;67(4):697–706.
4. Hollemans RA, Bakker OJ, Boermeester MA, et al. Superiority of step-up approach vs open necrosectomy in long-term follow-up of patients with necrotizing pancreatitis. Gastroenterology 2019;156(4):1016–26.
5. Onnekink AM, Boxhoorn L, Timmerhuis HC, et al. Endoscopic versus surgical step-up approach for infected necrotizing pancreatitis (ExTENSION): long-term follow-up of a randomized trial. Gastroenterology 2022;163(3):712–722 e14.
6. van Santvoort HC, Besselink MG, Bakker OJ, et al. A step-up approach or open necrosectomy for necrotizing pancreatitis. N Engl J Med 2010;362(16):1491–502.
7. Bakker OJ, van Santvoort H, van Brunschot S, et al. Endoscopic transgastric vs surgical necrosectomy for infected necrotizing pancreatitis: a randomized trial. JAMA 2012;307(10):1053–61.
8. Grimm H, Binmoeller KF, Soehendra N. Endosonography-guided drainage of a pancreatic pseudocyst. Gastrointest Endosc 1992;38(2):170–1.
9. Seifert H, Dietrich C, Schmitt T, et al. Endoscopic ultrasound-guided one-step transmural drainage of cystic abdominal lesions with a large-channel echo endoscope. Endoscopy 2000;32(3):255–9.
10. Seewald S, Groth S, Omar S, et al. Aggressive endoscopic therapy for pancreatic necrosis and pancreatic abscess: a new safe and effective treatment algorithm (videos). Gastrointest Endosc 2005;62(1):92–100.

11. Baron TH, DiMaio CJ, Wang AY, et al. American gastroenterological association clinical practice update: management of pancreatic necrosis. Gastroenterology 2020;158(1):67–75 e1.

12. Arvanitakis M, Dumonceau JM, Albert J, et al. Endoscopic management of acute necrotizing pancreatitis: European Society of Gastrointestinal Endoscopy (ESGE) evidence-based multidisciplinary guidelines. Endoscopy 2018;50(5):524–46.

13. Powers PC, Siddiqui A, Sharaiha RZ, et al. Discontinuation of proton pump inhibitor use reduces the number of endoscopic procedures required for resolution of walled-off pancreatic necrosis. Endosc Ultrasound 2019;8(3):194–8.

14. Messallam AA, Adler DG, Shah RJ, et al. Direct Endoscopic Necrosectomy With and Without Hydrogen Peroxide for Walled-off Pancreatic Necrosis: A Multicenter Comparative Study. Am J Gastroenterol 2021;116(4):700–9.

15. Mohan BP, Madhu D, Toy G, et al. Hydrogen peroxide-assisted endoscopic necrosectomy of pancreatic walled-off necrosis: a systematic review and meta-analysis. Gastrointest Endosc 2022;95(6):1060–1066 e7.

16. Ghabili K, Shaikh J, Pollak J, et al. Percutaneous chemical and mechanical necrosectomy for walled-off pancreatic necrosis. J Vasc Interv Radiol 2022. https://doi.org/10.1016/j.jvir.2022.11.011.

17. Larino-Noia J, de la Iglesia-Garcia D, Gonzalez-Lopez J, et al. Endoscopic drainage with local infusion of antibiotics to avoid necrosectomy of infected walled-off necrosis. Surg Endosc 2021;35(2):644–51.

18. Werge M, Novovic S, Roug S, et al. Evaluation of local instillation of antibiotics in infected walled-off pancreatic necrosis. Pancreatology 2018;18(6):642–6.

19. Bhargava V, Gupta R, Vaswani P, et al. Streptokinase irrigation through a percutaneous catheter helps decrease the need for necrosectomy and reduces mortality in necrotizing pancreatitis as part of a step-up approach. Surgery 2021;170(5):1532–7.

20. Gardner TB, Chahal P, Papachristou GI, et al. A comparison of direct endoscopic necrosectomy with transmural endoscopic drainage for the treatment of walled-off pancreatic necrosis. Gastrointest Endosc 2009;69(6):1085–94.

21. Hollemans RA, Bollen TL, van Brunschot S, et al. Predicting success of catheter drainage in infected necrotizing pancreatitis. Ann Surg 2016;263(4):787–92.

22. Cosgrove N, Shetty A, McLean R, et al. Radiologic predictors of increased number of necrosectomies during endoscopic management of walled-off pancreatic necrosis. J Clin Gastroenterol 2022;56(5):457–63.

23. Banks PA, Bollen TL, Dervenis C, et al. Classification of acute pancreatitis–2012: revision of the Atlanta classification and definitions by international consensus. Gut 2013;62(1):102–11.

24. Kapoor H, Issa M, Winkler MA, et al. The augmented role of pancreatic imaging in the era of endoscopic necrosectomy: an illustrative and pictorial review. Abdom Radiol (NY) 2020;45(5):1534–49.

25. Finkelmeier F, Sturm C, Friedrich-Rust M, et al. Predictive value of computed tomography scans and clinical findings for the need of endoscopic necrosectomy in walled-off necrosis from pancreatitis. Pancreas 2017;46(8):1039–45.

26. Fabbri C, Baron TH, Gibiino G, et al. The endoscopic ultrasound features of pancreatic fluid collections and their impact on therapeutic decisions: an interobserver agreement study. Endoscopy 2022;54(6):555–62.

27. Chandrasekhara V, Elhanafi S, Storm AC, et al. Predicting the need for step-up therapy after EUS-guided drainage of pancreatic fluid collections with lumen-apposing metal stents. Clin Gastroenterol Hepatol 2021;19(10):2192–8.

28. van Brunschot S, van Grinsven J, van Santvoort HC, et al. Endoscopic or surgical step-up approach for infected necrotising pancreatitis: a multicentre randomised trial. Lancet 2018;391(10115):51–8.

29. Facciorusso A, Amato A, Crino SF, et al. Definition of a hospital volume threshold to optimize outcomes after drainage of pancreatic fluid collections with lumen-apposing metal stents: a nationwide cohort study. Gastrointest Endosc 2022; 95(6):1158–72.

30. Zhai YQ, Ryou M, Thompson CC. Predicting success of direct endoscopic necrosectomy with lumen-apposing metal stents for pancreatic walled-off necrosis. Gastrointest Endosc 2022;96(3):522–529 e1.

31. Kedia P, Parra V, Zerbo S, et al. Cleaning the paracolic gutter: transcutaneous endoscopic necrosectomy through a fully covered metal esophageal stent. Gastrointest Endosc 2015;81(5):1252.

32. Thorsen A, Borch AM, Novovic S, et al. Endoscopic necrosectomy through percutaneous self-expanding metal stents may be a promising additive in treatment of necrotizing pancreatitis. Dig Dis Sci 2018;63(9):2456–65.

33. Laopeamthong I, Tonozuka R, Kojima H, et al. Percutaneous endoscopic necrosectomy using a fully covered self-expandable metal stent in severe necrotizing pancreatitis. Endoscopy 2019;51(2):E22–3.

34. Delmeule A, Jacques J, Lambin T, et al. Endoscopic necrosectomy using electric conductivity: anchoring the snare tip into a groove made with Endocut may improve necrosis grasping. Endoscopy 2021;53(6):E234–5.

35. Puri N, Hallac A, Srikureja W. Early experience with cap-assisted endoscopic pancreatic necrosectomy: a technique to enhance safe tissue extraction and decrease interventions. Endosc Int Open 2019;7(7):E912–5.

36. Brand M, Bachmann J, Schlag C, et al. Over-the-scope grasper: a new tool for pancreatic necrosectomy and beyond - first multicenter experience. World J Gastrointest Surg 2022;14(8):799–808.

37. Yachimski P, Landewee CA, Campisano F, et al. The waterjet necrosectomy device for endoscopic management of pancreatic necrosis: design, development, and preclinical testing (with videos). Gastrointest Endosc 2020;92(3):770–5.

38. Iwano K, Toyonaga H, Hayashi T, et al. Tunnel creation method in endoscopic necrosectomy for walled-off pancreatic necrosis. Endoscopy 2022;54(S 02): E828–9.

39. Aso A, Igarashi H, Matsui N, et al. Large area of walled-off pancreatic necrosis successfully treated by endoscopic necrosectomy using a grasping-type scissors forceps. Dig Endosc 2014;26(3):474–7.

40. van der Wiel SE, Poley JW, Grubben M, et al. The EndoRotor, a novel tool for the endoscopic management of pancreatic necrosis. Endoscopy 2018;50(9): E240–1.

41. Stassen PMC, de Jonge PJF, Bruno MJ, et al. Safety and efficacy of a novel resection system for direct endoscopic necrosectomy of walled-off pancreas necrosis: a prospective, international, multicenter trial. Gastrointest Endosc 2022; 95(3):471–9.

42. Rizzatti G, Rimbas M, De Riso M, et al. Endorotor-based endoscopic necrosectomy avoiding the superior mesenteric artery. Endoscopy 2020;52(11):E420–1.

43. Zeuner S, Finkelmeier F, Waidmann O, et al. Percutaneous endoscopic necrosectomy using an automated rotor resection device in severe necrotizing pancreatitis. Endoscopy 2022;54(7):E362–3.

44. Committee ASoP, Forbes N, Coelho-Prabhu N, et al. Adverse events associated with EUS and EUS-guided procedures. Gastrointest Endosc 2022;95(1): 16–26 e2.

45. Committee ASoP, Muthusamy VR, Chandrasekhara V, et al. The role of endoscopy in the diagnosis and treatment of inflammatory pancreatic fluid collections. Gastrointest Endosc 2016;83(3):481–8.

46. Seifert H, Biermer M, Schmitt W, et al. Transluminal endoscopic necrosectomy after acute pancreatitis: a multicentre study with long-term follow-up (the GEPARD Study). Gut 2009;58(9):1260–6.

47. Bonnot B, Nion-Larmurier I, Desaint B, et al. Fatal gas embolism after endoscopic transgastric necrosectomy for infected necrotizing pancreatitis. Am J Gastroenterol 2014;109(4):607–8.

48. Holmes I, Shinn B, Mitsuhashi S, et al. Prediction and management of bleeding during endoscopic necrosectomy for pancreatic walled-off necrosis: results of a large retrospective cohort at a tertiary referral center. Gastrointest Endosc 2022;95(3):482–8.

49. Kv A, Katukuri GR, Lakhtakia S, et al. Hemostasis during endoscopic necrosectomy: spray coagulation can be a savior. Am J Gastroenterol 2022;117(3):375–6.

50. Aburajab M, Smith Z, Khan A, et al. Safety and efficacy of lumen-apposing metal stents with and without simultaneous double-pigtail plastic stents for draining pancreatic pseudocyst. Gastrointest Endosc 2018;87(5):1248–55.

51. Puga M, Consiglieri CF, Busquets J, et al. Safety of lumen-apposing stent with or without coaxial plastic stent for endoscopic ultrasound-guided drainage of pancreatic fluid collections: a retrospective study. Endoscopy 2018;50(10): 1022–6.

52. Vanek P, Falt P, Vitek P, et al. Endoscopic ultrasound-guided transluminal drainage using lumen-apposing metal stent with or without coaxial plastic stent for treatment of walled-off necrotizing pancreatitis: a prospective bicentric randomized controlled trial. Gastrointest Endosc 2023. https://doi.org/10.1016/j.gie.2022.12.026.

Endoscopic Ultrasound Guided Walled-off Necrosis Drainage

Philippe Willems, MD[a,b], Shyam Varadarajulu, MD[a,b],*

KEYWORDS

- Walled-off necrosis • Endoscopic drainage • Endoscopic ultrasound
- Endoscopic necrosectomy • Minimally invasive surgery • Debridement
- Percutaneous drainage

KEY POINTS

- Walled-off necrosis is associated with significant morbidity and mortality, particularly in the presence of secondary infection.
- Endoscopy-based interventions are associated with less morbidity and costs compared to minimally invasive surgery.
- EUS-guided lumen-apposing metal stent placement followed by endoscopic necrosectomy is the current standard-of-care with treatment success greater than 90%.
- Evidence-based recommendations are needed to standardize post-procedure care to expedite recovery and reduce resource consumption.

INTRODUCTION

In the United States, acute pancreatitis is the third most common gastrointestinal disorder, requiring 291,915 hospitalizations annually.[1] Necrotizing pancreatitis occurs in about 20% of patients with acute pancreatitis and is associated with a mortality rate of 8% to 40%.[2] Mortality is more common in patients with secondary infection that may result in sepsis and multiorgan failure. Although traditional treatment has been open surgical necrosectomy, it is associated with high rates of adverse events (34%–95%) and mortality (11%–39%).[3,4] Recent studies suggest that minimally invasive techniques that incorporate a step-up approach of percutaneous drain placement in conjunction with video-assisted retroperitoneal debridement (VARD) are superior to open surgical necrosectomy with lower rates of postprocedural adverse events (40%) and long-term morbidity.[5] As an alternative to surgical methods, endoscopic interventions have gained increasing popularity for the treatment of necrotic collections,

---

[a] Center for Advanced Endoscopy, Research & Education; [b] Orlando Health Digestive Health Institute, 52 West Underwood Street, Orlando, FL 32806, USA
* Corresponding author.
E-mail address: svaradarajulu@yahoo.com

Gastrointest Endoscopy Clin N Am 33 (2023) 725–735
https://doi.org/10.1016/j.giec.2023.03.013
1052-5157/23/© 2023 Elsevier Inc. All rights reserved.

giendo.theclinics.com

with an adverse event rate between 10.4% and 24.5%, and a mortality rate of less than 10%.[6–9] In this review, we outline the approach to the management of walled-off necrosis (WON) with a particular focus on endoscopic treatment options. Additionally, the definition, indications for and timing of intervention, description of various procedural techniques, adverse events, and post-procedure management are reviewed.

DEFINITION OF WALLED-OFF NECROSIS

Acute necrotic collections and WON occur as a result of necrotizing pancreatitis and are characterized by the presence of solid, necrotic debris of varying quantities. Acute necrotic collections are present early in the course of necrotizing pancreatitis whereas WON develops a few weeks (usually > 4) after the onset of acute pancreatitis when a mature rim encapsulates the collection.[10] **Fig. 1** outlines the differences in characteristics between both fluid collections.

The distinction of a WON from a pseudocyst is important as the treatment outcome varies. Although the majority of pseudocysts can be treated successfully by endoscopic transmural drainage, WON may require multiple treatment sessions that include endoscopic necrosectomy or adjuvant interventions such as percutaneous drainage or VARD.[11] The most common initial imaging modality for evaluation of pancreatic fluid collection (PFC) is a contrast-enhanced computed tomography (CT)

Fluid collection	Pancreatitis	Duration in weeks	Wall Maturity	Necrosis	CT
Acute necrotic collection	Necrotizing	<4	Absent	Minimal	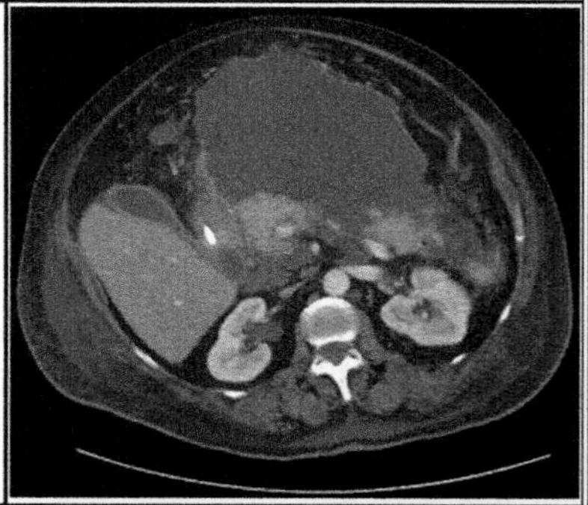
Walled-off necrosis	Necrotizing	>4	Present	Significant	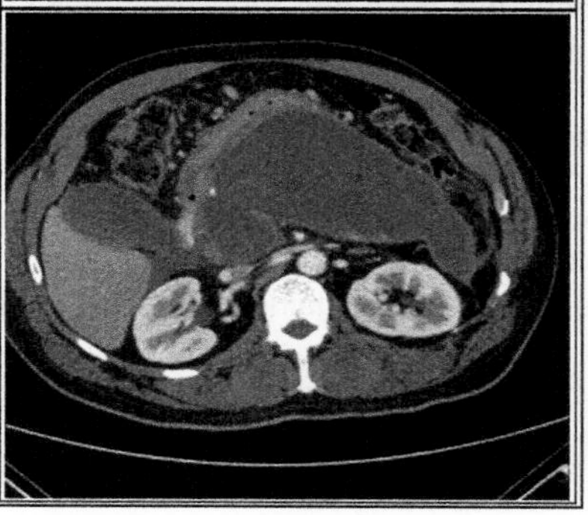

Fig. 1. Necrotic fluid collections. CT, computed tomogram; CT of acute necrotic collection reveals ill-defined fluid in the setting of parenchymal necrosis (*top image*); CT of WON reveals clear demarcation of the necrotic fluid collection that is conducive for drainage (*bottom image*).

scan of the abdomen, because it is readily available, relatively inexpensive, and can determine presence and extent of necrosis. MRI may be more sensitive for characterizing the contents (solid vs liquid) in a PFC and in determining pancreatic ductal integrity.[12,13]

Timing of Intervention

Drainage is indicated only for patients who are symptomatic, collections that compress vital structures, or have systemic illness that does not improve with medical management.[14] If patients meet the criteria for drainage, the next question is timing of intervention. Within the first 4 weeks after an acute attack of pancreatitis, the wall of the necrotic fluid collection is immature and so treatment should be temporized if possible,[15,16] with analgesics, enteral nutrition, and antibiotics. The most common reason for failure of conservative measures is infection, which can be managed by interventional radiology-guided placement of a percutaneous drainage catheter. Beyond the 3- to 4-week period, most collections develop a capsule and are prime for endoscopic drainage provided they are adherent or adjacent to the wall of the stomach or duodenum. In a recent randomized trial that compared immediate versus postponed drainage, no difference in complications was observed between treatment groups and patients with postponed drainage required fewer invasive interventions.[17]

IMPORTANT CONSIDERATIONS

Before embarking on a therapeutic intervention, the clinical history, and radiological and laboratory findings should be reviewed. The international normalized ratio and platelet counts should be corrected if abnormal to <1.5 and at least >50,000/mm^3, respectively. Prophylactic broad-spectrum antibiotics are administered to minimize the risk of infection and are to be continued after the procedure[18]; the choice of antibiotics and their duration is based on culture and sensitivity results or per infectious diseases recommendations. In cross-sectional imaging studies, evaluating the relationship of WON to the gastrointestinal lumen, presence of collateral vasculature, assessing from where in the pancreas the necrotic collection originates, and its extent, are all important to determine the type and site of potential intervention. Also, cystic pancreatic neoplasms, duplication cysts, and solid necrotic tumors can mimic a PFC on cross-sectional imaging, and therefore, need to be excluded.[19,20]

Choice of Intervention

Minimally Invasive Surgery: Treatment approaches include laparoscopic cystogastrostomy with transabdominal necrosectomy or VARD. In a recent randomized trial of 66 patients, an endoscopic transluminal approach for infected necrotizing pancreatitis, compared with minimally invasive surgery, significantly reduced major complications, lowered costs, and increased quality of life.[21] A recent meta-analysis evaluated three randomized trials involving 184 patients who underwent endoscopic or minimally invasive surgery-based interventions in patients with infective necrotizing pancreatitis.[22] Although there was no significant difference in mortality, new-onset multiple organ failure, enterocutaneous fistula/perforation, and pancreatic fistula were significantly lower for endoscopic interventions as compared to surgery. There was no significant difference in intraabdominal bleeding, and endocrine or exocrine pancreatic insufficiency between cohorts. The length of hospital stay was significantly shorter for endoscopic approach as compared to surgery. Therefore, when the requisite expertise is available, endoscopic intervention should be undertaken as the first-line therapy in the management of WON.

Percutaneous drainage: Percutaneous drain placement under radiological guidance is being increasingly practiced as initial treatment in the step-up surgical approach or as an adjunctive measure when the collections are not amenable to endoscopic drainage. An advantage of this approach is that necrosectomy can be obviated in up to 50% of patients following drain placement,[23] and in those requiring further interventions, the percutaneous tract can be utilized as a conduit for performing sinus tract necrosectomy or VARD. Adverse events associated with percutaneous drainage range from 22% to 50% and include bleeding, intestinal perforation, and pancreaticocutaneous or pancreaticoenteric fistula formation (**Fig. 2**A, B).[23–25] More recent data comparing endoscopic and percutaneous treatment approaches for PFC drainage have observed the percutaneous approach to be an independent risk factor for mortality.[26] Therefore, to expedite drainage of infected contents, we recommend the insertion of a large-bore percutaneous drain (16 Fr) as it can be used in conjunction with endoscopic internal transmural drainage as part of a "dual-modality" (endoscopic + percutaneous) approach to achieving optimal outcomes.[27]

Endoscopic interventions: Before performing an intervention, a thorough EUS examination should be undertaken as EUS has been shown to alter the management in up to 37.5% of patients referred for endoscopic drainage.[28] First, the suitability for endoscopic drainage as determined by the presence of a mature wall around the WON that is adherent to the gastric or duodenal wall can be confirmed on EUS, especially if less than 3 to 4 weeks have passed since the inciting event. Second, the presence of malignancy can be excluded as the etiology of the WON on EUS, which has been shown to occur in 1.25% of patients referred for endoscopic drainage.[20] Finally, other types of cysts, such as duplication cysts and mucinous cysts, can mimic a WON and can be excluded.[19]

There are two methods currently being adopted for performing EUS-guided drainage: multi-step technique using plastic stents and single-step technique using lumen-apposing metal stents (LAMS). However, before undertaking an intervention, it is important to perform a checklist to ensure successful technical and treatment outcomes (**Box 1**).

Plastic stents–Under EUS guidance, a 19-gauge fine needle aspiration (FNA) device is used to puncture the necrotic cavity. Suction is applied to sample the fluid to rule out infection (cultures, Gram stain) and for confirmation of diagnosis (tumor markers, cytology, biochemistry). A 0.025 inch or 0.035 inch guidewire is passed through the needle and coiled within the cavity. Transmural tract enlargement is performed with

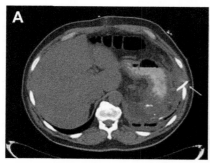
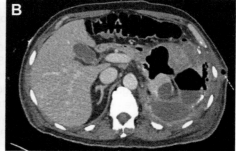

Fig. 2. Computed tomogram of the abdomen showing a percutaneous drain (*solid arrow*) into a WON (*A*). A pancreaticocutaneous fistula (*dotted arrow*) was observed (subcutaneous air bubble) on follow-up imaging (*B*).

> **Box 1**
> **Procedural checklist**
>
> - History and clinical examination, with review of vital signs and laboratory investigations to determine appropriateness of indication.
> - Review of the cross-sectional imaging to assess for presence of solid debris, confirmation of mature wall, exclusion of cyst neoplasm or intervening vasculature.
> - Optimization of coagulation parameters (INR $\leq$ 1.5, platelet count > 50,000/mm^3).
> - Assess nutritional status to determine need for enteral feeding
> - Administration of broad-spectrum intravenous antibiotics prior to instrumentation. Intravenous ciprofloxacin or piperacillin/tazobactam are the preferred antibiotics and should be continued for 3-5 days post-drainage.
> - Multidisciplinary care in consultation with pancreatic surgeons and interventional radiologists.

a graded dilation catheter or with the aid of electrocautery until it is large enough for passage of a dilating balloon (6–20 mm). WON drainage can usually be accomplished by the placement of two or more 7 F or 10 F double-pigtail plastic stents, 3 to 5 cm in length. In patients with WON that are non-communicating or very large in size (>10 cm), it is important to consider augmenting drainage adopting the multi-gate technique.[6]

LAMS: There has been growing interest in placing LAMS for WON drainage as the technique is much simpler than the placement of multiple plastic stents (**Fig. 3**A, B). LAMS are fully covered with a wide lumen (8–20 mm diameter) to expedite the drainage of necrotic contents and possess bilateral flanges at both ends to minimize the risk of stent migration. LAMS can be equipped with or without an electrocautery-enhanced delivery system. When using the non-electrocautery-based system, the WON is punctured under endosonographic guidance using a 19G FNA needle, followed by the insertion of a guidewire through the needle, which is looped inside the cavity. The transmural tract is then sequentially dilated using graded catheters or a cystotome, followed by a 4 to 6 mm dilating balloon. LAMS on a delivery system are then inserted over the guidewire into the necrotic cavity. The distal flange is deployed first under endosonographic guidance, followed by deployment of the proximal flange under either endosonographic or endoscopic view. When using the cautery-enhanced delivery system, the necrotic cavity is directly punctured using the electrocautery-enhanced tip of the stent delivery system under endosonographic guidance, without the need for a guidewire or pre-deployment dilation (**Fig. 4**A, B).

Outcomes of drainage: Although the majority of studies pertaining to LAMS for drainage of PFCs are retrospective, registry-based, case-control, or single-arm prospective series, three recent randomized trials comparing LAMS to plastic stents have yielded new information on treatment outcomes.[29–31] Although the procedural duration for LAMS placement is significantly shorter than for plastic stents, there was no significant difference in rates of technical or treatment success, adverse events, need for necrosectomy, hospital length of stay, or reinterventions between groups. However, the short procedural duration is clinically relevant, particularly when treating sicker patients who cannot withstand prolonged procedures. Another unique advantage pertaining to LAMS is the attribute of a wide lumen which facilitates easy access to the necrotic cavity to perform debridement. As initial reports suggested high rates of post-procedure bleeding (due to pseudoaneurysm) after LAMS

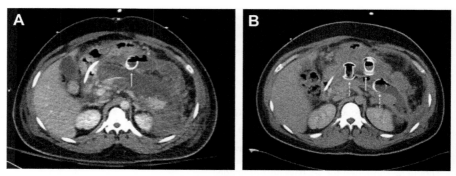

Fig. 3. Multi-gate technique using LAMS for a large WON collection. Despite successful drainage of a first collection using a single LAMS (*A, solid arrow*), the patient was persistently symptomatic. Two additional LAMS were subsequently placed to achieve optimal outcome (*B, dotted arrows* showing subsequent LAMS placed after index intervention; solid arrow showing LAMS from index procedure).

placement,[32–34] the consensus is that the endoprosthesis be removed within a 3- to 4-week time frame. Given the complexity of clinical presentation, varying extent and severity of disease, and frequent occurrence of pancreatic duct disconnection, we propose a comprehensive management protocol that yields a 6-month treatment success of greater than 95% (**Fig. 5**).[27]

Endoscopic necrosectomy: Nearly one-third of patients with WON respond well to transmural drainage alone and do not require direct endoscopic necrosectomy (DEN).[21,35] DEN is indicated when the WON cavity is filled with solid or infective debris and treatment response to transluminal stenting is suboptimal.[36,37] DEN is a labor-intensive and resource-consuming procedure involving non-standardized techniques. Consequently, the number of sessions required to achieve radiological resolution of WON ranges from 2 to 7, with a procedural morbidity of 14% to 25% and mortality of 5.6% to 7.5%.[8,22] Different aspects of the DEN procedure have been addressed with greater detail elsewhere in this issue. In this article, we have presented just a few salient aspects.

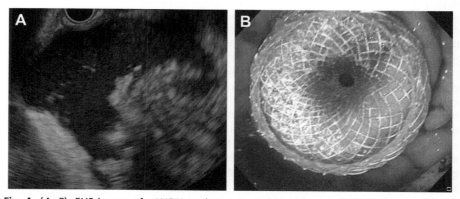

Fig. 4. (*A, B*). EUS image of a WON as demonstrated by an anechoic fluid collection with debris (*3A*), treated by deployment of a lumen-apposing metal stent as seen on endoscopic view (*3B*).

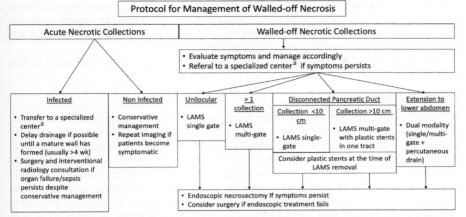

Fig. 5. Protocol-based management of WON. [a]A specialized center should have an experienced multidisciplinary team including therapeutic endoscopists, pancreaticobiliary surgeons, critical care specialists and interventional radiologists.

Technique: There are three critical steps to performing an efficient necrosectomy.[38]

Debridement (step 1): If the necrotic debris is non-adherent, 15 to 30 mm oval snares may be used. If the necrotic debris is adherent to the WON cavity, removal can be accomplished using 15 to 25 mm round, braided-wire snares. Only the cold snare technique is adopted for debridement unless the necrotic debris is adherent to the cavity. In such instances, electrocautery-assisted debridement may be performed. After placing the polypectomy snare around the base of the necrotic debris, it may be closed tightly and then lifted gently to ensure the absence of entangled vasculature. Electrocautery is administered and the necrotic material is peeled away from the walls of the necrotic cavity. In patients with extensive collateral vasculature, to minimize the risk of snaring a vessel, debridement is performed using wide-jaw, rat tooth forceps. Intra-procedural bleeding when encountered can be managed using the hemostatic forceps.

Extraction of debris (step 2): After necrosectomy, liquefied debris is suctioned using the gastroscope. Solid debris is extracted by suctioning necrotic chunks into the cap with the aid of wide-jaw, rat tooth forceps or polypectomy snares.

Irrigation (step 3): Normal saline can be used intermittently during the procedure for irrigation of the necrotic cavity. About 100 to 200 mL of half-strength hydrogen peroxide mixed in equal volume of normal saline is used to 'top-off' the irrigation step at the completion of each necrosectomy session with the intent of sterilizing the WON cavity. Hydrogen peroxide should be used only toward the end of the procedure because the emanating effervescence precludes adequate visualization of the necrotic cavity. A recent retrospective study demonstrated higher rates of treatment success with a shorter time to disease resolution when hydrogen peroxide was used for performing DEN.[39]

Special Considerations

Disconnected pancreatic duct syndrome (DPDS): DPDS is defined as the complete disruption of the main pancreatic duct with resultant disconnection of the viable upstream distal pancreatic gland from the main pancreatic duct downstream. Consequently, a symptomatic fluid collection can evolve in the disconnected gland. DPDS occurs in nearly 70% of patients with necrotizing pancreatitis.[40] In a randomized controlled trial of 46 patients who had successful transmural drainage, stent retrieval was associated with higher rates of PFC recurrence as compared to indwelling stents (38.4% vs 0%).[41] We, therefore, recommend indwelling plastic stents to minimize the chances of PFC recurrence in patients with DPDS.

Discussion of DPDS with greater details is available in an article dedicated to this entity in this issue.

Post-Procedure Care

Although a low-fat diet may be suitable for patients with minimal residual pancreatitis-related symptoms, enteral nutrition should be initiated for patients with ongoing pancreatic inflammation, particularly for those with persistent anorexia or abdominal pain.[42] There are no evidence-based recommendations for inpatient follow-up or indications for procedural reinterventions. In general, reinterventions are undertaken in patients with ongoing sepsis or systemic inflammatory response syndrome and when there is a suboptimal resolution of the WON on follow-up imaging. Following discharge, cross-sectional imaging study of the abdomen must be obtained at 6 to 8 weeks in patients treated with plastic stents or at 3 to 4 weeks in patients treated with LAMS to evaluate treatment response. If the collection measures less than 2 or 3 cm, and the main pancreatic duct is intact, the transmural stents may be removed. In patients with DPDS, indwelling transmural plastic stents have been shown to decrease the rates of PFC recurrence.[41]

SUMMARY

Endoscopic interventions are highly effective for the management of WON. However, outcomes are reliant on correct patient selection, risk stratification, practicing evidence-based procedural techniques, and more importantly pursuing a multidisciplinary treatment approach. Clinical studies to optimize post-procedure care and inpatient follow-up are required to shorten hospital length of stay and minimize resource utilization.

CLINICS CARE POINTS

- Before embarking on an intervention, a thorough EUS examination should be undertaken to exclude occult pancreatic tumor as a cause of acute pancreatitis.
- A protocol-based treatment strategy is important taking into consideration presence of a disconnected duct, the extent and number of fluid collections, as each of these factors determines the overall treatment outcome.
- Multidisciplinary care is an important requisite when caring for patients with necrotizing pancreatitis.

DISCLOSURES

P. Willems: None. S. Varadarajulu: Consultant for Boston Scientific, Medtronic, Fujifilm, Olympus.

REFERENCES

1. Peery AF, Crockett SD, Murphy CC, et al. Burden and cost of gastrointestinal, liver, and pancreatic diseases in the United States: update 2021. Gastroenterology 2022;162:621–44.

2. Tenner S, Baillie J, DeWitt J, et al. American college of gastroenterology guide-line: management of acute pancreatitis. Am J Gastroenterol 2013;108:1400–15, 1416.

3. Tsiotos GG, Luque-de Leon E, Sarr MG. Long-term outcome of necrotizing pancreatitis treated by necrosectomy. Br J Surg 1998;85:1650–3.

4. Rodriguez JR, Razo AO, Targarona J, et al. Debridement and closed packing for sterile or infected necrotizing pancreatitis: insights into indications and outcomes in 167 patients. Ann Surg 2008;247:294–9.

5. van Santvoort HC, Besselink MG, Bakker OJ, et al. A step-up approach or open necrosectomy for necrotizing pancreatitis. N Engl J Med 2010;362:1491–502.

6. Varadarajulu S, Phadnis MA, Christein JD, et al. Multiple transluminal gateway technique for EUS-guided drainage of symptomatic walled-off pancreatic necro-sis. Gastrointest Endosc 2011;74:74–80.

7. Gluck M, Ross A, Irani S, et al. Dual modality drainage for symptomatic walled-off pancreatic necrosis reduces length of hospitalization, radiological procedures, and number of endoscopies compared to standard percutaneous drainage. J Gastrointest Surg 2012;16:248–56 [discussion: 256-7].

8. Gardner TB, Coelho-Prabhu N, Gordon SR, et al. Direct endoscopic necrosec-tomy for the treatment of walled-off pancreatic necrosis: results from a multicenter U.S. series. Gastrointest Endosc 2011;73:718–26.

9. Bakker OJ, van Santvoort HC, van Brunschot S, et al. Endoscopic transgastric vs surgical necrosectomy for infected necrotizing pancreatitis: a randomized trial. JAMA 2012;307:1053–61.

10. Banks PA, Bollen TL, Dervenis C, et al. Classification of acute pancreatitis–2012: revision of the Atlanta classification and definitions by international consensus. Gut 2013;62:102.

11. Varadarajulu S, Bang JY, Phadnis MA, et al. Endoscopic transmural drainage of peripancreatic fluid collections: outcomes and predictors of treatment success in 211 consecutive patients. J Gastrointest Surg 2011;15:2080–111.

12. Hirota M, Kimura Y, Ishiko T, et al. Visualization of the heterogeneous internal structure of so-called "pancreatic necrosis" by magnetic resonance imaging in acute necrotizing pancreatitis. Pancreas 2002;25:63–7.

13. Morgan DE, Baron TH, Smith JK, et al. Pancreatic fluid collections prior to inter-vention: evaluation with MR imaging compared with CT and US. Radiology 1997; 203:773–8.

14. Committee ASoP, Muthusamy VR, Chandrasekhara V, et al. The role of endos-copy in the diagnosis and treatment of inflammatory pancreatic fluid collections. Gastrointest Endosc 2016;83:481–8.

15. Besselink MG, Verwer TJ, Schoenmaeckers EJ, et al. Timing of surgical interven-tion in necrotizing pancreatitis. Arch Surg 2007;142:1194–201.

16. van Santvoort HC, Bakker OJ, Bollen TL, et al. A conservative and minimally inva-sive approach to necrotizing pancreatitis improves outcome. Gastroenterology 2011;141:1254–63.

17. Boxhoorn L, van Dijk SM, van Grinsven J, et al. Immediate versus postponed intervention for infected necrotizing pancreatitis. N Engl J Med 2021;385: 1372–81.

18. Asge Standards of Practice C, Banerjee S, Shen B, et al. Antibiotic prophylaxis for GI endoscopy. Gastrointest Endosc 2008;67:791–8.

19. Varadarajulu S, Wilcox CM, Tamhane A, et al. Role of EUS in drainage of peri-pancreatic fluid collections not amenable for endoscopic transmural drainage. Gastrointest Endosc 2007;66:1107–19.

20. Holt BA, Varadarajulu S. EUS-guided drainage: beware of the pancreatic fluid collection (with videos). Gastrointest Endosc 2014;80:1199–202.

21. Bang JY, Arnoletti JP, Holt BA, et al. An Endoscopic Transluminal Approach, Compared With Minimally Invasive Surgery, Reduces Complications and Costs for Patients With Necrotizing Pancreatitis. Gastroenterology 2019;156: 1027–1040 e3.

22. Bang JY, Wilcox CM, Arnoletti JP, et al. Superiority of endoscopic interventions over minimally invasive surgery for infected necrotizing pancreatitis: meta-analysis of randomized trials. Dig Endosc 2020;32:298–308.

23. van Baal MC, van Santvoort HC, Bollen TL, et al. Systematic review of percutaneous catheter drainage as primary treatment for necrotizing pancreatitis. Br J Surg 2011;98:18–27.

24. Bradley EL 3rd, Howard TJ, van Sonnenberg E, et al. Intervention in necrotizing pancreatitis: an evidence-based review of surgical and percutaneous alternatives. J Gastrointest Surg 2008;12:634–9.

25. Adams DB, Anderson MC. Percutaneous catheter drainage compared with internal drainage in the management of pancreatic pseudocyst. Ann Surg 1992;215: 571–6 [discussion: 576-8].

26. Varadarajulu S. Endoscopic versus Percutaneous modalities for drainage of pancreatic fluid collections: assessment of clinical and economic outcomes. Available at: https://ueg.eu/library/endoscopic-versus-percutaneous-modalities-for-drainage-of-pancreatic-fluid-collections-assessment-of-clinical-and-economic-outcomes/252912.

27. Bang JY, Wilcox CM, Arnoletti JP, et al. Validation of the Orlando Protocol for endoscopic management of pancreatic fluid collections in the era of lumen-apposing metal stents. Dig Endosc 2022;34:612–21.

28. Fockens P, Johnson TG, van Dullemen HM, et al. Endosonographic imaging of pancreatic pseudocysts before endoscopic transmural drainage. Gastrointest Endosc 1997;46:412–6.

29. Bang JY, Navaneethan U, Hasan MK, et al. Non-superiority of lumen-apposing metal stents over plastic stents for drainage of walled-off necrosis in a randomised trial. Gut 2019;68:1200–9.

30. Boxhoorn L, Verdonk RC, Besselink MG, et al. Comparison of lumen-apposing metal stents versus double-pigtail plastic stents for infected necrotising pancreatitis. Gut 2023;72:66–72.

31. Karstensen JG, Novovic S, Hansen EF, et al. EUS-guided drainage of large walled-off pancreatic necroses using plastic versus lumen-apposing metal stents: a single-centre randomised controlled trial. Gut 2022. https://doi.org/10.1136/gutjnl-2022-328225.

32. Bang JY, Hasan M, Navaneethan U, et al. Lumen-apposing metal stents (LAMS) for pancreatic fluid collection (PFC) drainage: may not be business as usual. Gut 2017;66:2054–6.

33. Brimhall B, Han S, Tatman PD, et al. Increased Incidence of pseudoaneurysm bleeding with lumen-apposing metal stents compared to double-pigtail plastic stents in patients with peripancreatic fluid collections. Clin Gastroenterol Hepatol 2018;16:1521–8.

34. Bang JY, Hawes RH, Varadarajulu S. Lumen-apposing metal stent placement for drainage of pancreatic fluid collections: predictors of adverse events. Gut 2020; 69:1379–81.

35. van Brunschot S, van Grinsven J, van Santvoort HC, et al. Endoscopic or surgical step-up approach for infected necrotising pancreatitis: a multicentre randomised trial. Lancet 2018;391:51–8.
36. Bang JY, Holt BA, Hawes RH, et al. Outcomes after implementing a tailored endoscopic step-up approach to walled-off necrosis in acute pancreatitis. Br J Surg 2014;101:1729–38.
37. Seifert H, Biermer M, Schmitt W, et al. Transluminal endoscopic necrosectomy after acute pancreatitis: a multicentre study with long-term follow-up (the GEPARD Study). Gut 2009;58:1260–6.
38. Bang JY, Wilcox CM, Hawes R, et al. Outcomes of a structured, stepwise approach to endoscopic necrosectomy. J Clin Gastroenterol 2021;55:631–7.
39. Messallam AA, Adler DG, Shah RJ, et al. Direct endoscopic necrosectomy with and without hydrogen peroxide for walled-off pancreatic necrosis: a multicenter comparative study. Am J Gastroenterol 2021;116:700–9.
40. Bang JY, Wilcox CM, Navaneethan U, et al. Impact of disconnected pancreatic duct syndrome on the endoscopic management of pancreatic fluid collections. Ann Surg 2018;267:561–8.
41. Arvanitakis M, Delhaye M, Bali MA, et al. Pancreatic-fluid collections: a randomized controlled trial regarding stent removal after endoscopic transmural drainage. Gastrointest Endosc 2007;65:609–19.
42. Al-Omran M, Albalawi ZH, Tashkandi MF, et al. Enteral versus parenteral nutrition for acute pancreatitis. Cochrane Database Syst Rev 2010;2010:CD002837.

Percutaneous Endoscopic Necrosectomy

Soumya Jagannath Mahapatra, MD, DM,
Pramod Kumar Garg, MD, DM*

KEYWORDS

- Necrotizing pancreatitis • PEN • Necrosectomy • Sinus tract endoscopy

KEY POINTS

- Patients with infected necrotizing pancreatitis not responding to antibiotics require drainage and subsequent necrosectomy (Step-up approach).
- Percutaneous Endoscopic Necrosectomy (PEN) has evolved as a minimally invasive approach for necrosectomy through the percutaneous catheter route using a flexible endoscope and can be done under conscious sedation.
- It is best suited for predominantly laterally placed collections and also can be performed at the bedside for sick patients admitted to an ICU.
- PEN has a clinical success rate of 80% with minimal adverse events.

 Video content accompanies this article at http://www.giendo.theclinics.com.

INTRODUCTION

Acute pancreatitis (AP) is an acute inflammatory condition of the pancreas that can result in both local and systemic complications. AP is mild in the majority of patients but 20% to 30% of patients develop acute necrotizing pancreatitis leading to a more severe course of the disease.[1,2] Patients with significant pancreatic necrosis are prone to develop marked systemic inflammation which may even lead to organ failure. The mortality in this subgroup of patients with severe disease and organ failure may reach up to 40%.[3–5] Patients with acute necrotizing pancreatitis are susceptible to develop secondary infection of the necrotic tissue and fluid collections termed as infected necrotizing pancreatitis.

Infected necrotizing pancreatitis (INP) is a dreaded complication of AP. INP leads to significant morbidity and a mortality ranging from 23% to 39%.[3,4] Infection of the necrotic fluid collections occurs in up to 40% of patients with acute necrotizing pancreatitis and usually sets in after 2 to 3 weeks of the onset of illness. INP is suspected when a patient with acute necrotizing pancreatitis manifests with new onset

Department of Gastroenterology, All India Institute of Medical Sciences, New Delhi, India
* Corresponding author.
E-mail address: pkgarg@aiims.ac.in

Gastrointest Endoscopy Clin N Am 33 (2023) 737–751
https://doi.org/10.1016/j.giec.2023.04.011
giendo.theclinics.com

or persistent fever beyond the first week of illness, elevated leukocyte count, and deterioration or lack of improvement in his/her clinical condition without any other identifiable source of infection. The infection can be confirmed on the culture of the necrotic fluid. The presence of air foci in the necrotic (peri)pancreatic collection on a CT scan is also suggestive of INP.[6,7] Initial management of patients with INP involves the institution of broad-spectrum antibiotics, adequate nutrition, and supportive therapy. Subsequently, drainage of the infected collection is required if there is no response to antibiotics, and necrosectomy in case of nonresponse to drainage, the so-called "Step-up Approach."[5,8,9]

Over the past 2 decades, the management paradigm of INP has shifted from an open surgical debridement to the step-up approach.[8,10] Interventional treatment for INP is generally performed when the necrotic fluid collections are walled off, termed as 'Walled Off Necrosis (WON). In a randomized controlled trial, the primary composite outcome of major complications or death was 69% in the open surgical arm and 40% in the step-up approach ($P = .006$).[10] In the step-up approach, the initial management involves drainage of (peri)pancreatic fluid collection by either per-oral endoscopic transenteral drainage or percutaneous catheter drainage (PCD) preferably via the retroperitoneal route followed by necrosectomy if sepsis is not controlled. The step-up approach can avoid necrosectomy in 35% to 64% of patients.[10,11] If required, necrosectomy can be performed through the initial drainage tract that is, transenteral route by per-oral direct endoscopic necrosectomy (DEN) or a percutaneous approach through the PCD tract. This can be achieved by either video-assisted retroperitoneal debridement (VARD), which involves a 5 cm skin incision or minimal access retroperitoneal pancreatic necrosectomy (MARPN) via 2 to 3 ports using a nephroscope/laparoscope without the incision. Per-oral DEN has similar adverse events rate as compared to minimally invasive surgical necrosectomy but with lesser hospital stay and fistula rate as shown in two randomized trials.[12,13] Hence, per-oral transenteric drainage with DEN is preferred for walled-off necrosis (WON) located predominantly in the lesser sac. However, the majority of (peri)pancreatic fluid collections are not amenable for per-oral transenteral drainage either because their wall is not well-formed or they are located distant from the stomach or duodenum.[12,13]

Percutaneous Endoscopic Necrosectomy (PEN) is an important addition to our armamentarium of other modes of necrosectomy. It is an alternative to VARD and MARPN as necrosectomy is performed through the tract of percutaneous catheter that is, sinus tract using a flexible endoscope. Collections distant from the stomach and duodenum are most suitable for PEN as a minimally invasive endoscopic approach though it can be used in all types of collections which are drained by percutaneous catheter. In this article, we will review the indications, technique, and outcomes of PEN.

GENESIS AND EVOLUTION OF PERCUTANEOUS ENDOSCOPIC NECROSECTOMY

Pancreas being a retroperitoneal organ, the (peri)pancreatic necrotic fluid collections are predominantly retroperitoneal in location that is, deep seated in the pancreatic bed extending to paracolic gutters. Percutaneous catheter drainage (PCD) is considered the preferred modality of drainage in the majority of patients because of the following reasons: (a) distance between the collection and stomach/duodenum $\geq$ 3 to 4 cm (b) ongoing organ failure or general conditions making a patient unfit for general anesthesia which is required for per-oral DEN while PCD can be performed at the bedside in sicker patients under local anesthesia (c) multiple collections and/or deep extension of the collections requiring drainage, and (d) immature wall of the WON which is a relative contraindication for the per-oral endoscopic drainage.[14]

PCD tract acts as a guide to the deep-seated collections via the retroperitoneal route for minimally invasive necrosectomy thus avoiding the transperitoneal approach and collateral damage to the bowel. MARPN and VARD are done using this approach. However, these approaches involve the use of a rigid nephroscope or laparoscope which have limited maneuverability and require at least 2 ports, one for visualization and the other for necrosectomy. Following the success of per-oral DEN, endoscopists have developed a modality of necrosectomy using the percutaneous tract (also known as sinus tract) and this method of percutaneous endoscopic necrosectomy (PEN) is gaining popularity over the past several years.

The first description of "sinus tract endoscopy" was by Carter and colleagues[15] in 2000. In a series of 14 patients with INP, initial 4 patients underwent open necrosectomy followed by sinus tract endoscopy and through the tract necrosectomy for residual necrotic debris, and avoided additional surgery. In the next 10 patients, sinus tract endoscopy and necrosectomy were performed as the primary modality via the percutaneous tract using either a double-channel endoscope or a nephroscope. Incidentally, Seifert and colleagues[16] reported for the first time transgastric per-oral direct endoscopic debridement in the same year. Castellanos and colleagues[17] also described sinus tract necrosectomy in a prospective series of 11 patients in 2005. Over the next 10 years, this technique was not utilized much perhaps due to the development of VARD.[18] In 2015, Dhingra and colleagues[19] first described the usefulness of this procedure in a prospective series of patients with INP many of whom had ongoing organ failure and required ICU care, as a technique which could be done in the regular endoscopy suite and also at the patient's bedside under conscious sedation and local anesthesia. The authors coined the term "percutaneous endoscopic necrosectomy" (PEN). Subsequently, the feasibility and safety of the procedure as a step-up approach for necrosectomy as an alternative to VARD was demonstrated by Jain and colleagues in a prospective cohort of 177 patients with INP, 53 of whom underwent PEN as a step-up treatment protocol.[20] More recent case series have also shown its usefulness and successful outcome of patients treated with PEN.[21–24]

INDICATIONS OF PERCUTANEOUS ENDOSCOPIC NECROSECTOMY

The main indication of PEN is infected necrotic collections which are predominantly laterally placed (**Fig. 1**) and non-responding to conservative therapy including supportive treatment, antibiotics, and percutaneous drainage. An important caveat is

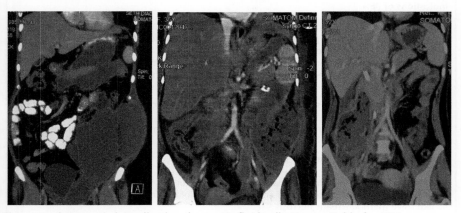

Fig. 1. Predominantly laterally placed necrotic fluid collections suitable for PEN.

that the PCD catheter should be upsized adequately before considering non-response. There is no definite guidance about the optimum size of the PCD catheter but in general 16 to 20 F size catheter is required to drain thick pus and bits of necrotic debris (the initial catheter size is usually 12 F).[25] First drainage with a large bore catheter (>20 Fr) is not preferred in view of higher risk of pancreatic bed hemorrhage.[26] The size of the catheter also depends on the size of the necrotic collection and the relative amount of necrotic debris. The judgment about upsizing the catheter is ideally made by the interventional radiologist based on the clinical response to the initial drainage. A few additional indications are summarized in **Box 1**.

TECHNIQUE OF PERCUTANEOUS ENDOSCOPIC NECROSECTOMY
Classification of Pancreatic Fluid Collections (PFCs)

For uniformity and ease of description, we propose the following classification system for pancreatic walled-off necrosis which requires intervention.

WON can be classified on the basis of location and amount of necrotic debris inside (**Fig. 2**).

On the basis of location.

1. Lesser sac only with or without subhepatic extension (L)
2. Paracolic gutter (G) only
   a. Right paracolic gutter (G_R)
   b. Left paracolic gutter (G_L)
3. Pelvis only (P)
4. A combination: such as lesser sac and left paracolic (L + G_L)
5. Others – perigastric, perihepatic, perisplenic, omentum, mesentery, mesocolon (O)
6. Extensive (E)

Quantification of Necrotic Debris

The amount of necrotic debris within the collection should be assessed before the drainage procedure either on abdominal USG or MRI scan and should be quantified as less than 30%, 30% to 50% or greater than 50%. In collections with predominantly solid debris and little fluid, PCD and subsequent minimally invasive procedure may not be the ideal approach and direct surgery may be a better option.

Box 1
Indications of PEN

Absolute Indications
1. Predominantly laterally placed necrotic fluid collections not amenable for transenteral drainage and no improvement/worsening sepsis after PCD
2. Ongoing organ failure or worsening organ failure (as a bedside technique in ICU)
3. Extensive gas in the collection resulting in poor visualization of the cavity on EUS

Relative Indications
1. Presence of multidrug resistant or extreme drug resistant bacteria in the first culture of the drained fluid
2. Poor nutritional status and general condition making patient unfit for general anesthesia

Contraindications
1. Large vessels coursing through the cavity
2. Suspected colonic fistula
3. Pancreatic bed hemorrhage (relative contraindication as PEN can be performed if a pseudoaneurysm is identified and embolized by radiologic intervention)
4. Extensive (peri)pancreatic necrosis

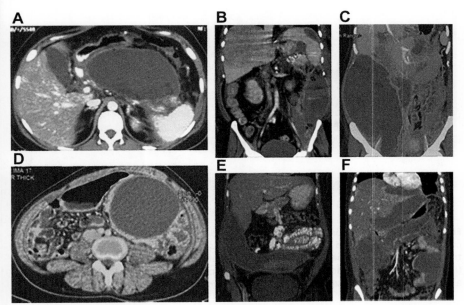

Fig. 2. (*A*) Lesser sac collection (L). (*B*) Left paracolic gutter collection (G$_L$). (*C*) Right paracolic gutter collection (G$_R$). (*D*) Collection in the omentum (O). (*E*) Right paracolic gutter and pelvic collection (G$_R$ + P). (*F*) Extensive collection in lesser sac with sub-hepatic extension and both paracolic gutter extension (*E*).

Prerequisites for Percutaneous Endoscopic Necrosectomy

Appropriate patient selection, prior PCD of the infected collection preferably through the retroperitoneal access, and adequate size of the percutaneous tract after gradual tract upsizing are important pre-requisites for PEN.

DRAINAGE OF THE COLLECTION

Percutaneous drainage should be performed for collections other than predominantly lesser sac collections, which may be better drained endoscopically by the per-oral route. Retroperitoneal access should be preferred for percutaneous drainage whenever feasible as it avoids peritoneal contamination, reduces the risk of bowel injury and facilitates the step-up approach. A minimum PCD catheter size of 16 F is required to start the PEN procedure.

Tract Size Upgradation and Endoscopic Lavage:

The authors prefer to do the procedure in the regular endoscopy theater under local anesthesia and conscious sedation but it can also be done under general anesthesia (GA) (**Fig. 3** and Video 1). First, the previously placed PCD is removed under strict aseptic precaution. An ultrathin flexible endoscope (outer diameter 4.9–5.5 mm) is introduced into the cavity. The prerequisite for the introduction of the ultrathin endoscope is a minimum 16 Fr PCD tract size. Pre-procedure, the endoscope should be thoroughly disinfected with glutaraldehyde for 30 minutes followed by additional cleaning of the biopsy channel with alcohol and betadine. The tract is entered under visual guidance by the instillation of normal saline and minimal CO_2 insufflation at a

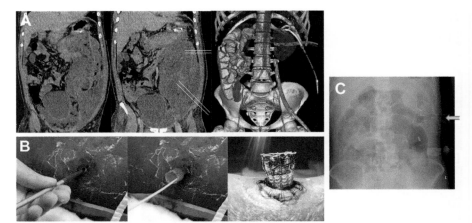

Fig. 3. (*A*) Large collection in the lesser sac extending to left paracolic gutter (L + G$_L$). The collection is distant from the stomach and wall is not well formed. Initial PCD was done through the retroperitoneal approach one in lesser sac and one in the left paracolic gutter. (*B*) Dilatation of the tract using covered self-expanding metal stent (16 mm). (*C*) X-ray abdomen showing the expanded SEMS (yellow *arrow*).

rate of 1.5 to 2.0 L/min. The WON cavity is inspected to determine the size, necrotic debris, and pus content. Liquid pus is washed with saline irrigation and sucked out till it clears off. Repeated gentle suctioning and endoscope withdrawal from the cavity is done so that the pressure in the collection doesn't increase. The cavity size and quantity of the necrotic debris determine whether the patient will need necrosectomy. After adequate lavage, a larger bore (2–4 Fr more than the previous catheter) straight PCD catheter (similar to a chest drainage tube) is placed using a Seldinger technique over a guidewire. In case of difficulty, the tract can be dilated with a CRE balloon. Tract dilatation with the upgradation of the PCD catheter and lavage of the cavity are done every alternate/third day till it reaches 30 Fr. The larger catheter can be inserted by back mounting it over the ultrathin endoscope which is used as a guide for proper placement. If tract dilatation to 30 Fr size is difficult to achieve for example, in the intercostal region, or if early necrosectomy is required due to sepsis, a fully covered self-expandable esophageal metal stent (16 mm diameter, length 8–12 cm) is placed.

ENDOSCOPIC NECROSECTOMY

After 48 hours of either a 30 Fr catheter or SEMS placement, necrosectomy is performed through the sinus tract/SEMS (**Fig. 4**). The procedure is performed under local anesthesia and conscious sedation with the monitoring of vital parameters. A regular upper gastrointestinal tract endoscope (diameter ~9 mm) is used for this procedure. The procedure can be performed at the patient's bedside if the patient is too sick to be moved to the endoscopy/operation theater. After inspecting the cavity, loose necrosum is removed using a snare and/or Roth-net basket as described previously by our group.[19,27] The cavity is irrigated well with saline. In addition, diluted hydrogen peroxide or povidone iodine may also be used for lavage. The duration of the procedure is guided by the patient's general condition and tolerance, and the amount of necrotic debris as judged by the endoscopist. The authors prefer to restrict the procedure time by not trying to remove all the necrotic debris in one go if the patient is sick. The duration of the procedure usually varies from 30 to 90 minutes.

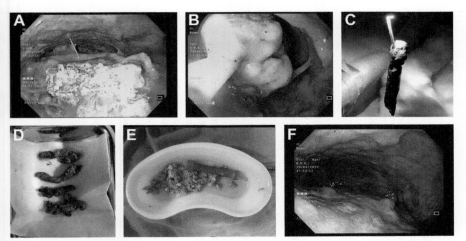

Fig. 4. (*A*) Inspection of the cavity shows extensive necrotic debris. (*B*) Debris removed with snare and Roth net during PEN. (*C*) Removed debris. (*D*) and (*E*) Debris with removed stent. (*F*) Residual clean cavity with granulation tissue.

Repeat Procedure

In case the cavity is not completely cleared off the debris, the next session of endoscopic debridement is undertaken after 2 to 3 days till complete clearance of the necrosum is achieved. Adherent debris should not be forcefully removed. After each session of necrosectomy, a 30-32 Fr drain tube is replaced into the cavity and the tract is lavaged twice daily with 500 mL normal saline through the percutaneous drain.

Downsizing the Tract

When the cavity is cleared off the debris and looks clean, the large bore tube is replaced with a smaller catheter of size 18 Fr (the authors prefer a nasogastric tube). When the draining fluid is clear after a few days, the catheter length is shortened and the collecting bag is replaced by an ostomy bag to prevent gravity-assisted drainage. These measures help prevent pancreatic fistula. The catheter is removed when the output decreases to less than 10 to 20 mL/d.

Based on the description above, there could be 2 approaches of PEN.

i. Endoscopic lavage and gradual upgradation of the PCD tract for necrosectomy: This approach is considered in relatively stable patients. First endoscopic lavage is done to remove the thick liquid pus and then gradual tract upgradation is done for subsequent necrosectomy in a phased manner depending upon the clinical course.

ii. Rapid tract dilatation and upfront necrosectomy: This approach is usually considered in patients with sepsis and persistent organ failure. If the patient doesn't improve after initial endoscopic lavage, rapid tract upgradation is done (usually using a SEMS) and upfront necrosectomy is performed.

OUTCOMES

Technical success is defined as successful clearance of the cavity by PEN. Clinical success is defined as the resolution of sepsis. The success rate and adverse events as reported in different series are summarized in **Table 1**.

Table 1
Summary of the results of major studies using PEN

Author, year	N	Technique	Success Rate	Adverse Events	Need for surgery and Mortality	Comments
Carter CR et al,[15] 2000	14	Rigid nephroscope alongside grasping forceps or a flexible endoscope was used along the percutaneous tract after dilatation	86%	Bleeding: 1 Prolonged ileus: 1 Recurrent collection: 2	Open surgery: 1 Mortality:2	Procedure done under GA over a median of 2 sessions
Castellanos et al,[17] 2005	11	Two large bore catheters placed in the collection through retroperitoneal route. Using a flexible endoscope, irrigation and suction were used to remove necrotic debris without insufflation.	73%	Not mentioned	Open surgery: 0 Mortality: 3	Procedure was completed under GA over a mean of 5 sessions (3–10)
Mui LM et al,[24] 2005	9	Initial 8.5 Fr percutaneous catheter was gradually upsized to 18 Fr Catheter. Choledochoscope (5 mm) was used for necrosectomy.	77%	Colonic Fistulization: 2 PCD related complication: 2	Open Surgery: 2 Mortality: 1	6 patients needed additional ERCP for CBD stone or pancreatic communication. It is not clear how necrosectomy was done using a choledochoscope which has a small working channel
Dhingra R et al,[19] 2015	15	After initial PCD was upsized gradually to 18 Fr catheter, an ultrathin endoscope was used for lavage and suction of liquid pus. Gradually, the catheter was upsized to 28–30Fr and necrosectomy was done using an adult gastroscope	93%	Bleeding: 1 Pancreatico-cutaneous fistula: 1	Open surgery: 1 Mortality: 1	Procedure done under conscious sedation without endotracheal intubation

Study	N	Technique	Success	Complications	Outcome	Comments
Mathers B et al,[30] 2016	10	After tract upsizing to 24–28 Fr, adult gastroscope was used for necrosectomy.	100%	Pancreatico-cutaneous fistula: 1	Open surgery: 0 Mortality: 0	Median time to resolution after intervention was 57 (10–210) days
Thorsen A et al,[22] 2018	5	Initial 7Fr catheter was upsized to 20 mm and a covered SEMS was placed. Debridement was done using a gastroscope through the SEMS.	80%	Severe abdominal pain: 5 Pancreatico-cutaneous fistula: 2	Open surgery: 0 Mortality: 1	Two patients underwent endoscopic transmural drainage and debridement prior to PEN. All patients had severe pain which might be attributable to rapid tract upgradation from 7Fr Catheter to 20 mm SEMS.
Tringali A et al,[31] 2018	3	SEMS placed through percutaneous tract and necrosectomy done using an adult gastroscope	100%	None	None	
Saumoy M et al,[21] 2018	9	Percutaneous catheter tract was dilated with 15 mm and 18 mm bougie dilator and a 18 mm covered SEMS was placed. Endoscopic necrosectomy was done through a SEMS using an adult gastroscope.	89%	None	Mortality: 1	Plastic stent placed through SEMS. Done under GA.
Goenka et al,[32] 2018	10	After initial percutaneous catheter placement, it was replaced with 32 Fr tube by blunt skin dissection. PEN was done using an adult gastroscope through the tract after 10 d.	90%	Pneumoperitoneum: 2	Surgery: 1	Two patients underwent transenteral LAMS placement in addition to PEN.

(continued on next page)

Table 1
(continued)

Author, year	N	Technique	Success Rate	Adverse Events	Need for surgery and Mortality	Comments
Ke Lu et al,[23] 2019	23	Endoscopic necrosectomy was done through a SEMS	65%	Major bleed: 10 Spontaneous enteric fistula: 5 Pancreatic fistula: 2	Mortality: 7 Surgery: 7	Transperitoneal approach was also used. Higher complication rate.
Jain et al,[20] 2020	53	After Initial PCD was upsized gradually to 18 Fr catheter, an ultrathin endoscope was used for lavage. Gradually, the catheter was upsized to 28–30Fr and necrosectomy was done using an adult gastroscope.	79%	Aspiration Pneumonia: 2 Peritonitis: 2 Paralytic Ileus: 1 Bleeding: 1 Subcutaneous emphysema: 1	Surgery: 8 Mortality: 11	Consecutive patients were included to avoid selection bias. A PEN centered step-up protocol was established. Independent predictors of mortality: Early OF and extensive necrosis

Abbreviations: Fr, French; GA, general anesthesia; OF, organ failure; PCD, percutaneous catheter; SEMS, self-expandable metal stent.

In the first series by Carter and colleagues[15] 10 of 14 patients with IPN were treated with necrosectomy through the sinus tract as a primary modality. A rigid nephroscope or flexible endoscope was used for necrosectomy by removing small bits of necrotic pieces with the help of grasping forceps. The procedure could be successfully performed in all the patients. Eight patients improved, 2 died due to worsening sepsis and one needed open surgery (gastrojejunostomy).

In a series of 11 patients by Castellanos and colleagues,[17] PEN was performed using a flexible endoscope. Two large bore catheters were placed into the cavity by retroperitoneal approach and loose bits of necrotic debris were removed by irrigation and suction using a flexible endoscope over a mean of 5 sessions (range 3–10 sessions). No formal necrosectomy was done. Eight patients improved and 3 died of worsening organ failure.

Dhingra and colleagues[19] described the procedure in detail and also used it as a bedside tool in patients with worsening sepsis. The authors used a regular flexible endoscope with a 2.8. mm channel which allowed the use of standard endoscopic accessories for formal necrosectomy. They showed that PEN could be done under local anesthesia and conscious sedation. The authors demonstrated improvement in sepsis and organ failure once the liquid pus was removed by endoscopic lavage. The procedure could be done successfully in all patients but one patient died of worsening sepsis and organ failure.

In a prospective series of 9 patients, Saumoy and colleagues[21] described PEN through a metal stent placed through the percutaneous tract. After a median of 3 endoscopic sessions, 8 patients had successful removal of all PCD catheters and resolution of sepsis. One patient died of multi-organ failure. Thorsen and colleagues[22] also described a similar technique in 5 patients with successful outcome in 4 of them. In a series of 23 patients with INP, Ke and colleagues[23] described PEN through the SEMS. Clinical success rate was 70% with 48% major complications or death. Jürgensen and colleagues[28] also described a series of 14 patients with INP who underwent PEN with success in 13 patients. In their series, 6 patients had also undergone endoscopic transenteral drainage and debridement.

The largest prospective series was published by Jain and colleagues who described a "PEN centered step-up protocol."[20] Of a total of 177 patients with IPN, 53 patients underwent PEN as a part of the step-up therapy. Of these, 42 (79.2%) patients could be treated successfully and 11 patients died. Independent predictors of mortality after PEN were greater than 50% necrosis and organ failure.

In a recently published systemic review and meta-analysis of PEN in 282 patients from 16 observational studies, the clinical success rate of PEN was 82% (95% CI 77%–87%) with a periprocedural morbidity rate of 10% and no procedure-related mortality. Based on the findings, the authors concluded PEN to be a safe and effective modality with a high success rate.[29]

ADVERSE EVENTS OF PERCUTANEOUS ENDOSCOPIC NECROSECTOMY

Adverse events following PEN are summarized in **Table 2**. Periprocedural major adverse events include bleeding, peritonitis, pneumoperitoneum, paralytic ileus and aspiration pneumonia. Long-term complications include the development of pancreatic fistula and recurrence of collections.

Bleeding during the procedure can be minor and self-limiting due to ooze from the granulation tissue or major due to injury to a vessel traversing through the cavity or a pseudo-aneurysm rupture. Major bleeding warrants radiologic or surgical intervention.

Table 2	
Adverse events	
Periprocedural Adverse Events	
Periprocedural bleeding	2%–3%
Peritonitis	1%–5%
Pneumoperitoneum	1%–3%
Aspiration pneumonia	1%–3%
Paralytic ileus	1%
Subcutaneous emphysema	1%
Colonic perforation	1%
Drain dislodgement	1%
Long term adverse events	
Pancreatic fistula	7%–13%
Recurrence of collection	1%–4%

Peritonitis may develop following leakage of the infected fluid into the peritoneal cavity during the procedure due to increased intra-cavitatary pressure. Usually, it is self-limiting but may require laparotomy. Excessive insufflation should therefore be avoided during the procedure.

SUMMARY

Over the past 20 years, PEN has emerged as a promising minimally invasive tool for necrosectomy in predominantly laterally placed infected WON with a very good success rate similar to other modalities of debridement that is, DEN and VARD. In comparison to DEN or VARD, it has the following added advantages: (a) It can be performed under conscious sedation as compared to the need for GA for VARD and DEN (b) Ability to maneuver through deeper pockets of the collection with the help of a flexibile endoscope as compared to rigid and non-flexible instruments used in VARD (c) Ease of using it as a bedside tool in very sick patients with ongoing organ failure in ICU and (d) Better patient tolerability and hence it can be repeated easily as compared to VARD. PEN may also be used as an adjunct to DEN for large extensive collections.

FUTURE PROSPECTS

Step-up intervention is the preferred modality for the management of INP. PEN has evolved as an effective minimally invasive approach as an alternative to VARD/MARPN with a good safety profile. Better tolerability by the patients and ease of performing the procedure multiple times under conscious sedation make it a preferred approach for patients with ongoing organ failure who are high risk for GA. Randomized trials comparing PEN with other minimally invasive techniques might provide further robust data in the future.

FUNDING

The authors gratefully acknowledge funding from Indian Council of Medical Research and JC Bose Fellowship to Pramod Kumar Garg from Science & Engineering Research Board.

CLINICS CARE POINTS

- Laterally placed infected necrotic fluid collections not responding to antibiotics and drainage are best suited for percutaneous endoscopic necrosectomy (PEN).
- Removal of thick liquid pus during endoscopic lavage helps in the improvement of sepsis and can be done bedside in sicker patient admitted in ICU prior to PEN.
- Rapid tract upgradation can be done with the balloon dilatation of tract or placement of fully covered metal stent.
- Procedure can be repeated as it can be done in an endoscopic theater under conscious sedation and is tolerated well.
- Post procedure patient should be monitored for signs of peritonitis and bleeding for 24 to 48 hours.

CONFLICT OF INTEREST

None.

SUPPLEMENTARY DATA

Supplementary data related to this article can be found online at https://doi.org/10.1016/j.giec.2023.04.011.

REFERENCES

1. Garg PK, Singh VP. Organ Failure Due to Systemic Injury in Acute Pancreatitis. Gastroenterology 2019;156(7):2008–23.
2. Forsmark CE, Vege SS, Wilcox CM. Acute Pancreatitis. N Engl J Med 2016; 375(20):1972–81.
3. Padhan RK, Jain S, Agarwal S, et al. Primary and Secondary Organ Failures Cause Mortality Differentially in Acute Pancreatitis and Should be Distinguished. Pancreas 2018;47(3):302–7.
4. Schepers NJ, Bakker OJ, Besselink MG, et al. Impact of characteristics of organ failure and infected necrosis on mortality in necrotising pancreatitis. Gut 2019; 68(6):1044–51.
5. van Dijk SM, Hallensleben NDL, van Santvoort HC, et al. Acute pancreatitis: recent advances through randomised trials. Gut 2017;66(11):2024–32.
6. IAP/APA evidence-based guidelines for the management of acute pancreatitis. Pancreatology 2013;13(4, Supplement 2):e1–15.
7. Banks PA, Bollen TL, Dervenis C, et al. Classification of acute pancreatitis–2012: revision of the Atlanta classification and definitions by international consensus. Gut 2013;62(1):102–11.
8. Mahapatra SJ, Garg PK. Management of pancreatic fluid collections in patients with acute pancreatitis. J Pancreatol 2019;2(3):82–90.
9. Boxhoorn L, van Dijk SM, van Grinsven J, et al. Immediate versus Postponed Intervention for Infected Necrotizing Pancreatitis. N Engl J Med 2021;385(15): 1372–81.
10. van Santvoort HC, Besselink MG, Bakker OJ, et al. A step-up approach or open necrosectomy for necrotizing pancreatitis. N Engl J Med 2010;362(16):1491–502.
11. Mouli VP, Sreenivas V, Garg PK. Efficacy of conservative treatment, without necrosectomy, for infected pancreatic necrosis: a systematic review and meta-analysis. Gastroenterology 2013;144(2):333–40.e2.

12. Bang JY, Arnoletti JP, Holt BA, et al. An Endoscopic Transluminal Approach, Compared With Minimally Invasive Surgery, Reduces Complications and Costs for Patients With Necrotizing Pancreatitis. Gastroenterology 2019;156(4): 1027–40.e3.

13. van Brunschot S, van Grinsven J, van Santvoort HC, et al. Endoscopic or surgical step-up approach for infected necrotising pancreatitis: a multicentre randomised trial. Lancet 2018;391(10115):51–8.

14. Freeman ML, Werner J, van Santvoort HC, et al. Interventions for necrotizing pancreatitis: summary of a multidisciplinary consensus conference. Pancreas 2012;41(8):1176–94.

15. Carter CR, McKay CJ, Imrie CW. Percutaneous necrosectomy and sinus tract endoscopy in the management of infected pancreatic necrosis: an initial experience. Ann Surg 2000;232(2):175–80.

16. Seifert H, Wehrmann T, Schmitt T, et al. Retroperitoneal endoscopic debridement for infected peripancreatic necrosis. Lancet 2000;356(9230):653–5.

17. Castellanos G, Piñero A, Serrano A, et al. Translumbar retroperitoneal endoscopy: an alternative in the follow-up and management of drained infected pancreatic necrosis. Arch Surg Chic Ill 1960 2005;140(10):952–5.

18. van Santvoort HC, Besselink MGH, Horvath KD, et al. Videoscopic assisted retroperitoneal debridement in infected necrotizing pancreatitis. HPB 2007;9(2): 156–9.

19. Dhingra R, Srivastava S, Behra S, et al. Single or multiport percutaneous endoscopic necrosectomy performed with the patient under conscious sedation is a safe and effective treatment for infected pancreatic necrosis (with video). Gastrointest Endosc 2015;81(2):351–9.

20. Jain S, Padhan R, Bopanna S, et al. Percutaneous Endoscopic Step-Up Therapy Is an Effective Minimally Invasive Approach for Infected Necrotizing Pancreatitis. Dig Dis Sci 2019. https://doi.org/10.1007/s10620-019-05696-2.

21. Saumoy M, Kumta NA, Tyberg A, et al. Transcutaneous Endoscopic Necrosectomy for Walled-off Pancreatic Necrosis in the Paracolic Gutter. J Clin Gastroenterol 2018;52(5):458–63.

22. Thorsen A, Borch AM, Novovic S, et al. Endoscopic Necrosectomy Through Percutaneous Self-Expanding Metal Stents May Be a Promising Additive in Treatment of Necrotizing Pancreatitis. Dig Dis Sci 2018;63(9):2456–65.

23. Ke L, Li G, Wang P, et al. The efficacy and efficiency of stent-assisted percutaneous endoscopic necrosectomy for infected pancreatic necrosis: a pilot clinical study using historical controls. Eur J Gastroenterol Hepatol 2021;33(1S Suppl 1): e435–41.

24. Mui LM, Wong SKH, Ng EKW, et al. Combined sinus tract endoscopy and endoscopic retrograde cholangiopancreatography in management of pancreatic necrosis and abscess. Surg Endosc 2005;19(3):393–7.

25. Gupta P, Bansal A, Samanta J, et al. Larger bore percutaneous catheter in necrotic pancreatic fluid collection is associated with better outcomes. Eur Radiol 2021;31(5):3439–46.

26. Elhence A, Mahapatra SJ, Madhusudhan KS, et al. Pancreatic hemorrhage contributes to late mortality in patients with acute necrotizing pancreatitis. Pancreatology 2022;22(2):219–25.

27. Jain S. Infected Pancreatic Necrosis due to Multidrug-Resistant Organisms and Persistent Organ failure Predict Mortality in Acute Pancreatitis. Clin Transl Gastroenterol 2018;9(10). Accessed July 10, 2019. insights.ovid.com.

28. Jürgensen C, Brückner S, Reichel S, et al. Flexible percutaneous endoscopic retroperitoneal necrosectomy as rescue therapy for pancreatic necroses beyond the reach of endoscopic ultrasonography: A case series. Dig Endosc 2017;29(3): 377–82.
29. Gjeorgjievski M, Bhurwal A, Chouthai AA, et al. Percutaneous endoscopic necrosectomy (PEN) for treatment of necrotizing pancreatitis: a systematic review and meta-analysis. Endosc Int Open 2023;11(3):E258–67.
30. Mathers B, Moyer M, Mathew A, et al. Percutaneous debridement and washout of walled-off abdominal abscess and necrosis using flexible endoscopy: a large single-center experience. Endosc Int Open 2016;4(1):E102–6.
31. Tringali A, Vadalà di Prampero SF, Bove V, et al. Endoscopic necrosectomy of walled-off pancreatic necrosis by large-bore percutaneus metal stent: a new opportunity? Endosc Int Open 2018;6(3):E274–8.
32. Goenka MK, Goenka U, Mujoo MY, et al. Pancreatic Necrosectomy through Sinus Tract Endoscopy. Clin Endosc 2018;51(3):279–84.

Management of Disconnected Pancreatic Duct

Jahangeer Basha, MD, DM, Sundeep Lakhtakia, MD, DM*

KEYWORDS

- Disconnected pancreatic duct • Acute necrotizing pancreatitis • Walled-off necrosis
- Pancreatic fluid collections • Pancreatic duct disruption

KEY POINTS

- Disconnected Pancreatic Duct is common after Acute Necrotising Pancreatitis (ANP); and its implications vary according to the clinical course.
- In the early phase of ANP, during evolution from acute necrotic collection (ANC) to mature Walled-Off Necrosis (WON), DPD can be detected; however, management largely revolves around drainage of WON
- In the later phase, after the resolution of WON, the presence of DPD becomes more evident and is most often confirmed by MRCP.
- Clinical implications of DPD include recurrent fluid collection, and external pancreatic fistula. Others being - asymptomatic, recurrent pain, obstructive chronic pancreatitis, and new-onset diabetes.
- Long-term indwelling plastic stents may prevent the recurrent PFC in DPD.

INTRODUCTION

Disconnected pancreatic duct (DPD) most often occurs following acute necrotizing pancreatitis (ANP) due to necrosis of the pancreatic parenchyma along with the involved pancreatic duct (PD), causing complete disconnection of proximal (i.e, downstream) part of the pancreas and its segmental PD from the distal (i.e, upstream) pancreas and its duct.[1,2] The other causes of pancreatic ductal disruptions are pancreatic trauma, pancreatic surgeries, and chronic pancreatitis.[2] DPD is a common complication of ANP but has not gained much importance until the recent past. Therefore, there are no standardized guidelines on how to diagnose and manage this clinical entity. Before discussing the management of DPD, understanding the pathophysiology of important events in the course of ANP is essential. This review discusses

Department of Gastroenterology, Asian Institute of Gastroenterology, AIG Hospitals, Gachibowli, Hyderabad 500032, Telangana, India
* Corresponding author.
E-mail address: drsundeeplakhtakia@gmail.com

Gastrointest Endoscopy Clin N Am 33 (2023) 753–770
https://doi.org/10.1016/j.giec.2023.04.004
1052-5157/23/© 2023 Elsevier Inc. All rights reserved.

giendo.theclinics.com

the sequential events and their management from the onset of ANP till the development of DPD and thereafter. These prominent events include pancreatic parenchymal necrosis, main PD disruptions, walled-off necrosis (WON) formation, drainage, pancreatic disconnection, and its clinical implications.

DISCONNECTED PANCREATIC DUCT

The term disconnected pancreatic duct was first coined by Kozarek in 1991.[3] The prevalence of DPD in ANP ranged from 10% to 75% among the reported studies.[4–6] This wide variation in reported prevalence could be due to earlier unawareness of the clinical condition among clinicians and radiologists, and the timing and diagnostic modalities used in the clinical course of ANP to diagnose DPD. In a recent study that included a large homogenous group of patients, the prevalence of DPD reported was 74%.[6]

The radiologic criteria proposed for the diagnosis of DPD included the following features.[7]

1. Area of necrotic pancreas measuring 2 cm or greater
2. Presence of viable pancreatic tissue in the disconnected upstream pancreas
3. Pancreatic duct total cutoff during endoscopic retrograde cholangiopancreatography (ERCP)
4. Pancreatic duct entering the fluid collection at 90° angle

Definition

We propose a more anatomical definition of DPD as "complete destruction of the segment of main pancreatic duct and the adjoining pancreatic parenchyma that leads to physical isolation or disconnection of the physiologically functioning upstream pancreas and its duct from the downstream pancreas."

Pathophysiology

ANP is characterized by variable degree of necrosis of the pancreas involving both the parenchyma and the pancreatic duct wall leading to PD disruption.[8,9]

These PD disruptions lead to spontaneous extravasation of pancreatic juice causing to pancreatic fluid collections (PFC). PD disruptions can be either partial or complete. A partial disruption is characterized by a segmental involvement of PD with defect in its wall involving only a part of the circumference. This manifests during ERCP as focal extravasation (leak) of contrast along with opacification of the upstream or distal PD. Complete disruption is characterized by total circumferential disruption of the pancreatic duct leading to disconnection of upstream or distal PD from proximal or downstream PD. During ERCP, the contrast leaks freely outside the main pancreatic duct without opacification of the upstream PD distal to the disruption site. A complete disruption leads to physically disconnected duct, that is, DPD.

During the early phase of ANP, the pancreatic duct is disrupted leading to the development of immature acute necrotic collection (ANC) that evolves during the next few weeks into mature WON (**Fig.** 1A). After the resolution of WON, either by drainage or spontaneously, the necrotic area involving pancreatic parenchyma and PD heals by fibrosis, which leads to disconnection or physical gap separating the downstream pancreas and its duct from the upstream pancreas and its PD. The pancreatic secretions from the downstream pancreas normally reach the duodenum through the intact downstream duct. However, the upstream viable pancreas that continues to secrete physiologically is unable to expel its juice due to disconnection of PD. Instead, they

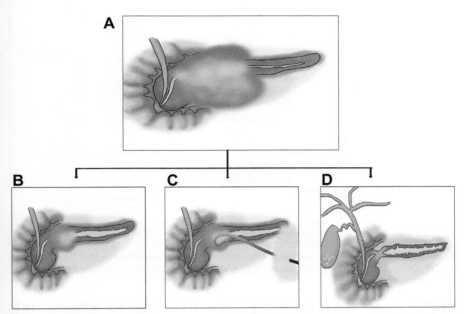

Fig. 1. Pathophysiology of events in ANP. Early phase of ANP with associated DPD causing WON (*A*); After resolution of WON, later phase showing persistent secretions from upstream pancreas causing recurrent PFC (*B*); EPF (*C*) in patients with prior PCD; and typical DPD with a gap of disconnection between downstream and upstream ducts (*D*). (*Courtesy of* Tanyaporn Chantarojanasiri, MD, Bangkok, TH.)

leak from the proximal end of the upstream duct into the surrounding space, causing persistent or recurrent fluid collections (**Fig. 1**B). In patients who are managed by percutaneous catheter drainage (PCD), the secretions from the upstream pancreas contribute to the persistence of external pancreatic fistulae (EPFs; **Fig. 1**C). In some patients as a part of natural course, the proximal end of the PD (**Fig. 1**D) gets fibrosed causing dilated upstream PD that can contribute to recurrent pain or recurrent pancreatitis, eventually leading to gradual atrophy of parenchyma of the upstream pancreas (**Fig. 2**).

DIAGNOSIS

Accurate diagnosis of DPD is a challenging task and not standardized.[10,11] The prominent reasons for this are lack of awareness of this clinical situation among radiologists and clinicians and the timing of imaging to label as DPD during the course of ANP. Trying to detect DPD in early phase may be inaccurate and affect the true prevalence. In the later phase of ANP, after the resolution of WON, DPD becomes more evident and clinically relevant. Finally, the choice of imaging for documenting DPD could also influence the diagnosis.

The various modalities used for diagnosing DPD are contrast-enhanced computed tomography (CECT), ERCP, endoscopic ultrasound (EUS), magnetic resonance cholangiopancreatography (MRCP), secretin MRCP (s-MRCP), and drain fluid amylase level.[12,13]

Timing of Imaging for Disconnected Pancreatic Duct

The ideal timing for diagnosing DPD is unclear, and there are no standard guidelines. Some studies reported DPD before the drainage of WON and others after the

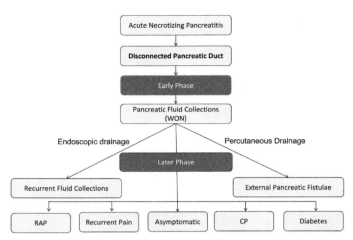

Fig. 2. Flowchart depicting the clinical implications of DPD according to the clinical course of ANP (DPD, disconnected pancreatic duct; ANP, acute necrotizing pancreatitis).

resolution.[6,14] Accurate assessment of DPD before drainage is challenging due to overlapping fluid collection and PD, especially if the collection is large. Moreover, extrinsic compression on the PD with upstream dilation can mimic DPD. Majority of the PFC in ANP have ductal injury leading to collections. The clinical relevance of labeling of DPD at the time of drainage is largely academic than clinically relevant. The only advantage it offers is the selection of a plastic stent in draining pseudocyst or WON having minimal debris and avoiding PCD if possible. However, most ANPs with duct disruption have significant necrosis and require metal stents due significant solid debris, than the presence of DPD. However, the advantage of diagnosing DPD after resolution of WON is better because resolved WON no longer interferes with the assessment of DPD.

Contrast-Enhanced Computed Tomography

CECT is a commonly used imaging modality used in AP and establishes the severity and associated fluid collections. CECT document the volume of parenchymal necrosis and location of collection that indirectly suggest the presence and site of DPD.[15] CECT also helps to assess the viability of the upstream pancreas. However, conventional CECT is suboptimal in evaluating the pancreatic ductal anatomy compared with MRCP. Current multirow detector CT scans can help better evaluate PD anatomy and hence DPD.[16]

There is scant literature of documenting DPD in ANP with high-resolution CT scan. Tann and colleagues compared CECT scan and ERCP with surgical findings. DPD was diagnosed at surgery in all patients that was missed on index CT. However, on reviewing the same CTs suggested the diagnoses of DPD.[15] In a study, Smoczynski and colleagues, evaluating transpapillary drainage for WON, observed a sensitivity of 80% for CT scan when ERCP was taken as the reference standard.[17]

Endoscopic retrograde cholangiopancreatography

ERCP, due to its dynamic nature, is considered the gold standard for evaluating pancreatic ductal anatomy. In early phase of ANP, ERCP demonstrates complete disruption of PD where injected contrast leaks freely outside the duct without opacification of distal or upstream PD. In the later phase of ANP, ERCP demonstrates complete cutoff PD without opacification of distal PD, suggesting DPD (**Fig. 3**).[9,15] Tann and colleagues observed complete correlation between ERCP and surgical findings in establishing DPD.[15]

Although ERCP is considered as the gold standard for diagnosing DPD, it has several inherent limitations. It is invasive and does not provide information about upstream disconnected PD, when compared with MRCP. Another disadvantage of ERCP is introduction of infection into a previous sterile collection and aggravation or inducing pancreatitis.

Magnetic Resonance Cholangiopancreatography and Secretin Magnetic Resonance Cholangiopancreatography

MRCP is the preferred imaging modality to evaluate the pancreatic ductal anatomy. The main advantage of MRCP is its noninvasive nature, despite being less sensitive compared with ERCP.[8,18,19] MRCP visualizes the site of disconnection, the downstream PD, and, importantly, the upstream disconnected duct (**Figs. 4**). This information best comes after the resolution of the fluid collection.[7,20]

Secretin, when injected during MRCP, augments the pancreatic secretions, providing the dynamic visualization of PD. Gillams and colleagues assessed the role of s-MRCP with surgical findings and observed a sensitivity of 83.3% in detecting DPD.[19] Drake and colleagues evaluated combined MRCP with s-MRCP and compared with ERCP as the reference standard. Combined MRCP with s-MRCP had high sensitivity (92%), specificity (100%), and overall accuracy (94%).[13,18] The main limitations of s-MRCP are limited availability and cost of secretin.

Endoscopic Ultrasound

EUS allows accurate visualization of pancreas and PD due to its proximity to stomach and duodenum. In ANP, EUS accurately evaluates the nature of PFC and is reasonable to assess its relationship with PD.

Bang and colleagues prospectively evaluated the role of EUS in DPD.[14] They observed that EUS had very-high sensitivity (100%) to diagnose DPD and matched with ERCP or surgery. However, few limitations of the study are inclusion of only WON greater than 6 cm in size and exclusion of 9 patients from the analysis due to

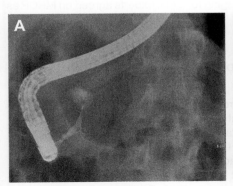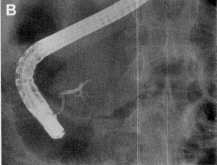

Fig. 3. ERCP-pancreatogram showing opacification of only downstream duct with leak of contrast into collection suggesting complete PD disruption in early phase (A); pancreatogram showing complete PD cut-off in later phase (B) (ERCP, endoscopic retrograde cholangiopancreatography).

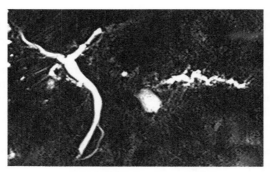

Fig. 4. MRCP showing DPD with both upstream and downstream ducts (MRCP, magnetic resonance cholangiopancreatography; DPD, disconnected pancreatic duct).

suboptimal assessment of distal pancreas, which could have affected the sensitivity. Overall, EUS is valuable for DPD diagnosis, and the accuracy depends on operators' expertise and PFC morphology.[13,14]

Drain Fluid Amylase

Fluid amylase measurement in PCD helps to identify the possibility of ductal communication in patients with EPF. A value of more than 3 times than the serum suggests ductal disruption.[13] Fluid amylase measurement has a sensitivity of 100%, specificity of 50%, and diagnostic accuracy of 65% when compared with ERCP to detect PD disruption.[21] However, it cannot differentiate between partial and complete PD disruptions.

Timmerhuis and colleagues in their systematic review of 8 studies compared 5 diagnostic modalities in 142 patients for the diagnosis of DPD.[13] The reported sensitivity of ERCP and EUS was 100% each. CT scan had lower sensitivity (range 0%–80%), MRCP or s-MRCP had a sensitivity of 83% each, and on combined sensitivity was 92%. Authors recommended that, due to their simple and noninvasive nature, MRCP or s-MRCP should be considered as the first choice of investigation for diagnosing DPD. In an international expert survey by Boxhoorn and colleagues, although there was a lack of consensus about the imaging for DPD, experts agreed on MRCP as the preferred diagnostic modality.[22]

CLINICAL IMPLICATIONS OF DISCONNECTED PANCREATIC DUCT AND MANAGEMENT

The clinical implications of DPD vary according to the disease course of ANP. In the early phase, the evolution of WON dominates the clinical picture. DPD usually exists from the onset of ANP, however, at this stage remains clinically insignificant. During the later phase, either at drainage or after the resolution of WON, the DPD is recognized on imaging as loss of pancreas replaced by fibrosis of variable length.

After establishment of DPD, the patient may remain asymptomatic or may have recurrent PFC and persistent EPFs if managed by PCD. Other presentations of DPD related to ductal hypertension and parenchymal atrophy include recurrent pain with or without pancreatitis, endocrine and exocrine insufficiency, and rarely chronic pancreatitis (see **Fig. 2**).

A. Early Phase

The main clinical implication of DPD at early phase is the development of WON and its management. The strategy of management of WON including the choice of the stent is mainly decided by its morphological characteristics rather than the presence of DPD in this phase. Few studies suggested using plastic stents for internal drainage if DPD is documented.[4,14] Plastic stents can be considered for draining pseudocyst or WON having minimal debris. However, WON with significant debris require metal stents for the effective drainage, even in the presence of DPD. The impact of DPD comes into the picture in the later phase after the resolution of collection. The only advantage of early diagnosis of DPD at this phase is that we can decide to avoid PCD to prevent EPF.[23]

Management of Walled-Off Necrosis with Disconnected Pancreatic Duct

Symptomatic WON are managed by drainage that can be done by endoscopic, percutaneous, or surgical methods. The choice of these drainage methods depends on maturity, access route, and extent of WON. Timmerhuis and colleagues evaluated the outcomes of large data of ANP with pancreatic ductal disruptions and disconnection and showed that patients with DPD required more pancreatic interventions than patients without DPD.[24] Recently, 3 meta-analyses were published based on studies evaluating treatment outcomes in DPD.[25–27] The details of the meta-analysis are mentioned in **Table 1**.

Percutaneous drainage

PCD is one of the common modalities for the drainage of PFC. Usually, PCD is performed as a part of a minimally invasive step-up approach or sole treatment of the drainage of PFC. PCD may be associated with risk of fistula formation in the setting of DPD and hence to be avoided as far as possible. In patients with symptomatic distant collections or infected pancreatic necrosis where endoscopic options are not feasible, PCD can be considered but must be cautioned about EPF formation. When PCD is necessary, dual modality drainage, combining both endoscopic transmural drainage and PCD, when possible, can be considered to prevent EPF.[28]

In a study by Meatman and colleagues, PCD in patients with DPD required more interventions, including upsizing catheter size and additional catheter placements.[29] Nealon and colleagues studied the pancreatic ductal anatomy and compared it with treatment outcomes in patients with pseudocyst and ANP. PCD was successful in none of the patients in type 3 duct, corresponding to DPD, and most require surgical debridement. EPF formation was also significantly high (85%) in patients with DPD.[30]

Transpapillary drainage

Transpapillary drainage can be attempted in small fluid collections with likely communication with PD. However, transpapillary drainage is not ideal in DPD because DPD is usually associated with WON with significant necrotic debris. Transpapillary stents, being small caliber plastic stents, may not effectively drain WON. Due to this ineffective drainage, they induce secondary infections and sometimes worsen the outcome.

A systematic review by Van Dijk and colleagues analyzed 6 studies evaluating transpapillary drainage in pancreatic ductal disruptions or disconnections, showed an overall success rate of 83%.[25] Later, Chong and colleagues published another meta-analysis and showed a success rate of only 58.5%.[26] The discrepancy between these 2 meta-analyses could be due to the differences in the studies included. An earlier meta-analysis by van Dijk and colleagues included studies reporting both partial and complete disruptions, whereas Chong and colleagues explicitly included studies

Table 1
Meta-analyses published on management outcomes of disconnected pancreatic duct

Authors	Studies Included	Total Patients	Study Selection Criteria	Success Rate of Trans-papillary drainage	Success Rate of Transmural drainage	Success Rate of Surgery
Van Dijk et al,[25] 2012	21 studies (1991–2017)	583	Studies reported treatment outcomes of DPD	81%	92%	DPS 80% RYID 84%
Chong et al,[26] 2021	30 studies (1995–2020)	1355	Studies reported treatment outcomes of DPD	58.5%	90.6%	DPS 86.6% RYID 85.8%
Hamada et al,[27] 2022	5 studies (2018–2021)	941	Studies reported outcomes of endoscopic drainage comparing DPD and non-DPD	-	OR - 0.77 (95% CI 0.33–1.81)	-

Abbreviations: DPS, distal pancreato-splenectomy; RYID, roux-en-y internal drainage

on DPD. Amin and colleagues conducted a meta-analysis of 9 studies, which evaluated the added advantage of transpapillary drainage to transmural drainage and found no additional benefit.[31]

Transmural drainage

Currently, EUS guided transmural drainage is considered the preferred modality for the drainage of WON. Choosing between plastic or lumen apposing metal stent (LAMS) largely depends of characteristics of PFC. LAMS being wider in caliber, provides effective drainage and allows endoscopic necrosectomy if required. In the setting of DPD, plastic stents can be kept long term to prevent the recurrence of fluid collection.

In a meta-analysis by Van Dijk and colleagues, the overall clinical success for transmural drainage was 92%.[25] The meta-analysis by Chong and colleagues, analyzed 11 studies, also showed a weighted clinical success rate of 90.6% for transmural drainage.[26]

Bang and colleagues retrospectively evaluated the impact of DPD on outcomes of endoscopic drainage of PFC among 361 patients. They observed no difference in treatment outcomes between patients with and without DPD. However, patients with DPD required more intervention, hybrid treatments, and rescue surgery.[4] Recently, Hamada and colleagues conducted a meta-analysis including 9 studies comprising 941 patients, which evaluated the treatment outcomes of EUS-guided drainage of PFC in patients with DPD. The meta-analysis showed no difference in the clinical success of WON between patients with DPD and no DPD.[27] Although, patients with DPD require more interventions than those without DPD, the overall clinical success, that is, the resolution of WON, remains same irrespective of DPD.

To summarize, in the early phase of ANP, the clinical outcome is more dependent on WON drainage rather addressing DPD. PCD should not be considered for drainage in DPD due to the risk of EPF formation. Transmural drainage is the choice of treatment of the drainage of WON, which also has an option of keeping long-term plastic stents to prevent a recurrence. Transpapillary drainage alone provides suboptimal drainage and has no added benefit to transmural drainage.

B. Later Phase

After the resolution of WON, it is imperative to evaluate PD anatomy and understand its roadmap including confirmation of DPD. The clinical outcome of DPD is variable depending on the volume of upstream disconnected pancreas and route of index drainage. A proportion of patients with DPD develop recurrent PFC.[6] Persistent EPF is in those who were drained by PCD.[23] Other manifestation of DPD include recurrent pain abdomen with or without pancreatitis or CP in evolution. In due course, pancreatic atrophy of the upstream-disconnected segment may lead to endocrine and exocrine dysfunction. Some patients remain asymptomatic in short-term to medium-term follow-up (see **Fig. 2**).

Recurrent Pancreatic Fluid Collections

Recurrent PFC is the most discussed clinical implication of DPD in literature. It occurs due to continued secretion of pancreatic juices from the leaking disconnected upstream pancreas. Studies have reported an incidence of 10% to 30%.[4,6,32] In a meta-analysis by Hamada and colleagues, the rate of recurrence reported among the 5 included studies ranged from 4.3% to 13%. The recurrence risk was more in DPD when compared with no DPD (pooled OR 6.72; 95% CI 2.72–16.6).[27]

After the complete resolution of PFC, it is advisable to obtain MRCP before removing the transmural stents to evaluate PD anatomy. If an ERCP performed at this juncture shows a "partial duct disruption," placing a bridging transpapillary plastic stent allows healing of the disruption and salvaging upstream pancreas. However, if ERCP shows a complete PD disruption or cutoff, a transpapillary plastic stent provides no benefit.

Prevention of Recurrent Pancreatic Fluid Collections

Keeping long-term indwelling double pigtail plastic stents has been proposed as a strategy to prevent recurrent PFC in presence of DPD. These stents allow continuous drainage of secretions from the upstream pancreas into the stomach either through its lumen or acting as wick.

In a randomized controlled trial including 28 patients, Arvanitakis and colleagues evaluated the role of keeping long-term plastic stents in PFC after index drainage. Stents were removed in 13 patients after the resolution of collection and remaining 15 patients had it in situ for the long term. After a median duration of 14 months, recurrent PFC was not observed among patients with long-term stents, whereas 5 developed recurrences in whom stents were removed ($P = .013$).[32] Subsequently, similar studies also demonstrated the benefit of long-term transmural plastic stents.[4,33,34]

The strategy of keeping long-term plastic stents would be appropriate when plastic stents are used for the initial drainage of WON. Currently, metal stents including lumen apposing metal stents (LAMS) or similar metal stents are preferred than plastic stents for the drainage of WON due to their efficacy.[35,36] However, unlike plastic stents, LAMS should be removed after 2 to 4 weeks of placement, due to adverse events, for example, bleeding and tissue embedment.[37]

Bang and colleagues attempted to address the strategy to prevent recurrence in WON drained by metal stents in their retrospective analysis that included 188 patients who underwent PFC drainage by LAMS.[38] DPD was observed in 94 (50%). At removal, LAMS were exchanged with plastic stents in 70 patients and in remaining 24 plastic stents could not be placed. There was only 1 recurrent PFC in the exchange group and 6 (25%) recurrences in the nonexchange group. This reconfirmed the strategy of keeping long-term indwelling plastic stents in DPD. **Table 2** illustrates studies that used metal stents for initial drainage and their subsequent strategy.[6,38–41]

Even though a majority of the publications reports the safety of long-term indwelling stents, there could be complications too. The reported complications include stent migration with associated small bowel obstruction and colon perforation, ulceration, and bleeding.[42,43] In a recent study by Gkolfakis and colleagues, the long-term outcomes of indwelling plastic stents were evaluated. During the mean follow-up of 80 months, plastic stents were spontaneously migrated in 90 out of 125 patients (72%); of these, 65 were asymptomatic migrations, and 12 had stent-induced complications including ulcers and erosions.[43] Overall recurrent PFC were observed in 35 out of 125 (28%) patients. The majority (92%) of recurrences occurred within 2 years. The main factors responsible for recurrent PFCs were stent migration, placement of long plastic stents, and chronic pancreatitis.

Another question in the given context is whether a metal stent be exchanged with plastic stent. Our group systematically evaluated the in a large homogenous group of 274 patients of WON drained initially using metal stents. DPD was confirmed in 189/256 (73.8%) patients by MRCP and ERCP. Metal stents were not exchanged with plastic stent at removal. During follow-up (median 5 months; range 1–19 months), the recurrent PFC was observed in only 34 (13.2%) patients of whom only half required intervention.[6]

Subsequently, we conducted a randomized controlled trial of 104 patients with DPD (52 in each arm), comparing exchange with plastic stents versus none, at the time of removal of metal stents. At 3 months follow-up, there was no statistical difference in the recurrence of PFC between the 2 groups. The same trend was observed at 6 and 12 months follow-up.[41] However, there was a trend of higher recurrence in patients without plastic stents at 12 months follow-up. Homogenous studies with long-term follow-up are likely to clarify this debate.

Treatment of recurrent pancreatic fluid collections

The clinical course of recurrent PFC in DPD can be variable. Some collections are small and asymptomatic that are likely to resolve spontaneously.[6,43] Symptomatic recurrent PFC require EUS-guided drainage using short-length double pigtail plastic stents that are kept indwelling for long term. Collections not amenable to endoscopic drainage can be considered for surgery.

External Pancreatic Fistulae

EPF occurs following PCD of PFC in setting of DPD. The upstream pancreas continues to secrete amylase rich pancreatic juices that continuously drain out via a PCD or the fistulous tract. EPF are debilitating and may persist for weeks to months even after the resolution of PFC.[5] In a study by Nealon and colleagues, DPD was associated with fistula formation in 85% of the patients who underwent PCD.[30]

EPF in the setting of DPD is challenging to manage because ERCP is usually unsuccessful due to - complete cutoff of PD. Various treatment options have been explored to address this challenging issue.

1. Combined radiologic and endoscopic approach—In this technique described by Irani and colleagues, first, the fistulous tract is demonstrated by contrast injection

Table 2
Clinical details of studies used metal stents for drainage of walled-off necrosis in disconnected pancreatic duct

Authors	Total Patients	Study Design	Patients with DPD	Metal Exchanged with Plastic Stent	Follow-up (Median)	Recurrent PFC with Exchange	Recurrent PFC without Exchange
Dhir et al,[39] 2018	88	Prospective	53 (60.9%)	0	22 mo	-	7 (13.2%)
Bang et al,[38] 2020	188	Prospective	94 (50%)	70 (74.5%)	6 mo	1 (1.4%)	6 (25%)
Basha et al,[6] 2020	274	Retrospective	189 (73.8%)	0	14 mo	-	13.2%
Pawa et al,[40] 2022	96	Retrospective	48 (50%)	21 (43.8%)	20 mo	1 (5%)	10 (37%)
Chavan et al,[41] 2022	236	RCT	104 (44%)	52 (50%)	12 mo	7 (13.5%)	13 (25%)

into the tract and visualized under fluoroscopy. Next, the needle used for Transjugular Intrahepatic Portosystemic shunt (TIPS) is advanced into the tract up to the stomach, and the gastric wall is punctured, confirmed by an endoscope inserted into the stomach. A guidewire is passed through the needle, which is grabbed by a snare passed through the endoscope. Then endoscopic dilatation of the tract by balloon catheter is done by passing through the scope over the guidewire. Finally, double pigtail plastic stents are placed into the tract to allow internal drainage. PCD catheter can be removed later.[44]

2. Complete endoscopic approach—Sometimes the fistulous tract could be seen close to the stomach under EUS guidance. EUS-guided transgastric needle puncture of the tract done; contrast injection can confirm the tract under fluoroscopy. Subsequently, the guidewire is passed into the tract and the tract is dilated with a balloon catheter over the guidewire. Finally, plastic stents can be placed into the fistula, which allows the PCD to be removed.[44]

3. EUS-guided drainage of upstream PD can be considered if the duct is sufficiently dilated DPD.[45]

4. Other techniques such as using fibrin and glue to close the fistulous tract have been reported.[46]

New Onset Diabetes

ANP is known to increase the risk of new-onset diabetes and the risk further increases with the severity of necrosis.[47] Recent data have shown that in patients with ANP, the presence of DPD further increases the risk.[4,5,34,48] **(Table 3)** This could be due to ductal hypertension in DPD, causing atrophy and loss of islet cell mass. Moreover, inflammation and fibrosis in the upstream pancreas contribute to the risk.

Thiruvengadam and colleagues evaluated the development of new-onset diabetes in DPD and observed that diabetes developed in 43% of patients with DPD, whereas only in 7.5% in those without.[48] Our group also observed that the risk of diabetes was significantly higher among patients with DPD when compared with patients without DPD. We also observed that risk is more in proximal disconnection (towards head) when compared with distal disconnection suggeasting a larger volume of pancreatic parenchyma at risk of atrophy in proximal disconnection.[6]

Recurrent Pain, Pancreatitis, Chronic Pancreatitis

Recurrent pain with or without pancreatitis can occur in some patients with DPD. The proximal end of upstream duct gets fibrosed causing ductal hypertension. Lawrence and colleagues, in a retrospective series, reported that half of the patients with DPD presented with recurrent symptoms.[5] In a recent study by Timmerhuis and colleagues, 30% of patients with DPD had recurrent pancreatitis during follow-up.[48]

Some patients due to subsequent slow atrophy of upstream pancreas may develop obstructive chronic pancreatitis. Pelaez-Luna and colleagues, in a retrospective study of 31 patients with DPD, reported that chronic pancreatitis was developed in 26% of patients.[34] Timmerhuis and colleagues also reported chronic pancreatitis in 17% of patients[48] **(Table 3)**.

Exocrine Insufficiency

Exocrine insufficiency can occur in DPD due to parenchymal atrophy of upstream pancreas and associated development of chronic pancreatitis. Studies reported a prevalence of 15% to 35% approximately[24,49] (see **Table 3**).

Table 3
Studies reporting long-term implications of disconnected pancreatic duct

Authors	Diabetes (%)	Recurrent Pain (%)	Recurrent Pancreatitis (%)	Chronic Pancreatitis (%)	Exocrine Insufficiency (%)
Chen et al,[49] 2019	14.3	-	-	-	21.4
Pelaez-Luna et al,[34] 2008	16	3	-	26	-
Tellez-Avina et al,[50] 2018	52	-	-	-	14
Lawrence et al,[5] 2007	53	53	-	-	-
Timmerhuis et al,[24] 2023	46	-	30	17	34

Asymptomatic Disconnected Pancreatic Duct

Not all patients with DPD present with symptoms. A proportion of patients remain asymptomatic during follow-up, despite DPD. Literature is sparse about the asymptomatic presentation of DPD. Factors that contribute for asymptomatic nature of DPD are unknown. There is a need for long-term follow-up study on the natural history of DPD.

Endoscopic Treatment of Symptomatic Disconnected Pancreatic Duct

EUS-guided drainage of DPD can be considered to drain the upstream-dilated PD in symptomatic patients (**Fig. 5**). This is similar to EUS-guided drainage of PD in chronic pancreatitis with difficult strictures. The drainage of upstream dilated PD can be performed using a plastic stent. The ideal setting being a sufficiently dilated PD with proximal disconnection. Few reports have shown successful EUS-guided drainage of DPD and stent placement.[45] Whenever EUS-guided drainge is not possible or available, surgery can be considered.

Role of Surgical Management in Disconnected Pancreatic Duct

The role of surgery in DPD in setting of ANP comes in 2 stages. In the early phase t some patients may require surgical drainage which is usually minimally invasive as step-up approach. In the later phase, the role of surgery in DPD is considered due to non-availability or failure of other non-surgical options (endoscopic or radiological). The 2 primary types of surgical options performed for patients with DPD are resection techniques or Roux-en-Y drainage procedures. The resection technique includes distal pancreatosplenectomy, generally considered when there is a small residual upstream segment in DPD. Roux-en-Y drainage procedures include cystojejunostomy, fistulojejunostomy or pancreatojejunostomy. DPD with the associated symptomatic collection, not feasible for endoscopic drainage, can be considered for cystojejunostomy. Patients with EPF in DPD can undergo fistulojejunostomy when other options fail. Pancreatojejunostomy can be considered when symptomatic DPD has a sizable upstream gland and dilated duct.

In the meta-analysis by Chong and colleagues, surgery was required after the failure of endoscopic treatment in about 22% of patients with DPD. The meta-analysis analyzed 10 studies reporting the outcomes of surgery in DPD.[26] The clinical success for distal pancreatosplenectomy observed was 86.6%, for Roux-en-Y drainage 85.8%, and the overall clinical success observed was 87.4%. Van Dijk and colleagues in their systematic review concluded that distal pancreatectomy when compared with

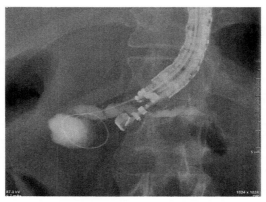

Fig. 5. EUS-guided drainage of DPD showing dilated disconnected duct communicating with small collection.

Roux-en-Y drainage procedures, had more intraoperative blood loss and incidence of pancreatic endocrine insufficiency were higher.[25]

Future Directions

1. Radiologists reporting MRCP should be able to differentiate DPD from the PD stricture of chronic pancreatitis with uniformity of descriptive terminologies.
2. Pancreatic volumetry assessment provides the natural course, especially of the upstream-disconnected segment, and may help select the patients for appropriate and timely interventions.
3. Long-term follow-up of DPD is necessary to see the evolution of clinical events and act accordingly.
4. Novel ERCP or EUS-based technologies need to be developed to reconnect and salvage the upstream-disconnected pancreas to prevent Diabetes and or exocrine dysfunction before it atrophies.

SUMMARY

DPD is common after ANP; however, its implications vary according to the clinical course. In the early phase of ANP, complete disruption of PD along with leakage of pancreatic secretions together with parenchymal necrosis cause ANC that matures and evolves into WON. During this phase, the management revolves around WON drainage, and the clinical significance of DPD is minimal. In the later phase, after the resolution of WON, the presence of DPD becomes evident, which can be confirmed by cross-sectional imaging with reconstruction, especially MRCP. Clinically DPD can have variable manifestation. Recurrent PFC (due to persistent significant secretion from the upstream viable pancreas) and EPF in patients with earlier percutaneous drainage of WON are the common clinical implications. The other implications are completely absence of symptoms, recurrent pain with or without recurrent pancreatitis, and obstructive chronic pancreatitis in upstream segment. Some patients present with new-onset diabetes. Long-term indwelling plastic stents have been proposed as an option to prevent the recurrent PFC.

CLINICS CARE POINTS

Pearls:
- Do not intervene in DPD even if radiologically evident, unless attributable symptoms are present.
- Consider long-term short-length DPT plastic stents for PFC/WON, if DPD is obvious radiologically.
- Avoid external drainage of central PFC "alone" to prevent EPF.
- Occasionally, ERP can confirm the communication between apparent MRCP-based diagnosis of DPD.

Pitfalls:
- MRCP can overdiagnose DPD.
- ERCP cannot bridge the DPD.
- Percutaneous drainage alone of centrally located PFC can lead to EPF. Combined or dual drainage should be considered in special situations.
- Failure to salvage disconnected pancreas can lead to diabetes and exocrine insufficiency.

ACKNOWLEDGMENTS

The authors thank Dr Tanyaporn Chantarojanasiri for preparing the diagrammatic illustrations and sketches.

DISCLOSURE

The authors have nothing to disclose.

REFERENCES

1. Kozarek RA. Endoscopic therapy of complete and partial pancreatic duct disruptions. Gastrointest Endosc Clin N Am 1998;8(1):39e53.
2. Devière J, Bueso H, Baize M, et al. Complete disruption of the main pancreatic duct: endoscopic management. Gastrointest Endosc 1995;42(5):445–51.
3. Kozarek RA, Ball TJ, Patterson DJ, et al. Endoscopic transpapillary therapy for disrupted pancreatic duct and peripancreatic fluid collections. Gastroenterology 1991;100(5 Pt 1):1362–70.
4. Bang JY, Wilcox CM, Navaneethan U, et al. Impact of disconnected pancreatic duct syndrome on the endoscopic man- agement of pancreatic fluid collections. Ann Surg 2018;267(3):561e8.
5. Lawrence C, Howell DA, Stefan AM, et al. Disconnected pancreatic tail syndrome: potential for endoscopic therapy and results of long-term follow-up. Gastrointest Endosc 2008;67(4):673–9.
6. Basha J, Lakhtakia S, Nabi Z, et al. Impact of disconnected pancreatic duct on recur- rence of fluid collections and new-onset diabetes: do we finally have an answer? Gut 2021;70(3):447–9.
7. Sandrasegaran K, Tann M, Jennings SG, et al. Disconnection of the pancreatic duct: an important but overlooked complication of severe acute pancreatitis. Radiographics 2007;27(5):1389–400.
8. Jang JW, Kim MH, Oh D, et al. Factors and outcomes associated with pancreatic duct disruption in patients with acute necrotizing pancreatitis. Pancreatology 2016;16(6):958–65.

9. Neoptolemos JP, London NJ, Carr-Locke DL. Assessment of main pancreatic duct integrity by endoscopic retrograde pancreatography in patients with acute pancreatitis. Br J Surg 1993;80(1):94–9.

10. Group W, Apa IAP, Pancreatitis A. IAP/APA evidence-based guidelines for the management of acute pancreatitis. Pancreatology 2013;13:e1–15.

11. Arvanitakis M, Dumonceau J-M, Albert J, et al. Endoscopic management of acute necrotizing pancreatitis: European society of gastrointestinal endoscopy (ESGE) evidence-based multidisciplinary guidelines. Endoscopy 2018;50:524–5.

12. Nadkarni NA, Kotwal V, Sarr MG, et al. Disconnected pancreatic duct syndrome: endoscopic stent or surgeon's knife? Pancreas 2015;44(1):16–22.

13. Timmerhuis HC, van Dijk SM, Verdonk RC, et al. Various modalities accurate in diagnosing a disrupted or disconnected pancreatic duct in acute pancreatitis: a systematic review. Dig Dis Sci 2020;66(5):1415–24.

14. Bang JY, Navaneethan U, Hasan MK, et al. EUS correlates of disconnected pancreatic duct syndrome in walled-of necrosis. Endosc Int Open 2016;4: E883–9.

15. Tann M, Maglinte D, Howard TJ, et al. Disconnected pancreatic duct syndrome: imaging findings and therapeutic implications in 26 surgically corrected patients. J Comput Assist Tomogr 2003;27(4):577–82.

16. Anderson SW, Soto JA. Pancreatic duct evaluation: accuracy of portal venous phase 64 MDCT. Abdom Imaging 2009;34:55–63.

17. Smoczyński M, Jagielski M, Jabłońska A, et al. Transpapillary drainage of walled-of pancreatic necrosis - a single center experience. Videosurg Other Miniinvasive Tech/Wideochirurgia i Inne Tech Malo Inwazyjne 2015;10:527–33.

18. Drake LM, Anis M, Lawrence C. Accuracy of magnetic resonance cholangiopancreatography in identifying pancreatic duct disruption. J Clin Gastroenterol 2012; 46(8):696–9.

19. Gillams AR, Kurzawinski T, Lees WR. Diagnosis of duct disruption and assessment of pancreatic leak with dynamic secretin-stimulated MR cholangiopancreatography. AJR Am J Roentgenol 2006;186(2):499–506.

20. Verma S, Rana SS. Disconnected pancreatic duct syndrome: updated review on clinical implications and management. Pancreatology 2020;20(6):1035–44.

21. Yokoi Y, Kikuyama M, Kurokami T, et al. Early dual drainage combining transpapillary endotherapy and percutaneous catheter drainage in patients with pancreatic fstula associated with severe acute pancreatitis. Pancreatology 2016;16: 497–507.

22. Boxhoorn L, Timmerhuis HC, Verdonk RC, et al. Diagnosis and treatment of pancreatic duct disruption or disconnection: an international expert survey and case vignette study. HPB 2021;23(8):1201–8.

23. Van Brunschot S, van Grinsven J, van Santvoort HC, et al. Endoscopic or surgical step-up approach for infected necrotising pancreatitis: a multicentre randomised trial. Lancet 2018;391(10115):51–8.

24. Timmerhuis HC, van Dijk SM, Robbert A, et al. Short-term and Long-term Outcomes of a Disruption and Disconnection of the Pancreatic Duct in Necrotizing Pancreatitis: A Multicenter Cohort Study in 896 Patients. Am J Gastroenterol 2022. https://doi.org/10.14309/ajg.0000000000002157.

25. van Dijk SM, Timmerhuis HC, Verdonk RC, et al. Treatment of disrupted and disconnected pancreatic duct in necrotizing pancreatitis: A systematic review and meta-analysis. Pancreatology 2019;19:905–15.

26. Chong E, Ratnayake CB, Saikia S, et al. Endoscopic transmural drainage is associated with improved outcomes in disconnected pancreatic duct syndrome: A systematic review and meta-analysis. BMC Gastroenterol 2021;21(1):87.

27. Hamada T, Iwashita T, Saito T, et al. Disconnected pancreatic duct syndrome and outcomes of endoscopic ultrasound-guided treatment of pancreatic fluid collections: Systematic review and meta-analysis Digestive. Endoscopy 2022;34: 676–86.

28. Ross A, Gluck M, Irani S, et al. Combined endoscopic and percutaneous drainage of organized pancreatic necrosis. Gastrointest Endosc 2010;71(1): 79–84.

29. Maatman TK, Mahajan S, Roch AM, et al. Disconnected pancreatic duct syndrome predicts failure of percutaneous therapy in necrotizing pancreatitis. Pancreatology 2020;20:362–8.

30. Nealon WH, Bhutani M, Riall TS, et al. A unifying concept: pancreatic ductal anatomy both predicts and determines the major complications resulting from pancreatitis. J Am Coll Surg 2009;208(5):790–801.

31. Amin S, Yang DJ, Lucas AL, et al. There is No advantage to transpapillary pancreatic duct stenting for the transmural endoscopic drainage of pancreatic fluid collections: a meta-analysis. Clin Endosc 2017;50(4):388–94.

32. Arvanitakis M, Delhaye M, Bali MA, et al. Pancreatic-fluid collections: a randomized controlled trial regarding stent removal after endoscopic transmural drainage. Gastrointest Endosc 2007;65(4):609–19.

33. Rana SS, Shah J, Sharma RK, et al. Clinical and morphological consequences of permanent indwelling transmural plastic stents in disconnected pancreatic duct syndrome. Endosc Ultrasound 2020;9(2):130e7.

34. Pelaez-Luna M, Vege SS, Petersen BT, et al. Disconnected pancreatic duct syndrome in severe acute pancreatitis: clinical and imaging characteristics and outcomes in a cohort of 31 cases. Gastrointest Endosc 2008;68(1):91–7.

35. Lakhtakia S, Basha J, Talukdar R, et al. Endoscopic "step-up approach" using a dedicated biflanged metal stent reduces the need for direct necrosectomy in walled- off necrosis (with videos). Gastrointest Endosc 2017;85:1243–52.

36. Sharaiha RZ, Tyberg A, Khashab MA, et al. Endoscopic therapy with lumen-apposing metal stents is safe and effective for patients with pancreatic walled-off necrosis. Clin Gastroenterol Hepatol 2016;14:1797–803.

37. Bang JY, Hasan M, Navaneethan U, et al. Lumen-apposing metal stents (LAMS) for pancreatic fluid collection (PFC) drainage: may not be business as usual. Gut 2017;66:2054–6.

38. Bang JY, Mel Wilcox C, Arnoletti JP, et al. Importance of disconnected pancreatic duct syndrome in recurrence of pancreatic fluid collections initially drained using Lumen-Apposing metal stents. Clin Gastroenterol Hepatol 2021;19(6): 1275–81.e2.

39. Dhir V, Adler DG, Dalal A, et al. Early removal of biflanged metal stents in the management of pancreatic walled-off necrosis: a prospective study. Endoscopy 2018;50:597–605.

40. Pawa R, Dorrell R, Russell G, et al. Long-term transmural drainage of pancreatic fluid collections with double pigtail stents following lumen-apposing metal stent placement improves recurrence-free survival in disconnected pancreatic duct syndrome. Dig Endosc 2022;34(6):1234–41.

41. Chavan R, Nabi Z, Lakhtakia S, et al. Impact of transmural plastic stent on recurrence of pancreatic fluid collection after metal stent removal in disconnected pancreatic duct: a randomized controlled trial. Endoscopy 2022;54(9):861–8.

42. Varadarajulu S, Wilcox CM. Endoscopic placement of permanent indwelling transmural stents in disconnected pancreatic duct syndrome: does benefit outweigh the risks? Gastrointest Endosc 2011;74(6):1408e12.
43. Gkolfakis P, Bourguignon A, Arvanitakia M, et al. Indwelling double-pigtail plastic stents for treating disconnected pancreatic duct syndrome-associated peri-pancreatic fluid collections: long-term safety and efficacy. Edoscopy 2021; 53(11):1141–9.
44. Irani S, Gluck M, Ross A, et al. Resolving external pancreatic fistulas in patients with disconnected pancreatic duct syndrome: using rendezvous techniques to avoid surgery Dwith video]. Gastrointest Endosc 2012;76D3:586–93.e1-3.
45. Will U, Fueldner F, Goldmann B, et al. Successful transgastric pancreaticography and endoscopic ultrasound-guided drainage of a disconnected pancreatic tail syndrome. Therap Adv Gastroenterol 2011;4(4):213–8.
46. Seewald S, Brand B, Groth S, et al. Endoscopic sealing of pancreatic fistula by using N-butyl-2-cyanoacrylate. Gastrointest Endosc 2004;59:463–70.
47. Tu J, Yang Y, Zhang J, et al. Effect of the disease severity on the risk of developing new-onset diabetes after acute pancreatitis. Medicine 2018;97:e10713.
48. Thiruvengadam NR, Forde KA, Miranda J, et al. Disconnected pancreatic duct syndrome: pancreatitis of the disconnected pancreas and its role in the development of diabetes mellitus. Clin Transl Gastroenterol 2022;13(2):e00457.
49. Chen Y, Jiang Y, Qian W, et al. Endoscopic transpapillary drainage in disconnected pancreatic duct syndrome after acute pancreatitis and trauma: long-term outcomes in 31 patients. BMC Gastroenterol 2019;19(1):54.
50. Tellez-Avina FI, Casasola-Sanchez LE, Ramirez-Luna MA, et al. Permanent indwelling transmural stents for endoscopic treatment of patients with disconnected pancreatic duct syndrome: long- term results. J Clin Gastroenterol 2018;52(1):85–90.

Postendoscopic Retrograde Cholangiopancreatography Pancreatitis Pathophysiology and Prevention

Venkata S. Akshintala, MD*, Vikesh K. Singh, MD, MSc

KEYWORDS

- ERCP • Complications • Pancreatitis • Prevention

KEY POINTS

- Careful patient selection is the most effective strategy to prevent post–endoscopic retrograde cholangiopancreatography (ERCP) pancreatitis (PEP), limiting ERCP exclusively as a therapeutic procedure.
- Understanding the patient and procedure-related risk factors for the development of PEP is necessary along with risk stratification to select the appropriate prophylaxis.
- Rectal nonsteroidal anti-inflammatory drugs and intravenous fluid should be considered in all patients undergoing ERCP.
- Prophylactic pancreatic duct stent placement should be considered in patients at high risk of developing PEP.

INTRODUCTION

Endoscopic retrograde cholangiopancreatography (ERCP) is performed to treat diseases of the pancreaticobiliary tract. Post-ERCP pancreatitis (PEP) is the most frequent complication of ERCP that occurs in 2% to 15% of cases and accounts for substantial morbidity, occasional mortality, and increased health-care expenditures.[1,2] PEP adds more than US$200 million annually to health-care costs in the United States and was found to be the most common reason for lawsuits related to ERCP.[3,4] There was a 15.3% increase in the rate of PEP admissions from 2011 to 2017 because ERCP is less frequently pursued for diagnostic indications and moved toward increasingly complex therapeutic indications.[5] Advances in our understanding of the pathophysiology of PEP, procedure technique, and patient selection along with improved PEP prophylaxis are expected to make the ERCP procedure safer and have been

Division of Gastroenterology, Johns Hopkins Medical Institutions, Baltimore, MD, USA
* Corresponding author. Johns Hopkins University School of Medicine, 600 North Wolfe Street, Blalock 411, Baltimore, MD 21205.
E-mail address: vakshin1@jhmi.edu

Gastrointest Endoscopy Clin N Am 33 (2023) 771–787
https://doi.org/10.1016/j.giec.2023.05.001
1052-5157/23/© 2023 Elsevier Inc. All rights reserved.

emphasized in the societal recommendations from the American Society for Gastrointestinal Endoscopy (ASGE) and the European Society of Gastrointestinal Endoscopy (ESGE).[3,6] In this article, we aim to present an evidence-based approach for the prevention of PEP and ongoing efforts to further reduce the incidence of PEP.

PATHOPHYSIOLOGY OF POST–ENDOSCOPIC RETROGRADE CHOLANGIOPANCREATOGRAPHY PANCREATITIS

The pathophysiology of PEP is poorly understood but numerous mechanisms have been hypothesized based on the injuries that occur during ERCP, including (1) mechanical injury to the papilla, pancreatic sphincter, and pancreatic duct (PD); (2) hydrostatic injury from injections; (3) chemical injury from contrast; (4) microbial injury from contamination by the gut flora; (5) thermal and electrical injury from electrosurgical current; and (6) neuronal injury.[7-10] Observations made to the risk factors for the development of PEP provided strength to these hypotheses and guided the development of PEP prophylaxis strategies. Animal models mimicking the true ERCP setting and the development of PEP are limited but the available models helped in identifying the inflammatory pathways involved, and therapeutic targets for prophylactic interventions.[11]

It is understood that the development of PEP is multifactorial and results in premature intrapancreatic activation of zymogens and downstream initiation of the inflammatory cascade.[12] One key pathway that has been well described to be causing PD outflow obstruction and activation of ductal trypsinogen is the edema in the papillary region.[12] Anatomical studies of the duodenal papilla and the ampullary region report the presence of onion skin-like pattern of numerous mucosal duplications within this space that are arranged as tongue-shaped flaps facing the papillary orifice (**Fig. 1**A).[13,14] Under these flaps are cul-de-sacs that along with the filamentous terminal septum can cause difficulty in cannulation due to the cannula or the guidewire being trapped within these spaces (**Fig. 1**B). Further, these mucosal flaps are highly vascularized and filled with seromucinous glands, and increase in the mucosal vasculature pressure, that is, edema in the mucosa, significantly increases the outflow pressure of the PD.[13] Established risk factors for PEP including difficult cannulation, pancreatic/precut sphincterotomy, among others are all suspected to cause peripapillary

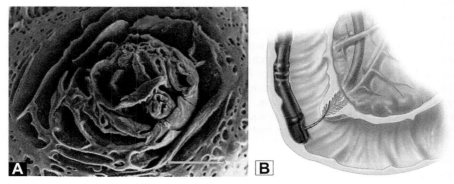

Fig. 1. (*A*) Electron microscopy view of the duodenal papilla demonstrating mucosal duplications within the ampulla. (*B*) Guidewire and sphincterotome trapped within the cul-de-sacs under the tongue-shaped mucosal flaps within the duodenal papilla or ampulla. ([*A*] *Adapted from* Paulsen FP, Bobka T, Tsokos M, Fölsch UR, Tillmann BN. Functional anatomy of the papilla Vateri: biomechanical aspects and impact of difficult endoscopic intubation. *Surg Endosc.* 2002;16(2):296-301; and [*B*] Illustration by Corinne Sandone © 2016 JHU AMM.)

edema and likely contributing to the development of PEP through this mechanism.[15,16] This also explains the difficult in cannulation of Type 3 or bulky protruding duodenal papillae, which are more densely filled by these mucosal flaps and was shown to increase the risk of PEP.[17,18]

Our understanding of these mechanistic features helped direct the PEP preventative strategies to address the difficulty in cannulation through improved techniques,[19,20] using pharmaceutic approaches to reduce papillary edema,[21,22] directly improve the PD flow using a stent, or alternatively through interventions that target the zymogen activation using protease inhibitors, downstream inflammatory pathways such as using nonsteroidal anti-inflammatory drugs (NSAIDs), calcineurin inhibitors, and intravenous fluids (IVFs).

DIAGNOSTIC CRITERIA FOR POST–ENDOSCOPIC RETROGRADE CHOLANGIOPANCREATOGRAPHY PANCREATITIS

A diagnosis of PEP and characterization of the severity is made either using Cotton's consensus criteria or the Atlanta criteria. Cotton's Consensus Criteria from 1991 defines PEP as new onset or increased upper abdominal pain, and pancreatic amylase (or lipase) elevation of 3 times greater than the upper limit of normal at 24 hours after ERCP and resulting hospitalization or prolongation of ongoing hospitalization of 2 or more nights.[23] The Atlanta classification of acute pancreatitis (AP) updated in 2012 defines PEP as the presence of 2 of the following 3 criteria: (1) abdominal pain consistent with AP (acute onset of a persistent, severe, epigastric pain often radiating to the back); (2) serum lipase (or amylase) level at least 3 times greater than the upper limit of normal; and (3) characteristic findings of AP on contrast-enhanced computed tomography or MRI or transabdominal ultrasonography.[24]

Although clinical trials reporting PEP have historically used varying definitions for the diagnosis of PEP, creating heterogeneity in reporting, the consensus criteria have become the most commonly used standard in the past 2 decades.[1] Smeets XJNM and colleagues,[25] comparing the consensus and the revised Atlanta criteria for defining PEP, found the revised Atlanta criteria to have a higher sensitivity (100% vs 55%), specificity (98% vs 72%), and positive predictive value (58% vs 5%). The revised Atlanta criteria were also found to be superior in characterizing the severity of PEP because the consensus criteria primarily rely on the length of hospitalization, which may be influenced by concomitant diseases.

Both these PEP definitions are, however, limited by the subjective nature of abdominal pain interpretation, varying practices of lipase or amylase checks, and routine hospitalizations following ERCP, which affect the diagnostic accuracy of PEP. This also introduces heterogeneity among the clinical studies reporting PEP, which mandates caution while interpreting these results. Further, it is also known that ERCP can cause abdominal pain without pancreatitis and lipase elevation may occur following ERCP due to mild irritation to the pancreas without full-blown activation of the inflammatory cascade.[26–28] All these factors affect the diagnostic accuracy of PEP and in the absence of a reliable biomarker for the diagnosis of PEP, cross-sectional imaging remains the gold standard. However, the radiation exposure and costs involved with cross-sectional imaging do not justify its routine use and a better diagnostic tool or biomarker that accurately diagnoses PEP especially early in the course of the disease is a need of the hour.

PATIENT SELECTION

Optimal patient selection and limiting the ERCP to when it is absolutely indicated is the best strategy to prevent PEP as recommended by societal guidelines.[3,6] There has been an increase in the utilization of ERCP in the past decade, and there was also a

15.3% increase in the PEP incidence from 2011 to 2017 within this period.[5,29,30] Choledocholithiasis remains the most common indication for the ERCP procedure but diagnostic ERCPs have been largely abandoned since the advent of magnetic resonance cholangiopancreatography (MRCP) and endoscopic ultrasound (EUS).[31–33] MRCP and EUS have also reduced the need for diagnostic ERCPs for the evaluation of PD pathologic conditions. ERCPs are appropriately and nearly exclusively currently being performed as therapeutic procedures and are becoming increasingly complex, which explains the increase in PEP incidence in the past decade. Interventional EUS also now provides an alternative to ERCP for biliary drainage in difficult-to-access anatomy and with obstructive pathologic conditions, potentially reducing the risk of PEP.[34,35] With improvement in EUS accessories such as the availability of steerable needles that makes the access to the ductal structures easier, safer will likely further reduce the risk of PEP.[36]

There, however, have continued to remain certain indications for the ERCP procedure where this is performed partly as a diagnostic procedure or as an "empiric trial" for therapeutic benefit. Sphincter of Oddi Dysfunction (SOD) is one such indication where an empiric sphincterotomy was performed when this was suspected to be causing the patient's symptoms. The evaluating predictors and interventions in sphincter of oddi sysfunction (EPISOD) trial has, however, conclusively proven the lack of benefit in performing a sphincterotomy for those with the formerly defined type 3 SOD, who are at an increased risk of developing PEP.[37] The results of this trial had a direct effect on the trends in the utilization of ERCP, with a sustained decrease in the rates of ERCP performed for SOD noted since 2013.[38] The utility of ERCP with empiric sphincterotomy for other similar conditions such as type 2 SOD and recurrent AP (pancreatic SOD) are still being studied.[39] A challenging feature among the pancreato-biliary pathologic conditions is differentiating between true ductal obstruction causing symptoms and ductal ectasia or benign dilation, and in this setting, ERCP with empiric stent placements are routinely performed as a trial monitoring for any change in patient's symptoms. These include certain posttransplant and chronic pancreatitis-related strictures, with highly variable clinical success rates ranging from 32% to 86%.[40] In recent years, considerable developments have been made in noninvasive pressure measurement technologies using ultrasound and computational fluid dynamics, reducing the need for diagnostic cardiovascular interventions.[41] Applications of these technologies in the pancreato-biliary space may help better identify the patients who will truly benefit from ERCP-based interventions and avoid diagnostic, empiric procedures, overall contributing to a reduction in PEP.

POST–ENDOSCOPIC RETROGRADE CHOLANGIOPANCREATOGRAPHY PANCREATITIS RISK STRATIFICATION

Risk factors: Understanding the factors contributing to an increase in the risk of PEP helps utilize the appropriate PEP prophylactic strategies and in modifying the procedure techniques to address these risk factors. Substantial research has been performed to recognize the patient and procedure-related risk factors for PEP, given this is the most common complication of the ERCP procedure (**Table 1**). ERCP procedures involving difficult or failed cannulation, guidewire cannulation, papillary, pancreatic sphincterotomy, precut sphincterotomy, PD brush cytology, pneumatic biliary dilation without biliary sphincterotomy, more than 2 PD guidewire passes, more than 2 PD contrast injections, pancreatic acinarization, and trainee involvement in the procedure have all been associated with an increased risk of developing PEP.[15,42–50] Patient-related risk factors have also been shown to increase the risk of PEP, such as female

Table 1
Patient and procedure related risk factors for the development of post-ERCP pancreatitis

Patient Related Risk Factors	Procedure Related Risk Factors
History of recurrent AP	Difficult cannulation
History of post-ERCP pancreatitis	Pancreatic or precut sphincterotomy
Suspected SOD	Multiple PD injections
Young age and female gender	Multiple PD guidewire passes
Chronic pancreatitis (protective)	Pancreatic acinarization
Pancreas head mass (protective)	Short-duration balloon dilation of an intact biliary
Earlier sphincterotomy (protective)	sphincter

gender, aged younger than 50 years, SOD, history of AP and history of PEP.[51,52] Primary sclerosing cholangitis was suspected to be an independent risk factor for PEP but larger studies did not identify this effect.[53] Patients with chronic calcified pancreatitis with severe pancreatic fibrosis and glandular atrophy, and those with pancreas head cancer have reduced acinar cell mass and were found to have reduced risk for the development of PEP.[49] Similarly, patients with earlier sphincterotomy will help reduce the risk of accidental PD cannulation and the risk of PEP. Heterogeneity among the studies defining these risk factors, limited sample size, and the observational nature of some of these studies limit the interpretation of the data pertaining to the PEP risk factors. However, the majority of the risk factors described here have consistently shown to be relevant and have been incorporated into ERCP quality reporting to improve the performance, and safety of the ERCP procedure.[54]

Risk Stratification Methods

Given the large number of risk factors for PEP that have a synergistic effect, and with varying importance to the overall PEP risk, it is challenging in a clinical situation to precisely determine a patient's risk for PEP. Several prognostic scoring systems have, therefore, been developed to stratify patients based on their risk of developing PEP, primarily using multivariable linear regression models, although none is in widespread clinical use or endorsed by professional society guidelines.[55-60] These have, however, been limited due to the use of retrospective and nonrandomized data, incorporation of a small number of risk factors, and limited ability to account for the interaction between risk factors.[56-58] Further, the previously described models were unable to predict risk reduction associated with PEP prophylaxis strategies such as rectal NSAIDs, aggressive hydration, or prophylactic PD stenting.[61] There, however, has been some promise in this regard, with the utilization of data from randomized controlled trials (RCTs) and the application of novel machine learning-based statistical techniques.[62] Web-based and other applications that can be integrated into the electronic medical records systems are being developed that will provide a real-time estimation of the PEP risk and will help in selecting the prophylactic strategy, and appropriate utilization of the resources.[58]

A priori understanding of the patient's risk profile based on the patient-related PEP risk factors will help in case selection, discussing the risks of the procedure with the patient and even with referral to a tertiary care center as applicable. Intraoperative PEP risk assessment based on the patient and procedure-related PEP risk factors will help identify patients who require prophylactic PD stent placement, which may be reserved for those who are at higher risk of PEP, due to the cost and technical challenges that are involved with PD stent. Similarly, NSAIDs may be reserved for those with moderate to high risk of PEP, avoiding those with low risk of PEP, especially considering the cost of rectal NSAIDs in countries such as the United States (see later discussion).[63] Practices pertaining to the postprocedure observation are highly variable across centers, with some centers admitting every patient, even after an uneventful elective ERCP procedure; however, this is cost prohibitive in most settings. Patients at the highest risk of developing PEP or those developing early signs of PEP during the immediate postoperative period may be considered to be admitted for observation or management. Lipase elevation more than 3 times the upper limit of normal within 2 to 4 hours of the ERCP procedure may be a useful biomarker to identify patients who may eventually develop PEP and would benefit from an inpatient admission but this requires large-scale prospective validation.[64] Other inflammatory biomarkers such as interleukin (IL)-6, IL-10, and tumor necrosis factor α did not however improve the early detection of PEP.[65] Further research using the biorepositories of ongoing large-scale PEP-related studies is needed to help identify biomarkers for risk stratification and early detection of PEP that may help appropriate patient, prophylaxis selection, and consideration for admission for observation after the ERCP procedure.

ENDOSCOPIC RETROGRADE CHOLANGIOPANCREATOGRAPHY PROCEDURE

Awareness of the pathophysiology and the risk factors for the development of PEP helps refining the ERCP procedure technique to reduce the risk of PEP. Below are some technical considerations for the appropriate selection of methods and technologies during the ERCP procedure.

Adverse events related to ERCP such as PEP are often reflectors of the quality of the procedure performed, including the appropriate patient selection, techniques used, recognition of the factors leading to the adverse events, and approaches applied to reduce these adverse events. ERCP has a steep learning curve, is technically demanding, and requires adequate training in the relevant cognitive aspects described above to reduce the risk of adverse events. Societal recommendations have heavily emphasized the importance of having well-defined and validated competency thresholds during training evaluations to ensure competency in performing the ERCP procedure.[66] In addition, transparent reporting and auditing of the quality indicators were shown to reduce the risk of procedural complications.[67,68] Standardized quality report cards have been developed for the ERCP procedure, and at our institution, we use an automated system that captures the quality metrics related to ERCP for each endoscopist.[69,70]

As previously described, papillary edema resulting in an increase in the PD pressure is suspected to be a key pathophysiological mechanism for the development of PEP. Difficult cannulation causing trauma to the duodenal papilla is one such aspect increasing the risk of PEP and is often due to an inadequate understanding of the anatomy of the papilla, including the papillary projections within (see **Fig. 1**). Maneuvering the ERCP catheter or other instruments using an appropriate technique such as the compact disc method described by Takenaka and colleagues,[19] address these anatomical aspects of the papilla, with selective biliary cannulation and reducing the risk of trauma to the PD. In the setting of difficult cannulation when initial cannulation attempts are unsuccessful, alternate techniques such as double-wire cannulation, needle-knife fistulotomy, transpancreatic septotomy, and precut sphincterotomy should be considered.[71] Although these maneuvers were suspected to be increasing the risk of PEP, it is now established that it is the preceding difficult cannulation, papillary edema that truly increases the PEP risk and each additional minute spent attempting cannulation increased the odds ratio (OR) for PEP by 1.072.[72] Early use of precut sphincterotomy is one such example to validate this hypothesis because it was found to reduce the risk of PEP when compared with late precut after repeated papillary cannulation attempts.[20] Adequate training in such alternate cannulation techniques and recognition of the point to switch to these, typically after 5 to 10 minutes of standard cannulation, along with the use of intense PEP prophylactic strategies should be considered. Use of blended over pure-cut current and iso-osmolar over hyperosmolar contrast agents have been recognized to be the safer options and become the standard of care.[73,74]

Historically, contrast-assisted cannulation involving the engagement of a cannula into the papilla followed by injection of contrast in the direction of the desired duct has been the standard cannulation technique. During the past several years, guidewire-assisted cannulation into the desired duct without the aid of contrast injection has become the most widely practiced technique with higher cannulation success rates and found to be safer.[75] However, Freeman and colleagues[76] noted that 1 or more deep guidewire passes into the PD significantly increased PEP risk and also when the pancreatic guidewire is manipulated during stent placement attempts or if stent placement is unsuccessful. We made a similar observation in an RCT, with the PEP risk increasing when there were more than 2 guidewire passes into the PD and the PEP risk increasing with an increasing number of guidewire passes into the PD, or when pancreatic brush cytology was performed.[77] This suggests an important effect of the trauma from guidewire or ERCP accessories in the PD or its side branches in the etiopathogenesis of PEP (**Fig. 2**). We also found that 13.7% of patients with more than 2 guidewire passes into the PD developed PEP despite receiving rectal indomethacin. This suggests that these patients and will need additional PEP prophylaxis, and it seems logical to place a PD stent when the guidewire is inserted into the PD as recommended by the ESGE guidelines.[78] Double guidewire is another common alternate technique to achieve biliary cannulation in the setting of repeat unintentional passage of the guidewire into the PD, where the guidewire is left in the PD to straighten the common channel and repeat the biliary cannulation attempts. Use of PD stent similarly in this context was also found to reduce the risk of PEP while increasing the cannulation success.[79]

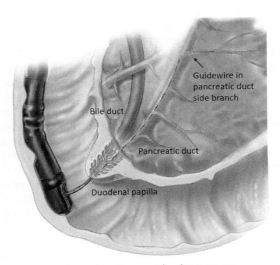

Fig. 2. Trauma to the PD side branches from guidewire passage.

In patients with large bile duct stones, mechanical lithotripsy may be required, which increases the risk of PEP.[50] Endoscopic papillary large balloon dilation (EPLBD) is an alternative that involves focal dilation of the biliary sphincter with or without preceding sphincterotomy.[80] Biliary sphincterotomy in this setting causes "controlled disruption" of the biliary sphincter and less papillary edema, and is the preferred approach.[81] ASGE and ESGE guidelines recommend using EPLBD combined with limited sphincterotomy as the first-line approach for large bile duct stones.[82,83]

POSTENDOSCOPIC RETROGRADE CHOLANGIOPANCREATOGRAPHY PANCREATITIS PROPHYLAXIS

Numerous prophylactic agents for PEP prophylaxis have been investigated in RCTs since 1977.[84] However, the strongest evidence is in favor of rectal NSAIDs,[85] high-volume IVF administration,[86,87] and PD stent placement-based prophylaxes.[88] More recently, the role of combinations of these prophylaxes has been with cumulative additive benefit has been recognized but few head-to-head RCTs exist.[61] ESGE guidelines recommend the routine use of rectal NSAIDs for all patients, PD stent for those deemed high risk, and IVF for those unable to receive rectal NSAIDs.[78] The recently revised ASGE guidelines similarly recommend the use of rectal NSAIDs for all patients, along with aggressive periprocedural and postprocedural IVF while limiting PD stent use for those identified to be at high risk for developing PEP.[6]

Nonsteroidal Anti-inflammatory Drugs

Although it is well established that PEP is a result of uncontrolled activation of the inflammatory cascade following injury related to the PEP procedure, less is known regarding the key inflammatory mediators involved. Cyclooxygenase-2 is one such proinflammatory mediator that has been implicated and animal models with pharmacologic inhibition or selective genetic deletion reduced the severity of pancreatitis.[89] Numerous clinical trials have been performed evaluating the efficacy of NSAIDs for PEP prevention and a recent comprehensive review and network meta-analysis (NMA) has identified at least 11 different NSAID regimens using diclofenac, indomethacin, celecoxib, naproxen, or ketoprofen in various doses and routes of delivery (**Fig. 3**).[61] There was heterogeneity in the results due to differences in patient population, along with the type, route, and dose of NSAIDs used. Another source of heterogeneity is likely the polymorphisms in cytochrome P450 2C9 enzyme levels that are involved in the metabolism of NSAIDs.[90] However, the overall rectal route for the delivery of NSAIDs was identified to be superior to the oral route. This is likely to better bioavailability of NSAIDs when delivered through the rectal route that avoids the first-pass metabolism in the liver and with only 50% to 60% of the drug reaching systemic circulation when delivered orally.[91] Pharmacokinetic studies demonstrated a sustained availability of peak concentration of indomethacin when delivered rectally, compared with intravascular and intramuscular administration.[92]

Within the United States (US), rectal indomethacin became widely used as prophylaxis following the publication of a landmark clinical trial in 2012.[93,94] Rectal indomethacin was found to be effective and reduced the PEP risk by approximately 50%.[93] Given the expenditures involved and implications of PEP, all prophylactic strategies including rectal indomethacin use were found to be cost-effective for PEP prophylaxis.[95] However, there has been an exorbitant increase in the cost of rectal indomethacin in the US (from US$2 in 2005 to US$340 for 100 mg in

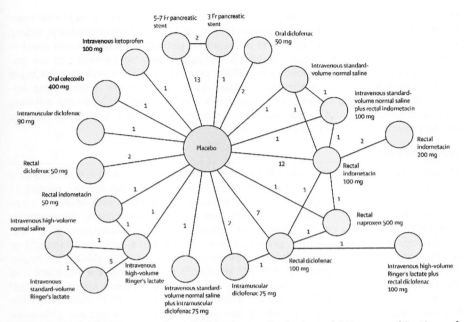

Fig. 3. Network of RCTs comparing NSAIDs, pancreatic stents, and IVFs, or combinations of these. (Reprinted with permission from Elsevier. The Lancet Gastroenterol Hepatol 2021;6(9):733-742.)

2021).[63] This price increase adds a burden to the health-care system and often results in out-of-pocket charges to the patient. Other NSAIDs or alternative agents have been explored to be used in lieu of rectal indomethacin. There were at least 15 RCTs that evaluated rectal indomethacin 100 mg while another 9 RCTs evaluated rectal diclofenac 100 mg. Interestingly, rectal diclofenac 100 mg was found to be more efficacious than rectal indomethacin 100 mg (OR 0.59; 95% CI: 0.40–0.89) or at least as effective.[61] Two recent RCTs attempted to increase the total dose of rectal indomethacin administered to 200 mg but did not find this strategy to be superior to 100 mg of rectal indomethacin.[61]

Intravenous Fluid

The use of intravenous fluid remains the central therapy in the management of AP and for PEP prophylaxis IVF plays an essential role in potentially limiting the inflammation generated in the pancreas following the ERCP procedure. Lactated ringer (LR) was especially found to be superior to normal saline in this setting, potentially due to the anti-inflammatory effect of lactate through immunomodulatory mechanisms and the effect of lactate on the acidosis being developed in the setting of AP.[96] In a recent NMA, we found aggressive hydration with LR or NS to be more efficacious for PEP prophylaxis compared with placebo or standard volume hydration.[61] Various regimens for IVF have been considered in these RCTs, which differed based on the practice of admitting the patient for observations following the ERCP procedure. In one recent RCT, an aggressive hydration for 8 hours following the ERCP was not found to be superior to a moderate hydration.[97] Prolonged duration of aggressive hydration was also shown to increase the risk of fluid overload and third spacing of fluid.[98] Optimal regimen for hydration is yet to be identified but may be reasonable to consider 2 to 3L of LR in the periprocedural setting for all patients undergoing ERCP and adjusted for patients with associated renal or cardiopulmonary comorbidities. Additional hydration may be provided to the patients admitted with pain following the ERCP procedure while monitoring for signs of fluid overload. About combinations of IVF and NSAIDs, there is conflicting evidence on the additive benefits of using these combinations.[97] Given the differing mechanisms of action, it is plausible that a combination of IVF and rectal NSAIDs would provide cumulative additive benefit.

Pancreatic Duct Stent

Prophylactic PD stent placement is expected to improve the ductal flow, avoiding ductal hypertension in the setting of papillary edema and other factors related to PEP pathogenesis described previously. Multiple RCTs and meta-analyses have consistently shown PD stents to be effective for PEP prophylaxis, especially in reducing the severity of PEP and other associated PEP consequences.[61,99] PD stents vary in diameter, length, presence of internal flanges, and type (straight or single pigtail). NMAs have compared various dimensions of PD stents and found 5-Fr PD stents to be superior to 3-Fr PD stents.[100] The length of the PD stent and the duration for which the PD stent has to remain, which is most suitable for PEP prophylaxis is not known.[100] Although some reported lower PEP rates when the PD stent reached the body or tail of the pancreas, others did not find any difference among various lengths of PD stents used.[88,101] PD stents however have several disadvantages given the costs and inconveniences involved in follow-up imaging and repeat endoscopy for stent removal, which is required in 5% to 10% of the procedures.[102,103] Further, PD stent placement is often technically challenging and additional attempts to cannulate the PD only to place the PD stent may further increase the PEP risk.[104] However, in the settings where a guidewire has already entered the PD, especially with multiple guidewire passes into the PD, the placement of a PD stent is likely to provide a clear benefit with PEP prophylaxis. Pharmacoprophylaxis has several advantages over PD stents due to the reasons described above, and about combination regimens, the indirect comparison did not identify a significant difference between the use of a 5 to 7-Fr PD stent and a combination of IVF and rectal NSAIDs.[61] This however needs to be answered with a prospective RCT, if a combination of NSAIDs and IVF can be used in lieu of PD stent, and is the topic of a large ongoing RCT that is awaiting results.[105] Currently, societal guideline recommendations remain to use PD stents for patients at high risk of developing PEP.[6,78]

A multitude of other PEP prophylactic strategies has been explored, including more than 40 different pharmaco-prophylactic agents with only a few demonstrating consistently promising results.[84] However, recent studies using animal models have identified potential new mediators involved in PEP pathogenesis such as calcium-dependent serine, threonine phosphatase calcineurin (Cn) and Cn inhibitors such as tacrolimus are being considered for PEP prophylaxis.[11,106] In conclusion, the incidence of PEP remains high despite our improvement in understanding of PEP pathophysiology and prophylactic strategies being available. Future research should continue to focus on identifying better PEP prophylaxis, especially pharmacological, refine procedural techniques, and improve risk stratification approaches, with a personalized prophylactic strategy for each patient. The primary approach to PEP prevention should be through careful patient selection, appropriate ERCP technique, and the use of recommended PEP prophylaxis.

CLINICS CARE POINTS

- When considering an ERCP procedure, ensure there is an appropriate indication that is exclusively therapeutic.
- Review the patient and procedure-related risk factors for the development of post-ERCP pancreatitis, to select the appropriate prophylaxis.
- Consider rectal NSAIDs, intravenous fluid in all patients undergoing ERCP, and PD stent among high-risk patients.

DISCLOSURE

The authors have no disclosures relevant to this publication.

REFERENCES

1. Kochar B, Akshintala VS, Afghani E, et al. Incidence, severity, and mortality of post-ERCP pancreatitis: a systematic review by using randomized, controlled trials. Gastrointest Endosc 2015;81:143–149 e9.
2. Akshintala VS, Kanthasamy K, Bhullar FA, et al. Incidence, severity and mortality of post ERCP pancreatitis: an updated systematic review and meta-analysis of 145 randomized controlled trials. Gastrointest Endosc 2023. https://doi.org/10.1016/j.gie.2023.03.023.
3. Dumonceau JM, Kapral C, Aabakken L, et al. ERCP-related adverse events: European Society of Gastrointestinal Endoscopy (ESGE) Guideline. Endoscopy 2020;52:127–49.
4. Cotton PB. Analysis of 59 ERCP lawsuits; mainly about indications. Gastrointest Endosc 2006;63:378–82 [quiz: 464].
5. Mutneja HR, Vohra I, Go A, et al. Temporal trends and mortality of post-ERCP pancreatitis in the United States: a nationwide analysis. Endoscopy 2020.
6. Buxbaum JL, Freeman M, Amateau SK, et al. American society for gastrointestinal endoscopy guideline on post-ERCP pancreatitis prevention strategies: summary and recommendations. Gastrointest Endosc 2023;97:153–62.
7. Freeman ML, Guda NM. Prevention of post-ERCP pancreatitis: a comprehensive review. Gastrointest Endosc 2004;59:845–64.
8. Pezzilli R, Romboli E, Campana D, et al. Mechanisms involved in the onset of post-ERCP pancreatitis. JOP 2002;3:162–8.
9. Akashi R, Kiyozumi T, Tanaka T, et al. Mechanism of pancreatitis caused by ERCP. Gastrointest Endosc 2002;55:50–4.
10. Li C, Zhu Y, Shenoy M, et al. Anatomical and functional characterization of a duodeno-pancreatic neural reflex that can induce acute pancreatitis. Am J Physiol Gastrointest Liver Physiol 2013;304:G490–500.
11. Wen L, Javed TA, Yimlamai D, et al. Transient high pressure in pancreatic ducts promotes inflammation and alters tight junctions via calcineurin signaling in mice. Gastroenterology 2018;155:1250–1263 e5.
12. Rinderknecht H. Activation of pancreatic zymogens. Normal activation, premature intrapancreatic activation, protective mechanisms against inappropriate activation. Dig Dis Sci 1986;31:314–21.
13. Paulsen FP, Bobka T, Tsokos M, et al. Functional anatomy of the papilla Vateri: biomechanical aspects and impact of difficult endoscopic intubation. Surg Endosc 2002;16:296–301.

14. Brown JO, Echenberg RJ. Mucosal reduplications associated with the ampullary portion of the major duodenal papilla in humans. Anat Rec 1964;150:293–301.

15. Cheng CL, Sherman S, Watkins JL, et al. Risk factors for post-ERCP pancreatitis: a prospective multicenter study. Am J Gastroenterol 2006;101:139–47.

16. Wang P, Li ZS, Liu F, et al. Risk factors for ERCP-related complications: a prospective multicenter study. Am J Gastroenterol 2009;104:31–40.

17. Haraldsson E, Kylanpaa L, Gronroos J, et al. Macroscopic appearance of the major duodenal papilla influences bile duct cannulation: a prospective multicenter study by the Scandinavian Association for Digestive Endoscopy Study Group for ERCP. Gastrointest Endosc 2019;90:957–63.

18. Mohamed R, Lethebe BC, Gonzalez-Moreno E, et al. Morphology of the major papilla predicts ERCP procedural outcomes and adverse events. Surg Endosc 2021;35:6455–65.

19. Takenaka M, Yoshikawa T, Minaga K, et al. A novel teaching tool for visualizing the invisible bile duct axis in 3 dimensions during biliary cannulation (Compact Disc method). VideoGIE 2020;5:389–94.

20. Mariani A, Di Leo M, Giardullo N, et al. Early precut sphincterotomy for difficult biliary access to reduce post-ERCP pancreatitis: a randomized trial. Endoscopy 2016;48:530–5.

21. Ohno T, Katori M, Nishiyama K, et al. Direct observation of microcirculation of the basal region of rat gastric mucosa. J Gastroenterol 1995;30:557–64.

22. Igawa M, Miyaoka M, Saitoh T. Influence of topical epinephrine application on microcirculatory disturbance in subjects with ulcerative colitis evaluated by laser doppler flowmetry and transmission electron microscopy. Dig Endosc 2000;12:126–30.

23. Cotton PB, Lehman G, Vennes J, et al. Endoscopic sphincterotomy complications and their management: an attempt at consensus. Gastrointest Endosc 1991;37:383–93.

24. Banks PA, Bollen TL, Dervenis C, et al. Classification of acute pancreatitis–2012: revision of the Atlanta classification and definitions by international consensus. Gut 2013;62:102–11.

25. Smeets X, Bouhouch N, Buxbaum J, et al. The revised Atlanta criteria more accurately reflect severity of post-ERCP pancreatitis compared to the consensus criteria. United European Gastroenterol J 2019;7:557–64.

26. Hameed AM, Lam VW, Pleass HC. Significant elevations of serum lipase not caused by pancreatitis: a systematic review. HPB (Oxford) 2015;17:99–112.

27. Prat F, Amaris J, Ducot B, et al. Nifedipine for prevention of post-ERCP pancreatitis: a prospective, double-blind randomized study. Gastrointest Endosc 2002;56:202–8.

28. Shah R, Raphael KL, Mekaroonkamol P, et al. Non-pancreatitis-Related Abdominal Pain Following ERCP in Patients With Pancreas Divisum: 91. Official Journal of the American College of Gastroenterology | ACG 2017;112:S42–4.

29. Coelho-Prabhu N, Shah ND, Van Houten H, et al. Endoscopic retrograde cholangiopancreatography: utilisation and outcomes in a 10-year population-based cohort. BMJ Open 2013;3:e002689.

30. Kroner PT, Bilal M, Samuel R, et al. Use of ERCP in the United States over the past decade. Endosc Int Open 2020;8:E761–9.

31. Moffatt DC, Yu BN, Yie W, et al. Trends in utilization of diagnostic and therapeutic ERCP and cholecystectomy over the past 25 years: a population-based study. Gastrointest Endosc 2014;79:615–22.

32. Huang RJ, Thosani NC, Barakat MT, et al. Evolution in the utilization of biliary interventions in the United States: results of a nationwide longitudinal study from 1998 to 2013. Gastrointest Endosc 2017;86:319–326 e5.

33. Ahmed M, Kanotra R, Savani GT, et al. Utilization trends in inpatient endoscopic retrograde cholangiopancreatography (ERCP): A cross-sectional US experience. Endosc Int Open 2017;5:E261–71.

34. Kakked G, Salameh H, Cheesman AR, et al. Primary EUS-guided biliary drainage versus ERCP drainage for the management of malignant biliary obstruction: a systematic review and meta-analysis. Endosc Ultrasound 2020; 9:298–307.

35. Logiudice FP, Bernardo WM, Galetti F, et al. Endoscopic ultrasound-guided vs endoscopic retrograde cholangiopancreatography biliary drainage for obstructed distal malignant biliary strictures: a systematic review and meta-analysis. World J Gastrointest Endosc 2019;11:281–91.

36. Lakhtakia S, Chavan R, Ramchandani M, et al. EUS-guided rendezvous with a steerable access needle in choledocholithiasis. VideoGIE 2020;5:359–61.

37. Cotton PB, Durkalski V, Romagnuolo J, et al. Effect of endoscopic sphincterotomy for suspected sphincter of Oddi dysfunction on pain-related disability following cholecystectomy: the EPISOD randomized clinical trial. JAMA 2014; 311:2101–9.

38. Smith ZL, Shah R, Elmunzer BJ, et al. The Next EPISOD: trends in utilization of endoscopic sphincterotomy for sphincter of oddi dysfunction from 2010-2019. Clin Gastroenterol Hepatol 2022;20:e600–9.

39. Cote GA, Durkalski-Mauldin VL, Serrano J, et al. SpHincterotomy for acute recurrent pancreatitis randomized trial: rationale, methodology, and potential implications. Pancreas 2019;48:1061–7.

40. Dumonceau JM, Delhaye M, Tringali A, et al. Endoscopic treatment of chronic pancreatitis: European Society of Gastrointestinal Endoscopy (ESGE) guideline - updated August 2018. Endoscopy 2019;51:179–93.

41. Min JK, Taylor CA, Achenbach S, et al. Noninvasive fractional flow reserve derived from coronary CT angiography: clinical data and scientific principles. JACC Cardiovasc Imaging 2015;8:1209–22.

42. Vandervoort J, Soetikno RM, Tham TC, et al. Risk factors for complications after performance of ERCP. Gastrointest Endosc 2002;56:652–6.

43. Rabenstein T, Schneider HT, Bulling D, et al. Analysis of the risk factors associated with endoscopic sphincterotomy techniques: preliminary results of a prospective study, with emphasis on the reduced risk of acute pancreatitis with low-dose anticoagulation treatment. Endoscopy 2000;32:10–9.

44. Christoforidis E, Goulimaris I, Kanellos I, et al. Post-ERCP pancreatitis and hyperamylasemia: patient-related and operative risk factors. Endoscopy 2002; 34:286–92.

45. Hookey LC, RioTinto R, Delhaye M, et al. Risk factors for pancreatitis after pancreatic sphincterotomy: a review of 572 cases. Endoscopy 2006;38:670–6.

46. Boender J, Nix GA, de Ridder MA, et al. Endoscopic papillotomy for common bile duct stones: factors influencing the complication rate. Endoscopy 1994; 26:209–16.

47. Christensen M, Matzen P, Schulze S, et al. Complications of ERCP: a prospective study. Gastrointest Endosc 2004;60:721–31.

48. Masci E, Toti G, Mariani A, et al. Complications of diagnostic and therapeutic ERCP: a prospective multicenter study. Am J Gastroenterol 2001;96:417–23.

49. Freeman ML, DiSario JA, Nelson DB, et al. Risk factors for post-ERCP pancreatitis: a prospective, multicenter study. Gastrointest Endosc 2001;54:425–34.

50. Freeman ML. Complications of endoscopic sphincterotomy. Endoscopy 1998; 30:A216–20.

51. Chen JJ, Wang XM, Liu XQ, et al. Risk factors for post-ERCP pancreatitis: a systematic review of clinical trials with a large sample size in the past 10 years. Eur J Med Res 2014;19:26.

52. Ding X, Zhang F, Wang Y. Risk factors for post-ERCP pancreatitis: a systematic review and meta-analysis. Surgeon 2015;13:218–29.

53. Natt N, Michael F, Michael H, et al. ERCP-related adverse events in primary sclerosing cholangitis: a systematic review and meta-analysis. Chin J Gastroenterol Hepatol 2022;2022:2372257.

54. Keswani RN, Duloy A, Nieto JM, et al. Interventions to improve the performance of ERCP and EUS quality indicators. Gastrointest Endosc 2023;97(5):825–38.

55. Friedland S, Soetikno RM, Vandervoort J, et al. Bedside scoring system to predict the risk of developing pancreatitis following ERCP. Endoscopy 2002;34: 483–8.

56. Park CH, Park SW, Yang MJ, et al. Pre- and post-procedure risk prediction models for post-endoscopic retrograde cholangiopancreatography pancreatitis. Surg Endosc 2021.

57. Chiba M, Kato M, Kinoshita Y, et al. The milestone for preventing post-ERCP pancreatitis using novel simplified predictive scoring system: a propensity score analysis. Surg Endosc 2020.

58. Rodrigues-Pinto E, Morais R, Sousa-Pinto B, et al. Development of an online app to predict post-endoscopic retrograde cholangiopancreatography adverse events using a single-center retrospective cohort. Dig Dis 2021;39:283–93.

59. Development and validation of a risk stratification score for post-endoscopic retrograde cholangiopancreatography (ERCP) pancreatitis Kamal A., Akshintala V.S., Elmunzer B.J., Lehman G.A., et al. Gastrointestinal Endoscopy 2018 87:6 Supplement 1 (AB573-).

60. Rex DK, Schoenfeld PS, Cohen J, et al. Quality indicators for colonoscopy. Gastrointest Endosc 2015;81:31–53.

61. Akshintala VS, Sperna Weiland CJ, Bhullar FA, et al. Non-steroidal anti-inflammatory drugs, intravenous fluids, pancreatic stents, or their combinations for the prevention of post-endoscopic retrograde cholangiopancreatography pancreatitis: a systematic review and network meta-analysis. Lancet Gastroenterol Hepatol 2021;6(9):733–42.

62. Akshintala VS, Kuo A, Kamal A, et al. Development, validation of a post-ERCP pancreatitis risk calculator and machine learning based decision making tool for prophylaxis selection. Gastroenterology 2019;156:S-116.

63. McKee K, Singh VK, Akshintala VS. Rectal nonsteroidal anti-inflammatory drugs for post-endoscopic retrograde cholangiopancreatography pancreatitis prophylaxis: a case study in a price-escalation era. Gastroenterology 2022;163:543–6.

64. Goyal H, Sachdeva S, Sherazi SAA, et al. Early prediction of post-ERCP pancreatitis by post-procedure amylase and lipase levels: a systematic review and meta-analysis. Endosc Int Open 2022;10:E952–70.

65. Concepcion-Martin M, Gomez-Oliva C, Juanes A, et al. IL-6, IL-10 and TNFalpha do not improve early detection of post-endoscopic retrograde cholangiopancreatography acute pancreatitis: a prospective cohort study. Sci Rep 2016;6:33492.

66. Wani S, Hall M, Wang AY, et al. Variation in learning curves and competence for ERCP among advanced endoscopy trainees by using cumulative sum analysis. Gastrointest Endosc 2016;83:711–719 e11.

67. Adler DG, Lieb JG 2nd, Cohen J, et al. Quality indicators for ERCP. Gastrointest Endosc 2015;81:54–66.

68. Shao H, Fonseca V, Furman R, et al. Impact of quality improvement (QI) program on 5-year risk of diabetes-related complications: a simulation Study. Diabetes Care 2020;43:2847–52.

69. Cote GA, Elmunzer BJ, Forster E, et al. Development of an automated ERCP quality report card using structured data fields. Tech Innov Gastrointest Endosc 2021;23:129–38.

70. Singh A, Brenner TA, Bujnak B, et al. Development of an automated real-time ercp quality report card. Gastrointest Endosc 2022;95:AB100–1.

71. Elmunzer BJ. Reducing the risk of post-endoscopic retrograde cholangiopancreatography pancreatitis. Dig Endosc 2017;29:749–57.

72. Canena J, Lopes L, Fernandes J, et al. Efficacy and safety of primary, early and late needle-knife fistulotomy for biliary access. Sci Rep 2021;11:16658.

73. Verma D, Kapadia A, Adler DG. Pure versus mixed electrosurgical current for endoscopic biliary sphincterotomy: a meta-analysis of adverse outcomes. Gastrointest Endosc 2007;66:283–90.

74. Ogura T, Imoto A, Okuda A, et al. Can iodixanol prevent post-endoscopic retrograde cholangiopancreatography pancreatitis? A prospective, randomized, controlled trial. Dig Dis 2019;37:255–61.

75. Tse F, Liu J, Yuan Y, et al. Guidewire-assisted cannulation of the common bile duct for the prevention of post-endoscopic retrograde cholangiopancreatography (ERCP) pancreatitis. Cochrane Database Syst Rev 2022;3(3):CD009662.

76. Freeman ML, Overby C, Qi D. Pancreatic stent insertion: consequences of failure and results of a modified technique to maximize success. Gastrointest Endosc 2004;59:8–14.

77. Kamal A, Akshintala VS, Talukdar R, et al. A randomized trial of topical epinephrine and rectal indomethacin for preventing post-endoscopic retrograde cholangiopancreatography pancreatitis in high-risk patients. Am J Gastroenterol 2019; 114:339–47.

78. Dumonceau JM, Andriulli A, Elmunzer BJ, et al. Prophylaxis of post-ERCP pancreatitis: European Society of Gastrointestinal Endoscopy (ESGE) Guideline - updated June 2014. Endoscopy 2014;46:799–815.

79. Ito K, Fujita N, Noda Y, et al. Can pancreatic duct stenting prevent post-ERCP pancreatitis in patients who undergo pancreatic duct guidewire placement for achieving selective biliary cannulation? A prospective randomized controlled trial. J Gastroenterol 2010;45:1183–91.

80. Draganov PV, Evans W, Fazel A, et al. Large size balloon dilation of the ampulla after biliary sphincterotomy can facilitate endoscopic extraction of difficult bile duct stones. J Clin Gastroenterol 2009;43:782–6.

81. Attasaranya S, Cheon YK, Vittal H, et al. Large-diameter biliary orifice balloon dilation to aid in endoscopic bile duct stone removal: a multicenter series. Gastrointest Endosc 2008;67:1046–52.

82. Committee ASoP, Buxbaum JL, Abbas Fehmi SM, et al. ASGE guideline on the role of endoscopy in the evaluation and management of choledocholithiasis. Gastrointest Endosc 2019;89:1075–1105 e15.

83. Manes G, Paspatis G, Aabakken L, et al. Endoscopic management of common bile duct stones: European Society of Gastrointestinal Endoscopy (ESGE) guideline. Endoscopy 2019;51:472–91.
84. Akshintala VS, Hutfless SM, Colantuoni E, et al. Systematic review with network meta-analysis: pharmacological prophylaxis against post-ERCP pancreatitis. Aliment Pharmacol Ther 2013;38:1325–37.
85. Serrano JPR, de Moura DTH, Bernardo WM, et al. Nonsteroidal anti-inflammatory drugs versus placebo for post-endoscopic retrograde cholangiopancreatography pancreatitis: a systematic review and meta-analysis. Endosc Int Open 2019;7:E477–86.
86. Choi JH, Kim HJ, Lee BU, et al. Vigorous periprocedural hydration with lactated ringer's solution reduces the risk of pancreatitis after retrograde cholangiopancreatography in hospitalized patients. Clin Gastroenterol Hepatol 2017;15:86–92 e1.
87. Park CH, Paik WH, Park ET, et al. Aggressive intravenous hydration with lactated Ringer's solution for prevention of post-ERCP pancreatitis: a prospective randomized multicenter clinical trial. Endoscopy 2018;50:378–85.
88. Phillip V, Pukitis A, Epstein A, et al. Pancreatic stenting to prevent post-ERCP pancreatitis: a randomized multicenter trial. Endosc Int Open 2019;7:E860–8.
89. Ethridge RT, Chung DH, Slogoff M, et al. Cyclooxygenase-2 gene disruption attenuates the severity of acute pancreatitis and pancreatitis-associated lung injury. Gastroenterology 2002;123:1311–22.
90. Bruno A, Tacconelli S, Patrignani P. Variability in the response to non-steroidal anti-inflammatory drugs: mechanisms and perspectives. Basic Clin Pharmacol Toxicol 2014;114:56–63.
91. Willis JV, Kendall MJ, Flinn RM, et al. The pharmacokinetics of diclofenac sodium following intravenous and oral administration. Eur J Clin Pharmacol 1979;16:405–10.
92. Jensen KM, Grenabo L. Bioavailability of indomethacin after intramuscular injection and rectal administration of solution and suppositories. Acta Pharmacol Toxicol 1985;57:322–7.
93. Elmunzer BJ, Scheiman JM, Lehman GA, et al. A randomized trial of rectal indomethacin to prevent post-ERCP pancreatitis. N Engl J Med 2012;366:1414–22.
94. Avila P, Holmes I, Kouanda A, et al. Practice patterns of post-ERCP pancreatitis prophylaxis techniques in the United States: a survey of advanced endoscopists. Gastrointest Endosc 2020;91:568–573 e2.
95. Thiruvengadam NR, Saumoy M, Schneider Y, et al. A cost-effectiveness analysis for post-endoscopic retrograde cholangiopancreatography pancreatitis prophylaxis in the United States. Clin Gastroenterol Hepatol 2022;20:216–226 e42.
96. de-Madaria E, Herrera-Marante I, Gonzalez-Camacho V, et al. Fluid resuscitation with lactated Ringer's solution vs normal saline in acute pancreatitis: A triple-blind, randomized, controlled trial. United European Gastroenterol J 2018;6:63–72.
97. Sperna Weiland CJ, Smeets X, Kievit W, et al. Aggressive fluid hydration plus non-steroidal anti-inflammatory drugs versus non-steroidal anti-inflammatory drugs alone for post-endoscopic retrograde cholangiopancreatography pancreatitis (FLUYT): a multicentre, open-label, randomised, controlled trial. Lancet Gastroenterol Hepatol 2021;6:350–8.
98. de-Madaria E, Buxbaum JL, Maisonneuve P, et al. Aggressive or moderate fluid resuscitation in acute pancreatitis. N Engl J Med 2022;387:989–1000.

99. Mazaki T, Mado K, Masuda H, et al. Prophylactic pancreatic stent placement and post-ERCP pancreatitis: an updated meta-analysis. J Gastroenterol 2013.
100. Afghani E, Akshintala VS, Khashab MA, et al. 5-Fr vs. 3-Fr pancreatic stents for the prevention of post-ERCP pancreatitis in high-risk patients: a systematic review and network meta-analysis. Endoscopy 2014;46:573–80.
101. Sugimoto M, Takagi T, Suzuki R, et al. Pancreatic stents for the prevention of post-endoscopic retrograde cholangiopancreatography pancreatitis should be inserted up to the pancreatic body or tail. World J Gastroenterol 2018;24: 2392–9.
102. Brackbill S, Young S, Schoenfeld P, et al. A survey of physician practices on prophylactic pancreatic stents. Gastrointest Endosc 2006;64:45–52.
103. Chahal P, Baron TH, Petersen BT, et al. Pancreatic stent prophylaxis of post endoscopic retrograde cholangiopancreatography pancreatitis: spontaneous migration rates and clinical outcomes. Minerva Gastroenterol Dietol 2007;53: 225–30.
104. Choksi NS, Fogel EL, Cote GA, et al. The risk of post-ERCP pancreatitis and the protective effect of rectal indomethacin in cases of attempted but unsuccessful prophylactic pancreatic stent placement. Gastrointest Endosc 2015;81:150–5.
105. Elmunzer BJ, Serrano J, Chak A, et al. Rectal indomethacin alone versus indomethacin and prophylactic pancreatic stent placement for preventing pancreatitis after ERCP: study protocol for a randomized controlled trial. Trials 2016; 17:120.
106. Akshintala VS, Husain SZ, Brenner TA, et al. Rectal INdomethacin, oral TacROlimus, or their combination for the prevention of post-ERCP pancreatitis (INTRO Trial): Protocol for a randomized, controlled, double-blinded trial. Pancreatology 2022;22:887–93.

Endotherapy for Pancreas Divisum

Sumant Inamdar, MD, MPH[a],*, Gregory A. Cote, MD, MS[b],
Dhiraj Yadav, MD, MPH[c]

KEYWORDS

- Pancreatic divisum • Minor papilla intervention • Minor sphincterotomy

KEY POINTS

- Pancreas divisum (PD) is an anatomic variant of the pancreatic duct, which occurs in ~10% of the general population.
- PD is associated with several pancreatitis susceptibility mutations (eg, CFTR gene mutations).
- Increased intraductal pressure due to suboptimal drainage of pancreatic juice through a smaller opening in individuals with PD is hypothesized to increase the risk of pancreatitis and used as the rationale for minor papilla sphincterotomy (miES).
- In clinical practice, miES is offered to patients with idiopathic acute recurrent pancreatitis. An ongoing multicenter, international randomized sham-controlled clinical trial (SpHincterotomy in Acute Recurrent Pancreatitis) is evaluating the role of miES in patients with idiopathic acute recurrent pancreatitis who have PD.
- Endoscopic therapy for pain relief has limited to no benefit in patients with chronic abdominal pain or chronic pancreatitis who have PD and is not recommended.

 Video content accompanies this article at http://www.giendo.theclinics.com.

CASE SUMMARIES

Clinical presentation in patients with pancreas divisum (PD) varies from incidental diagnosis to being highly symptomatic. The authors highlight two cases of PD and acute recurrent pancreatitis (ARP) to highlight differences in management approaches based on the presence of associated findings.

---

[a] Division of Gastroenterology and Hepatology, Department of Medicine, University of Arkansas for Medical Sciences, Shorey Building, 8th Floor, 4301 West Markham Street, Little Rock, AR 72205, USA; [b] Division of Gastroenterology, Oregon Health and Science University, 3181 SW Sam Jackson Park Road, Mail Code L461, Portland, OR, USA; [c] Division of Gastroenterology, Hepatology and Nutrition, University of Pittsburg Medical Center, 200 Lothrop Street, M2, C-wing, Pittsburgh, PA 15213, USA
* Corresponding author.
E-mail addresses: sinamdar@uams.edu; sumant.c.inamdar@gmail.com
Twitter: @SumantInamdar (S.I.)

Gastrointest Endoscopy Clin N Am 33 (2023) 789–805
https://doi.org/10.1016/j.giec.2023.04.012
1052-5157/23/© 2023 Elsevier Inc. All rights reserved.

Case 1

A 49-year old woman was hospitalized for her first episode of acute pancreatitis (AP). She drinks alcohol socially, denies smoking, takes no medications, and has no family history of pancreas problems, cystic fibrosis, or celiac disease. Serum lipase was several folds above normal, and liver chemistries and calcium and triglyceride levels were normal. Abdominal ultrasound showed a normal gallbladder. A contrast-enhanced computed tomography (CECT) scan of the abdomen revealed peripancreatic stranding consistent with interstitial AP and is suspicious for PD, which was confirmed by a magnetic resonance cholangiopancreatography (MRCP). Over the next 8 months, she had two more episodes of mild AP. Genetic testing for mutations in PRSS1, SPINK1 genes, and cystic fibrosis screen was negative. She was offered an endoscopic retrograde cholangiopancreatography (ERCP) with minor papilla sphincterotomy (miES).

Case 2

A 42-year-old man is hospitalized for his third episode of AP. He has a history of heavy alcohol consumption and smokes one pack of cigarettes per day. He has no family history of pancreatitis and takes no medications associated with AP. Serum liver chemistries are elevated with an AST 122, ALT 100, and bilirubin 1.8 mg/dL. Serum calcium and triglycerides are normal. An abdominal ultrasound shows sludge in the gallbladder. An MRI with contrast with MRCP shows a normal common bile duct, an area of necrosis in the tail of the pancreas, and the presence of PD. He is managed conservatively and advised to abstain from alcohol and smoking.

EPIDEMIOLOGY AND DISEASE BURDEN

Pancreatitis is among the most common gastrointestinal disorders. In the United States, annually there are over 250,000 hospitalizations, over 400,000 emergency room visits, and health care expenditure of ~$5 billion for pancreatitis.[1] Identifying and addressing the etiology of pancreatitis is the key to prevent recurrent episodes of AP (RAP) and progression to and of chronic pancreatitis (CP).

PD is common in the general population. In a systematic review of 23 autopsy studies, the pooled prevalence of PD in 2895 persons without pancreatic disease was 7.8% (95% confidence interval 6.8–8.8).[2] Pooled estimate for secretin-enhanced MRCP (sMRCP) was higher but the sample size was small ($n = 156$). In a more recent large representative study of 929 volunteers, the prevalence of PD on sMRCP was 9.6%.[3]

Whether PD has a causal association with pancreatitis is an ongoing debate and conclusive evidence for this has not been established.[2,4] In PD, most of the pancreas drains through the minor papilla which is a smaller opening. This is believed to result in functional obstruction to the flow of pancreatic juice and thereby increase the risk of AP.[5] Mechanistically, this is plausible as obstruction to the pancreatic duct is an established cause of AP in several situations, such as gallstones, pancreatic ductal adenocarcinoma, and pancreatic duct strictures. In experimental studies, an increase in ductal pressure is shown to trigger pancreatitis by a variety of mechanisms.[6-8]

As noted in the above case summaries, assigning PD as the etiology of pancreatitis in individual cases can be challenging, especially in patients with other potential risk factors. In clinical practice, the association is usually reserved for patients with no obvious etiology. The prevalence of PD in patients who have experienced their first episode of AP is not well-defined, as MRCP, endoscopic ultrasound (EUS), and ERCP (imaging studies most likely to identify PD and other pancreatic ductal abnormalities) is usually reserved for patients with unexplained RAP or CP. Evidence has also been presented for a potential synergistic role for PD in the presence of other etiologic factors, for example, certain genetic mutations.[9,10]

ANATOMY AND EMBRYOLOGY

At around 5 weeks of embryonic development, the dorsal and ventral portions of the pancreas seem as separate outpouchings of the endodermal lining of the duodenum. The dorsal pancreas grows faster than the ventral pancreas, which undergoes rotation toward the dorsal pancreas followed by fusion of the two along with realignment of their ductal systems.[11] In the majority, the ventral duct (duct of Wirsung) fuses with the dorsal duct (duct of Santorini) to become the main pancreatic duct, whereas the dorsal duct becomes the minor (lesser) duct.

In about 10% individuals, fusion of the ductal systems is incomplete leading to the dorsal duct draining most of the pancreas through the minor papilla which is significantly smaller than the major ampulla.[3] In complete PD, there is a total failure of fusion of the dorsal and ventral ducts. Less common is incomplete PD, where a small communication exists between the dorsal and ventral ducts, but the drainage is primarily through the minor papilla.[3] Clinically, the term PD should be reserved for patients who have dorsal duct dominant drainage, where most of the pancreas drains into the duodenum through the minor papilla.

CLINICAL PRESENTATION

PD can be detected incidentally in patients with no pancreatic symptoms on cross-sectional abdominal imaging (eg, CECT or MRCP) performed for evaluation of unrelated symptoms or conditions. In symptomatic patients, the clinical presentation spans the spectrum of exocrine pancreatic diseases including abdominal pain, pancreatitis (AP, ARP, and CP) and less often pancreatic neoplasms.

DIAGNOSIS

In patients with an unexplained single episode of AP, ARP, or CP, an MRCP (preferably with secretin) is the best noninvasive test to evaluate for ductal abnormalities, such as PD (**Fig. 1**). In PD, rather than going toward the major papilla, the main pancreatic duct crosses the common bile duct to open at the minor papilla. EUS can also diagnose PD. The presence of PD on EUS is suggested by an absence of the "stack sign" (common bile duct, ventral pancreatic duct and portal vein running in parallel through the pancreatic head), presence of "crossed ducts" (dorsal pancreatic duct crosses over the bile duct anteriorly and superiorly),[12] and inability to follow the pancreatic duct from major papilla to the pancreatic body.[13,14] It is important to remember that the identification of PD on EUS is variable, even in expert hands. Less commonly, PD can be identified on a CECT[15] (**Fig. 2**). Among cross-sectional studies, an sMRCP has the best accuracy to detect PD.[15–17] In a systematic review and meta-analysis comparing the performance of MRCP, sMRCP, and EUS, the area under the receiver operating curve (ROC) was the highest for sMRCP (0.99, 95% CI 0.97–0.99) when compared with MRCP (0.90, 95% CI 0.87–0.92) and EUS (0.97, 95% CI 0.96–0.98). The corresponding sensitivity and specificity for the three modalities were 83% and 99% (sMRCP), 59% and 99% (MRCP), and 85% and 97% (EUS).[16]

INDICATIONS FOR THERAPY OF PANCREAS DIVISUM

Minor papilla cannulation and sphincterotomy (aka papillotomy) can be grouped into two categories: (1) the sphincterotomy itself is intended to be the therapeutic

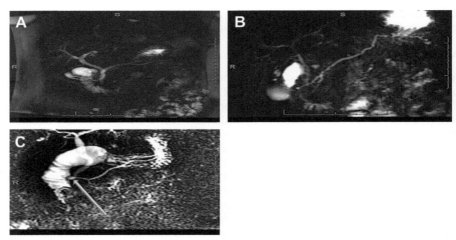

Fig. 1. Secretin-enhanced MRCP images in patients with—(A) complete PD; (B) incomplete PD; and (C) PD with santorinicele

intervention, such as in a patient with idiopathic acute recurrent pancreatitis (iRAP) and PD (with or without santorinocele) and (2) to facilitate access to the pancreatic duct for main duct interventions, such as removal of a pancreatic stone, dilation/stenting of a stricture or treatment of complications from AP needing dorsal duct drainage.[18]

In this article, the authors focus on endotherapy for PD in the setting of ARP. For patients with PD and CP who have main pancreatic duct stricture and/or intraductal stone(s), the techniques for pancreatic duct endoscopic therapy through the minor and major papillae are identical. Sometimes the minor papilla and the dorsal pancreatic duct can be used to gain access to the main pancreatic duct when cannulation

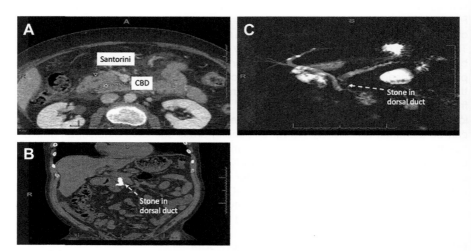

Fig. 2. (A) CT scan in a patient with PD. (B) CT scan in a patient with PD with stone in the dorsal duct. (C) MRCP in a patient with PD with a stone in the dorsal duct and upstream dilatation of the pancreatic duct.

through the major papilla is unsuccessful.[19] This technique is useful in patients who have a patent dorsal duct but still have a ventral dominant drainage or codominant drainage of the pancreas.

ENDOSCOPIC THERAPY FOR PANCREAS DIVISUM

Endoscopic therapy options for PD in the setting of ARP include miES, balloon orifice dilation (eg, balloon sphincteroplasty), and serial stenting to encourage remodeling of the minor papilla. The intent is to increase the size of the minor papilla opening to reduce pressure gradient between the pancreatic duct and the duodenum. In recent times, miES has emerged as the favored technique as repeated stenting may lead to pancreatic ductal abnormalities and balloon dilatation of the minor papilla is associated with more frequent and severe post-ERCP pancreatitis (PEP).[20–23] There are no comparative efficacy studies of miES with minor papilla balloon orifice dilation.

PREPARING THE PATIENT
Informed Consent

Owing to the complexity of minor papilla therapy, it should be performed only by endoscopists with sufficient training and expertise. Moreover, the lack of strong data supporting the outcomes makes a high-quality informed consent discussion essential. The discussion should occur in a relaxed environment where the patient does not feel rushed, and all the potential alternate approaches should be explored. The risk benefit discussion should be individualized and the endoscopist should be cognizant of the high rate of PEP in these patients.[24] In short, the consent should be honest in presenting the potential (not conclusive) benefit (elimination of AP episodes or reduction in their frequency) as well as the risks (short-term risk of PEP even with use of currently used prophylactic measures, post-sphincterotomy restenosis, bleeding, and perforation). There are no empirical data to suggest that endoscopic intervention slows the progression to CP. So, caution is advised in suggesting that there is a clear benefit without supporting empirical data.

Perioperative Fluid Administration

Perioperative intravenous hydration, preferably with Lactated Ringer's solution may reduce the risk of PEP by preventing microvascular hypoperfusion of the pancreas and has been suggested in society guidelines[25] or in patients with contraindication to nonsteroidal anti-inflammatory drugs (NSAIDs), provided that they are not at risk of fluid overload and that a prophylactic pancreatic duct stent is not placed.[26] A recent network meta-analysis of 55 randomized control trials noted that the use of intravenous hydration along with other interventions (eg, pancreatic duct stenting) may be more efficacious in preventing PEP than individual interventions alone.[27] Although specific recommendations for the amount and duration of fluid administration have been made,[25,26] with results of the recent randomized trial in patients with AP, this may need to be revisited.[28]

Sedation and Patient Positioning

ERCP in general can be performed in various positions such as prone, supine, left lateral, or oblique. The choice of position is based on the endoscopist's preference, anesthetic considerations, and patient factors such as abdominal distention due to ascites, severe obesity, recent abdominal surgery, or cervical spinal injury/surgery restricting neck mobility. For minor papilla cannulation, either supine or prone position is optimal, though some experts prefer supine position as it gives a true anatomic visualization instead of the inverted image in prone position on fluoroscopy.[29,30] As ERCP in these patients may be prolonged and often requires a long scope position, sedation administered by an anesthesiologist via either deep sedation or general anesthesia is preferred.

Positioning of the Endoscope

As ERCP in PD is performed primarily for therapeutic purposes, most endoscopists use the standard large channel duodenoscope. Duodenoscopes are essentially designed for interventions at the major papilla; hence, slight modifications to the technique with positioning of the duodenoscope in a "long" or "semi-long" position aid in the visualization of the minor papilla (**Fig. 3**).

IDENTIFYING THE MINOR PAPILLA

Identification of the minor papilla can be challenging as its location and appearance differ from the more familiar major papilla. Therefore, it is essential to recognize landmarks for the minor papilla. The minor papilla is usually located proximal and slightly lateral to the major papilla (1 o'clock position relative to the major papilla), anywhere from 2 cm to as far proximal as the duodenal bulb (**Fig. 4**). It is much smaller than the major papilla and typically lacks a longitudinal fold. Occasionally, the minor papilla appears like a tiny dimple with no mound or obvious opening. In some patients, the minor papilla is below a duodenal fold or even hiding within a shallow diverticulum and might require retraction with a catheter or other device for visualization.[31,32] Sometimes gentle probing might be necessary to visualize the minor papilla, though care should be taken not to perform excessive manipulation as it might lead to edema and interfere with precise localization and cannulation of the minor papillary orifice. When the minor papilla is not easily visualized, additional maneuvers or techniques such as secretin administration with or without dye-enhanced visualization may be used for localization.[32]

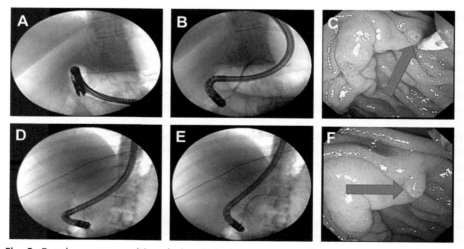

Fig. 3. Duodenoscope position during ERCP in a patient with PD in (*A*) long position; (*B*) semi-long position; (*C*) minor papilla appearance on long/semi-long position; (*D*) near short position; (*E*) short position; and (*F*) minor papilla appearance on near short/short position.

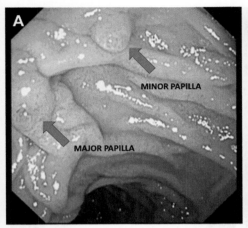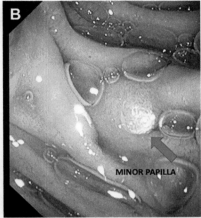

Fig. 4. Endoscopic images of the minor papilla in relation to the major papilla.

Secretin Stimulation

The administration of intravenous secretin at a dose of 0.2 μg/kg (typically with a maximum dose of 16 μg) over 1 minute can stimulate pancreatic exocrine function leading to increased pancreatic juice secretion making the minor papilla more prominent and easier to identify,[33] facilitate cannulation rate, and reduce cannulation time.[33,34] The effect of secretin is usually noted in 1 to 3 min after the administration with temporary dilation of the duct for about 15 minutes. The efficacy of secretin is reduced in patients with severe CP or when the pancreatic duct is very dilated or obstructed.

Dye-Enhanced Visualization

Just like chromoendoscopy, methylene blue or indigo carmine can be sprayed in the expected area of the minor papilla. This is typically used in conjunction with secretin. After spraying the dye, the area is carefully examined to see if the clear pancreatic juice washes the dye away and aid in the identification of the minor papillary orifice.[32,35] In cases of incomplete PD, the ventral pancreatic duct can be cannulated and injected with methylene blue-tinted iodinated contrast which then exits through the minor papillary orifice[36,37] (**Fig. 5**).

CANNULATION OF THE MINOR PAPILLA

Foundational techniques for minor papilla intervention have been well described.[18,38,39] The success rate of minor papilla cannulation is variable, ranging from 73% to 95% with higher technical success when performed by an experienced endoscopist.[38,40,41]

Cannulation Technique

Once the minor papillary orifice is identified, cannulation can be achieved using a tapered cannula or a sphincterotome (Video 1). Most experts prefer a narrow tip sphincterotome (3–4 Fr) but even a standard size sphincterotome can be used (5–6 Fr). Cannulation is usually attempted with a hydrophilic or a partially hydrophilic straight guidewire with the size of the wire depending on the cannula or sphincterotome used. Owing to the smaller opening of the minor papilla, experts usually prefer

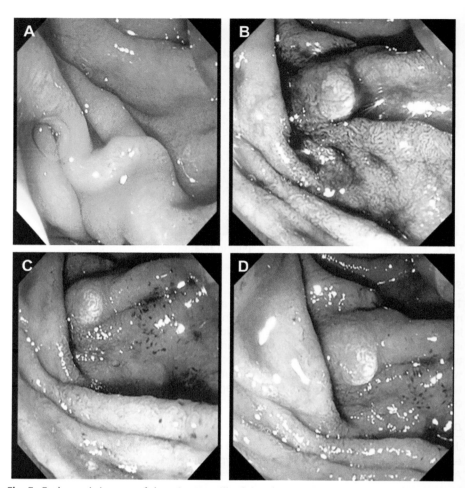

Fig. 5. Endoscopic images of the minor papilla. (*A*) Before methylene blue is sprayed. (*B*) After methylene blue is sprayed. (*C*) and (*D*) Minor papilla seen after administration of secretin.

smaller caliber wires (0.018 or 0.021 inch) over larger ones (0.025 inch or 0.035 inch). Less experienced endoscopists may find manipulating the smaller caliber wires difficult as they may be too floppy.

Cannulation can be achieved by one of two methods: guidewire first approach or cannula or sphincterotome first approach. Most experts prefer guidewire first approach because the minor papillary orifice is usually less than 1 mm (3Fr) in diameter and the smallest cannulating devices are 3Fr making them suboptimal in many cases.

1. Guidewire first approach
In this approach, about 3 to 4 mm of the guidewire is extended out from the tip of the accessory and used to insinuate into the minor papillary orifice. Once the wire has gripped the minor orifice, the endoscopist or the assistant gently probes the guidewire under fluoroscopic guidance. If the guidewire advances with minimal resistance, then about 5 cm of the wire is advanced into the duct which is then followed with the

cannula or sphincterotome (over the wire). After the catheter is advanced into the duct, the guidewire can be advanced into the tail by one of two techniques: (1) guidewire-directed: This method is ideal when a soft tipped small caliber wire (0.018 or 0.025 inch) is used for cannulation as the tip frequently "knuckles" on itself preventing side branch entry. If the wire passage is easy with a leading "knuckle" then the wire can be passed to the tail of the pancreas under fluoroscopy before contrast injection and (2) Contrast-directed: This method is ideal if there is any resistance in passing the wire or fails to "knuckle". Contrast is injected before the guidewire is advanced deep into the body or the tail of the pancreas to avoid a side branch puncture. If overly exuberant, the branch duct could be perforated or acinarization may follow contrast injection of the impacted acinar group resulting in increasing the risk of complications. Contrast injection must be used judiciously to minimize the risk of PEP.

2. Cannula/sphincterotome first approach

In this approach, the cannula or the sphincterotome is inserted gently into the minor orifice followed by probing with the guidewire. This technique must be performed very cautiously as it can lead to trauma-related edema of the minor papilla which makes subsequent cannulation attempts more difficult.

If the minor papillary orifice is stenotic then only the wire might pass into the duct and inserting the catheter over the wire is not possible. In such situations, options include (1) using a tapered push catheter next to guidewire, (2) performing a precut using the guidewire as reference, or (3) performing a precut over the guidewire. One should avoid attempting minor papilla therapies until completely confident that the pancreatic duct will be cannulated. It is exceedingly uncommon to achieve guidewire cannulation without being able to then insinuate a tapered cannula tip into the orifice to perform a pancreatogram.

Once deep cannulation is achieved with the guidewire it should be advanced carefully through the pancreatic duct into the body and tail of the pancreas. This provides support over which the catheter can be advanced into the duct. Gently maneuvering the endoscope into a short position might provide the mechanical advantage needed to advance the catheter through the minor papillary orifice, allowing for further interventions.[18,42]

ADVANCED TECHNIQUES FOR MINOR PAPILLA CANNULATION

Despite efforts outlined above, minor papilla cannulation can fail even in expert hands. Cannulation might be difficult due to minor papilla-related (opening not identifiable, minor papilla in a diverticulum, scarring from prior interventions), duodenum-related (duodenal stenosis, vigorous duodenal motility, altered anatomy from surgery) or operator-related issues (inexperienced endoscopist, inappropriate equipment such as the use of large caliber catheters or wires). In such situations, reassessing the indication and a repeat attempt on another day (and depending on expertise, by another endoscopist) should be a consideration. Advanced techniques to achieve cannulation in case conventional approaches fail have been described, are associated with the increased risk of complications, and are discussed below.

Free-Hand Precut Needle Knife Sphincterotomy

When conventional techniques are unsuccessful, precut of the minor papilla with the needle knife without guidewire passage or stent placement can be performed. Even though the technique involved in free-hand precut needle knife of the minor papilla is similar to that of the major papilla, there are a few modifications and adjustments that need to be made. The minor papilla is first identified and then the needle knife is inserted about 1 to 2 mm into the minor papilla at the upper rim. A 2-to-4 mm free-hand incision is then made at 10 to 12 o'clock position, followed by short 1 to 2 mm deeper cuts until pancreatic juice is seen and the papillary orifice is open. Once the minor papilla is open, a guidewire is used for deep cannulation. This technique has been found to be safe and efficacious, though it carries an increased risk of PEP.[18,38,43] It is important to remember that failure to achieve cannulation with this technique further increases the risk of PEP.

Endoscopic Ultrasound-Assisted Technique

Although empirical data are not available, the EUS-guided approach, especially if the pancreatic duct is dilated, is preferable over precut as unclear landmarks of the minor papilla make precut challenging. Two potential approaches on EUS can aid in gaining access to the minor papilla. For both, a linear echoendoscope is used to identify the pancreatic duct in the body or tail of the pancreas. In the first technique, a 19- or 22-gauge fine-needle aspiration (FNA) needle is introduced into the pancreatic duct and methylene blue tinted iodinated contrast is injected into the duct. The echoendoscope is then removed and a duodenoscope is passed to identify the minor papilla using endoscopic (methylene blue at the papilla) and fluoroscopic (contrast injection) assistance. Then, conventional minor papilla cannulation techniques or the precut technique can be used to achieve cannulation. This technique is preferred if the pancreatic duct is non-dilated and a 22-gauge needle is preferred.[37,44,45] Secretin administration may help to transiently dilate the pancreatic duct making it easier to perform selective FNA. The second technique is the EUS-guided rendezvous technique where a 19- or 22-gauge FNA needle is passed into the pancreatic duct. A 0.035-inch (if 19-gauge needle is used) or a 0.018-inch (if 22-gauge needle is used) long guidewire (450 cm) is then passed from the pancreatic duct antegrade into the duodenum. The echoendoscope is then replaced with a duodenoscope to identify the wire exiting the minor papilla. The wire is then held with a snare or rat tooth forceps and pulled out from the mouth of the patient. The minor papilla can be cannulated adjacent to the wire using conventional techniques or a precut sphincterotomy can be performed using the wire as a guide. If unsuccessful, the wire can be backloaded onto the duodenoscope and a sphincterotome can be introduced over the guidewire into the duct.[18,46–48]

MINOR PAPILLARY ORIFICE INTERVENTIONS
Minor Papilla Sphincterotomy

Unlike major papilla sphincterotomy, miES is not standardized. The depth of cut and the direction of extension are not well-defined or studied due to the lack of consistent and clear landmarks.[49] Most endoscopists use their experience and judgment to gauge the adequacy of the cut. Only in cases where the minor papilla is protruding, such as in a patient with a santorinicele, the direction of the cut is clear. miES can be performed with either a standard sphincterotome or a needle knife.[18,42,49] When miES is performed with a sphincterotome, the device is inserted into the minor papilla and bowed to create moderate tension on the tissue and cut using electrocautery. The aim is to cut about 3 to 4 mm deep to avoid incomplete incision; ideally the pancreatic duct lumen can be visualized endoscopically with insufflation once the incision is completed. The direction of the cut depends on the scope position; in a long position, the cut is made at around 10 to 11 o'clock position, whereas in a short position the cut is made around 11 to 12 o'clock position. Blended current with Endocut mode 120W with effect 3 or pure cut can be used. Pure cut has a lower risk of PEP but a higher risk of bleeding.[18,42,50] If a needle knife is used, then the sphincterotomy can be performed over a guidewire or pancreatic duct stent using a needle knife sphincterotome. This technique is thought to have a lower risk of perforation but may be associated with higher rates of restenosis due to incomplete incision.[18,42]

Balloon Dilation

Balloon dilation of the minor papillary orifice was used in the past and was thought to have comparable outcomes to miES.[22] More recent studies have shown that this is associated with a higher risk of adverse events and severe PEP even with placement of prophylactic pancreatic duct stents. This technique has fallen out of favor, and the currently acceptable treatment for ARP with PD is miES.[23,51] If a satisfactory miES cannot be achieved due to challenging scope position, it is reasonable to supplement a partial/small miES with balloon orifice dilation immediately thereafter. In cases of post-miES restenosis, sometimes balloon orifice dilation is easier and more effective when the scarred area involves the terminal pancreatic duct.

Stent Placement

Small-caliber stents (3–5 Fr) are used regularly in minor papillary interventions for prophylaxis of PEP and as a scaffold over which miES is performed. Most experts recommend temporary pancreatic duct stents. The use of longer pancreatic duct stents gained favor in the 1990s based on a small randomized trial ($n = 19$) which demonstrated significant reduction in hospitalization and emergency room visits for abdominal pain in patients receiving serial stents when compared with controls.[52] The practice of serial stenting has now become obsolete due to the increased risk of PEP and the potential for iatrogenic stent-related pancreatic duct strictures.[21]

POSTPROCEDURE MANAGEMENT

ERCP for minor papilla intervention is usually performed as an outpatient procedure with most patients discharged after 1 to 2 hours of observation. Patients may have postprocedure pain or nausea, the latter likely related to anesthesia, which resolve quickly with symptomatic treatment. Depending on the difficulty of the procedure, most patients are kept nil per mouth for 2 to 4 hours postprocedure and then advanced to clear liquids. If there are no complications, patients are advised to advance diet as tolerated over the next 24 hours. Patients with significant postprocedure pain may need overnight admission for observation, intravenous hydration, and pain management. Minor papilla intervention is among the highest risk indication for ERCP and is associated with 10% to 15% risk of PEP.[24,53,54] These patients need admission to the hospital for appropriate management (see below).

ADVERSE EVENTS

The risk of post-sphincterotomy bleeding, perforation, and infection after minor papilla intervention is the same as for ERCP performed for other indications.[54–56]

Post-Endoscopic Retrograde Cholangiopancreatography Pancreatitis

PEP is the most common adverse event after minor papilla manipulation.[53–55,57] PEP risk is exacerbated by technically challenging and longer procedures, presumably due to increased periampullary edema. Studies have shown that younger age (<40 years), miES, female gender, and previous history of PEP are independent risk factors associated with a higher rate of PEP, whereas calcific CP is associated with a lower rate.[53,54,58] In a systematic review by Kanth and colleagues, it was found that PD increased the risk of PEP by about twofolds (odds ratio [OR] 2.2, 95% CI 1.4–3.4).[24]

The risk of PEP can be reduced by the administration of periprocedural fluids (discussed previously), short-term pancreatic duct stenting and the use of NSAIDs.[27,59,60] Small-caliber pancreatic duct stents (3–5 Fr) reduce PEP presumably by reducing intraductal pressure, promoting early duct flushing and protecting drainage, whereas iatrogenic papillary edema resolves. These stents frequently migrate spontaneously within 2 weeks which can be confirmed by abdominal x-ray. In 10% to 30% of patients, depending on the size of the stents used, an upper endoscopy is needed to remove the retained stent.[18,38,42] Periprocedural NSAIDs such as rectal indomethacin are recommended to prevent PEP in all high-risk cases[42,59] and encouraged to prevent PEP in patients without prior sphincterotomy.[25,26] Unless there is chronic calcific pancreatitis, all cases involving the minor papilla are high risk. The medication (100 mg in adults; 50 mg in children [dose adjusted based on weight]) can be administered either before, during, or after the completion of ERCP.[61–64]

Bleeding

miES can lead to bleeding in less than 1% cases which can be subclassified as immediate, early or late based on the timing, or as mild, moderate, or severe based on the severity.[54] The management of bleeding after minor papilla therapy is similar to major papilla bleeding. The application of epinephrine, cautery, or clip might increase the risk of PEP and stenosis of the minor papilla due to its smaller size when compared with the major papilla. To prevent adverse events, a prophylactic pancreatic duct stent should be placed before any hemostasis therapy.

OUTCOMES AFTER MINOR PAPILLA INTERVENTIONS

Technical success in minor papilla interventions is defined as successful performance of miES and/or deployment of a stent in the minor papilla and is achieved in about 76%. This meta-analysis, published in 2017, included 17 studies had aimed to evaluate the clinical efficacy of endoscopic therapy for PD (miES with prophylactic stent placement in most studies). Clinical efficacy was noted in patients with ARP (pooled efficacy 76%, 95% CI 71.2%–80.3%).[41] Results were less promising among patients with chronic abdominal pain (pooled efficacy 48%, 95% CI 37.1%–59.0%) and CP (pooled efficacy 52.4%, 95% 40.6%–64.0%).[24,65] In a single-center study published more recently, the clinical efficacy of miES in 81 patients with ARP and PD who were followed for at least 12 months was much lower (46%).[66] Several limitations of published studies make interpretation of results difficult; most importantly, only one small published study has included a control group (n = 19),[52] whereas others have evaluated patients who were followed after endoscopic therapy without a comparison group. Other limitations included variable definitions for inclusion, outcome of interest, and duration of follow-up. A multicenter, international sham-controlled randomized clinical trial (SpHincterotomy in Acute Recurrent Pancreatitis [SHARP]) is ongoing to evaluate the impact of miES with prophylactic stent placement in patients with idiopathic RAP who also have PD. This study is powered to detect a 33% relative risk reduction in the development of subsequent AP. The investigators selected 33% as the lowest acceptable benefit of miES considering the known risks of ERCP. Results from the SHARP trial are anticipated to provide empirical data to make firm recommendations on the role of endotherapy in these patients.[67] A recent publication also outlines challenges in designing endoscopic therapy trials for AP including the SHARP trial and ways to address them.[68]

SUMMARY

PD is commonly encountered in a variety of clinical settings ranging from patients who are incidentally diagnosed to those with a high burden of symptoms including ARP or CP. In the past decades, advances have been made in approaches to endoscopic therapy for PD and measures to reduce the risk of procedure-related complications. The need for endoscopic therapy in some patients is obvious and clear (eg, those with local complications of AP), whereas in others, the available data are not definitive to make firm recommendations (eg, iRAP with PD). Hopefully, results from an ongoing clinical trial will provide empirical data on the role of miES in such patients. Until then, physicians should carefully counsel patients about available data and how best to balance the risks and benefits of endoscopic therapy.

CLINICS CARE POINTS

- In patients with unexplained recurrent acute or chronic pancreatitis, a magnetic resonance cholangiopancreatography (preferably with secretin) should be considered for evaluation of pancreatic ductal abnormalities such as pancreas divisum (PD).
- Empirical evidence for beneficial effect of minor papilla sphincterotomy (miES) in patients with idiopathic acute recurrent pancreatitis (iRAP) and PD is lacking.
- Although miES in clinical practice is often considered in patients with iRAP, a thorough discussion for current evidence, pros and cons should be discussed with the patient before performing the procedure.
- miES should be performed only by endoscopists with adequate training and expertise.

FUNDING

National Institute of Diabetes and Digestive and Kidney Diseases (NIDDK) under award number U01DK116743 (Gregory A Cote; Dhiraj Yadav). The content is solely the responsibility of the authors and does not necessarily represent the official views of the National Institutes of Health.

DISCLOSURE

S. Inamdar: None. G.A Cote: Consultant, Interpace Diagnostics and Olympus America. D. Yadav: None.

ACKNOWLEDGMENT

The authors thank Evan L Fogel, MD, for a critical review of the manuscript and helpful suggestions.

SUPPLEMENTARY DATA

Supplementary data related to this article can be found online at https://doi.org/10.1016/j.giec.2023.04.012.

REFERENCES

1. Peery AF, Crockett SD, Murphy CC, et al. Burden and Cost of Gastrointestinal, Liver, and Pancreatic Diseases in the United States: Update 2021. Gastroenterology 2022;162(2):621–44.

2. Fogel EL, Toth TG, Lehman GA, et al. Does endoscopic therapy favorably affect the outcome of patients who have recurrent acute pancreatitis and pancreas divisum? Pancreas 2007;34(1):21–45.

3. Bülow R, Simon P, Thiel R, et al. Anatomic variants of the pancreatic duct and their clinical relevance: an MR-guided study in the general population. Eur Radiol 2014;24(12):3142–9.

4. DiMagno MJ, Wamsteker EJ. Pancreas divisum. Curr Gastroenterol Rep 2011; 13(2):150–6.

5. Cotton PB. Congenital anomaly of pancreas divisum as cause of obstructive pain and pancreatitis. Gut 1980;21(2):105–14.

6. Romac JMJ, Shahid RA, Swain SM, et al. Piezo1 is a mechanically activated ion channel and mediates pressure induced pancreatitis. Nat Commun 2018;9(1): 1715.

7. Wen L, Javed TA, Yimlamai D, et al. Transient High Pressure in Pancreatic Ducts Promotes Inflammation and Alters Tight Junctions via Calcineurin Signaling in Mice. Gastroenterology 2018;155(4):1250–63.e5.

8. Lerch MM, Weidenbach H, Hernandez CA, et al. Pancreatic outflow obstruction as the critical event for human gall stone induced pancreatitis. Gut 1994; 35(10):1501–3.

9. Bertin C, Pelletier AL, Vullierme MP, et al. Pancreas divisum is not a cause of pancreatitis by itself but acts as a partner of genetic mutations. Am J Gastroenterol 2012;107(2):311–7.

10. Gelrud A, Sheth S, Banerjee S, et al. Analysis of cystic fibrosis gener product (CFTR) function in patients with pancreas divisum and recurrent acute pancreatitis. Am J Gastroenterol 2004;99(8):1557–62.

11. Pandol SJ. In: Pandol SJ, editor. Pancreatic embryology and development. San rafael (CA): Morgan & Claypool Life Sciences; 2010.

12. Rana SS, Bhasin DK, Sharma V, et al. Role of endoscopic ultrasound in the diagnosis of pancreas divisum. Endosc ultrasound 2013;2(1):7–10.

13. Lai R, Freeman ML, Cass OW, et al. Accurate diagnosis of pancreas divisum by linear-array endoscopic ultrasonography. Endoscopy 2004;36(8):705–9.

14. Bhutani MS, Hoffman BJ, Hawes RH. Diagnosis of pancreas divisum by endoscopic ultrasonography. Endoscopy 1999;31(2):167–9.

15. Kushnir VM, Wani SB, Fowler K, et al. Sensitivity of endoscopic ultrasound, multidetector computed tomography, and magnetic resonance cholangiopancreatography in the diagnosis of pancreas divisum: a tertiary center experience. Pancreas 2013;42(3):436–41.

16. Shen Z, Munker S, Zhou B, et al. The Accuracies of Diagnosing Pancreas Divisum by Magnetic Resonance Cholangiopancreatography and Endoscopic Ultrasound: A Systematic Review and Meta-analysis. Sci Rep 2016;6:35389.

17. Wan J, Ouyang Y, Yu C, et al. Comparison of EUS with MRCP in idiopathic acute pancreatitis: a systematic review and meta-analysis. Gastrointest Endosc 2018; 87(5):1180–8.e9.

18. Testoni PA, Mariani A. 21 - Minor Papilla Cannulation and Sphincterotomy. In: Baron TH, Kozarek RA, editors. Carr-locke DLBTE. Third E. Elsevier; 2019. p. 182–95.e1.

19. Kwon CI, Gromski MA, Sherman S, et al. Clinical response to dorsal duct drainage via the minor papilla in refractory obstructing chronic calcific pancreatitis. Endoscopy 2017;49(4):371–7.

20. Lehman GA, Sherman S. Pancreas divisum. Diagnosis, clinical significance, and management alternatives. Gastrointest Endosc Clin N Am 1995;5(1):145–70. Available at: http://www.ncbi.nlm.nih.gov/pubmed/7728342.
21. Bakman YG, Safdar K, Freeman ML. Significant clinical implications of prophylactic pancreatic stent placement in previously normal pancreatic ducts. Endoscopy 2009;41(12):1095–8.
22. Yamamoto N, Isayama H, Sasahira N, et al. Endoscopic minor papilla balloon dilation for the treatment of symptomatic pancreas divisum. Pancreas 2014; 43(6):927–30.
23. Heyries L, Barthet M, Delvasto C, et al. Long-term results of endoscopic management of pancreas divisum with recurrent acute pancreatitis. Gastrointest Endosc 2002;55(3):376–81.
24. Kanth R, Samji NS, Inaganti A, et al. Endotherapy in symptomatic pancreas divisum: a systematic review. Pancreatology 2014;14(4):244–50.
25. ASGE Standards of Practice Committee, Chandrasekhara V, Khashab MA, Muthusamy VR, et al. Adverse events associated with ERCP. Gastrointest Endosc 2017;85(1):32–47.
26. Dumonceau JM, Kapral C, Aabakken L, et al. ERCP-related adverse events: European Society of Gastrointestinal Endoscopy (ESGE) Guideline. Endoscopy 2020;52(2):127–49.
27. Akshintala VS, Sperna Weiland CJ, Bhullar FA, et al. Non-steroidal anti-inflammatory drugs, intravenous fluids, pancreatic stents, or their combinations for the prevention of post-endoscopic retrograde cholangiopancreatography pancreatitis: a systematic review and network meta-analysis. lancet Gastroenterol Hepatol 2021;6(9):733–42.
28. de-Madaria E, Buxbaum JL, Maisonneuve P, et al. Aggressive or Moderate Fluid Resuscitation in Acute Pancreatitis. N Engl J Med 2022;387(11):989–1000.
29. Mashiana HS, Jayaraj M, Mohan BP, et al. Comparison of outcomes for supine vs. prone position ERCP: a systematic review and meta-analysis. Endosc Int Open 2018;6(11):E1296–301.
30. Maydeo A, Patil GK. ERCP: does patient position count? Endosc Int Open 2018; 6(11):E1302–3.
31. Benage D, McHenry R, Hawes RH, et al. Minor papilla cannulation and dorsal ductography in pancreas divisum. Gastrointest Endosc 1990;36(6):553–7.
32. Park SH, de Bellis M, McHenry L, et al. Use of methylene blue to identify the minor papilla or its orifice in patients with pancreas divisum. Gastrointest Endosc 2003; 57(3):358–63.
33. Devereaux BM, Lehman GA, Fein S, et al. Facilitation of pancreatic duct cannulation using a new synthetic porcine secretin. Am J Gastroenterol 2002;97(9): 2279–81.
34. Devereaux BM, Fein S, Purich E, et al. A new synthetic porcine secretin for facilitation of cannulation of the dorsal pancreatic duct at ERCP in patients with pancreas divisum: a multicenter, randomized, double-blind comparative study. Gastrointest Endosc 2003;57(6):643–7.
35. Ohshima Y, Tsukamoto Y, Naitoh Y, et al. Function of the minor duodenal papilla in pancreas divisum as determined by duodenoscopy using indigo carmine dye and a pH sensor. Am J Gastroenterol 1994;89(12):2188–91. Available at: http://www.ncbi.nlm.nih.gov/pubmed/7977239.
36. Elmunzer BJ, Piraka CR. EUS-Guided Methylene Blue Injection to Facilitate Pancreatic Duct Access After Unsuccessful ERCP. Gastroenterology 2016; 151(5):809–10.

37. Aneese AM, Ghaith G, Cannon ME, et al. EUS-guided methylene blue injection to facilitate endoscopic cannulation of an obscured pancreatic duct orifice after ampullectomy. Am J Gastroenterol 2018;113(5):782–3.

38. Gutta A, Fogel E, Sherman S. Identification and management of pancreas divisum. Expert Rev Gastroenterol Hepatol 2019;13(11):1089–105.

39. Klein SD, Affronti JP. Pancreas divisum, an evidence-based review: part II, patient selection and treatment. Gastrointest Endosc 2004;60(4):585–9.

40. Wang W, Gong B, Jiang WS, et al. Endoscopic treatment for pancreatic diseases: Needle-knife-guided cannulation via the minor papilla. World J Gastroenterol 2015;21(19):5950–60.

41. Michailidis L, Aslam B, Grigorian A, et al. The efficacy of endoscopic therapy for pancreas divisum: a meta-analysis. Ann Gastroenterol 2017;30(5):550–8.

42. Adams DB, Coté GA. Current surgical therapy. 13th edition (Cameron, John L. CAM, ed.).; 2020.

43. Sahin B, Parlak E, Ciçek B, et al. Precutting of the minor papilla for pancreatic duct cannulation in pancreas divisum patients. Endoscopy 2005;37(8):779.

44. Dewitt J, McHenry L, Fogel E, et al. EUS-guided methylene blue pancreatography for minor papilla localization after unsuccessful ERCP. Gastrointest Endosc 2004;59(1):133–6.

45. Carrara S, Arcidiacono PG, Diellou AM, et al. EUS-guided methylene blue injection into the pancreatic duct as a guide for pancreatic stenting after ampullectomy. Endoscopy 2007;39(Suppl 1):E151–2.

46. Papachristou GI, Gleeson FC, Petersen BT, et al. Pancreatic endoscopic ultrasound-assisted rendezvous procedure to facilitate drainage of nondilated pancreatic ducts. Endoscopy 2007;39(Suppl 1):E324–5.

47. Nakai Y, Kogure H, Isayama H, et al. Endoscopic ultrasound-guided pancreatic duct drainage. Saudi J Gastroenterol 2019;25(4):210–7.

48. Will U, Meyer F, Manger T, et al. Endoscopic ultrasound-assisted rendezvous maneuver to achieve pancreatic duct drainage in obstructive chronic pancreatitis. Endoscopy 2005;37(2):171–3.

49. Attwell A, Borak G, Hawes R, et al. Endoscopic pancreatic sphincterotomy for pancreas divisum by using a needle-knife or standard pull-type technique: safety and reintervention rates. Gastrointest Endosc 2006;64(5):705–11.

50. Elta GH, Barnett JL, Wille RT, et al. Pure cut electrocautery current for sphincterotomy causes less post-procedure pancreatitis than blended current. Gastrointest Endosc 1998;47(2):149–53.

51. Ertan A. Long-term results after endoscopic pancreatic stent placement without pancreatic papillotomy in acute recurrent pancreatitis due to pancreas divisum. Gastrointest Endosc 2000;52(1):9–14.

52. Lans JI, Geenen JE, Johanson JF, et al. Endoscopic therapy in patients with pancreas divisum and acute pancreatitis: a prospective, randomized, controlled clinical trial. Gastrointest Endosc 1992;38(4):430–4.

53. Ojo AS. Pancreatic Duct Variations and the Risk of Post-Endoscopic Retrograde Cholangiopancreatography Pancreatitis. Cureus 2020;12(9):e10445.

54. Moffatt DC, Coté GA, Avula H, et al. Risk factors for ERCP-related complications in patients with pancreas divisum: a retrospective study. Gastrointest Endosc 2011;73(5):963–70.

55. Chacko LN, Chen YK, Shah RJ. Clinical outcomes and nonendoscopic interventions after minor papilla endotherapy in patients with symptomatic pancreas divisum. Gastrointest Endosc 2008;68(4):667–73.

56. Gerke H, Byrne MF, Stiffler HL, et al. Outcome of endoscopic minor papillotomy in patients with symptomatic pancreas divisum. JOP 2004;5(3):122–31. Available at: http://www.ncbi.nlm.nih.gov/pubmed/15138333.

57. Cheng CL, Sherman S, Watkins JL, et al. Risk factors for post-ERCP pancreatitis: a prospective multicenter study. Am J Gastroenterol 2006;101(1):139–47.

58. Freeman ML, Guda NM. Prevention of post-ERCP pancreatitis: a comprehensive review. Gastrointest Endosc 2004;59(7):845–64.

59. Inamdar S, Han D, Passi M, et al. Rectal indomethacin is protective against post-ERCP pancreatitis in high-risk patients but not average-risk patients: a systematic review and meta-analysis. Gastrointest Endosc 2017;85(1):67–75.

60. Elmunzer BJ, Scheiman JM, Lehman GA, et al. A randomized trial of rectal indomethacin to prevent post-ERCP pancreatitis. N Engl J Med 2012;366(15): 1414–22.

61. Wan J, Ren Y, Zhu Z, et al. How to select patients and timing for rectal indomethacin to prevent post-ERCP pancreatitis: a systematic review and meta-analysis. BMC Gastroenterol 2017;17(1):43.

62. Serrano JPR, Jukemura J, Romanini SG, et al. Nonsteroidal anti-inflammatory drug effectivity in preventing post-endoscopic retrograde cholangiopancreatography pancreatitis: A systematic review and meta-analysis. World J Gastrointest Endosc 2020;12(11):469–87.

63. Yang C, Zhao Y, Li W, et al. Rectal nonsteroidal anti-inflammatory drugs administration is effective for the prevention of post-ERCP pancreatitis: An updated meta-analysis of randomized controlled trials. Pancreatology 2017;17(5):681–8.

64. Fogel EL, Lehman GA, Tarnasky P, et al. Rectal indometacin dose escalation for prevention of pancreatitis after endoscopic retrograde cholangiopancreatography in high-risk patients: a double-blind, randomised controlled trial. lancet Gastroenterol Hepatol 2020;5(2):132–41.

65. Liao Z, Gao R, Wang W, et al. A systematic review on endoscopic detection rate, endotherapy, and surgery for pancreas divisum. Endoscopy 2009;41(5):439–44.

66. de Jong DM, Stassen PM, Poley JW, et al. Clinical outcome of endoscopic therapy in patients with symptomatic pancreas divisum: a Dutch cohort study. Endosc Int Open 2021;9(7):E1164–70.

67. Coté GA, Durkalski-Mauldin VL, Serrano J, et al. SpHincterotomy for Acute Recurrent Pancreatitis Randomized Trial: Rationale, Methodology, and Potential Implications. Pancreas 2019;48(8):1061–7.

68. Cote GA, Durkalski-Mauldin V, Williams A, et al. Design and execution of sham-controlled endoscopic trials in acute pancreatitis: Lessons learned from the SHARP trial. Pancreatology 2023;23(2):187–91.

Management of Pancreatic Duct Stones: Extracorporeal Approach

Manu Tandan, MD, DM*, Partha Pal, MD, DNB, MRCP (UK),
Duvvuru Nageshwar Reddy, MD, DM

KEYWORDS

- Extracorporeal shock wave lithotripsy • Chronic pancreatitis • Pancreatic calculi
- Endoscopic retrograde cholangiopancreatography

KEY POINTS

- Extracorporeal shock wave lithotripsy (ESWL) is a safe and effective procedure for large pancreatic calculi in the head and body not extractable by standard endoscopic retrograde cholangiopancreatography techniques as an alternative to surgery.
- ESWL in properly selected patients can lead to long-term pain relief in two-thirds of patients with a need for re-intervention in less than half on long-term follow-up.

INTRODUCTION

Chronic pancreatitis (CP), a disease of diverse etiology, is associated with progressive and irreversible changes leading to the destruction of functional pancreatic tissue with resulting loss of exocrine and endocrine function. Of the many etiologies, alcohol and smoking are the commonest in most industrialized nations. In India, an idiopathic variety of CP is prevalent in young adults who do not consume any alcohol.[1,2] Predisposition due to genetic mutation is a likely major contributing factor in these patients with idiopathic CP.[3,4] Irrespective of the etiology, pancreatic calculi (PC) are common sequelae of this disease. They are seen in over 50% of patients.[1,5] The incidence of calculi increases with time and may even reach 100% at 14 years.[6,7] These calculi eventually obstruct the main pancreatic duct (MPD) resulting in upstream ductal hypertension with subsequent development of parenchymal hypertension. This ductal hypertension is responsible for the recurring pain, often excruciating, which is a dominant symptom in patients with CP.

As CP is an irreversible disease, the aim of all therapies, both endoscopic and surgical is to remove the calculi and reduce the ductal hypertension with a resultant

Asian Institute of Gastroenterology, 6-3-661, Somajiguda, Hyderabad, TG 500082, India
* Corresponding author. Clinical Services.
E-mail address: mantan_05@rediffmail.com

Gastrointest Endoscopy Clin N Am 33 (2023) 807–820
https://doi.org/10.1016/j.giec.2023.04.006
1052-5157/23/© 2023 Elsevier Inc. All rights reserved.

decrease in the pain.[2] Pain in CP is, however, multifactorial and can be secondary to tissue and neural ischemia, neural entrapment, nociception, or visceral and central sensitization.[8] These multiple mechanisms of pain explain the persistence of pain in some patients despite complete clearance of the MPD.[2,8] Pancreatic stone extraction can be done endoscopically with or without the use of lithotripsy or by surgical methods. Lithotripsy can be extracorporeal shock wave lithotripsy (ESWL) or intraductal lithotripsy using a pancreatoscope. For intraductal lithotripsy either electrohydraulic lithotripsy (EHL) or laser lithotripsy (LL) is used to fragment the calculi. In this article, we will discuss in detail the extracorporeal approach to clear the stones from the MPD in patients with CP.

CLASSIFICATION OF PANCREATIC CALCULI

PC are classified based on type, density, numbers, and location.

1. PC may be radio opaque, radiolucent, or mixed type. The majority of PC are radio opaque. In our experience with over 5000 patients, 79.2% of calculi were radio opaque, 16% were radiolucent while the rest (4.7%) were of the mixed type.[2] Radio opaque calculi were seen in 62% of patients in a multi-center survey of 879 patients. Stones were more frequent in men who were heavy alcohol consumers (>80 g/day) and heavy smokers (>20 cig/day).[9]
2. PC may be single or multiple. In the above-mentioned study of over 5000 patients, 75.1% of PC were single while the rest were multiple (**Table 1**).[2]
3. Stones were also classified based on their location, that is, in the head, body, or tail. In 51.5% of patients in our study, PC were located in the head region, 21.4% in the body, and 7.4% in the tail area; 15.9% were extensive and located in multiple areas, that is, head, body, and tail regions (see **Table 1**).[2]
4. PC may be intraductal, either MPD, in secondary branches, or in the parenchyma.

PC > 5 mm in size, located in the MPD are difficult to extract by the standard procedure of endoscopic retrograde cholangiopancreatography (ERCP) and pancreatic sphincterotomy. Balloon trawl or baskets are used to clear the pancreatic duct (PD) of calculi. PC, especially those in idiopathic CP are dense, spiculated, and adherent to the ductal mucosa. This makes their extraction challenging. Besides, the relatively thin diameter of the MPD, as well as its tortuosity, makes the passage of endoscopic accessories difficult. The European Society of Gastrointestinal Endoscopy (ESGE) in its clinical guidelines states that for uncomplicated and painful CP with calculi >5 mm in MPD, ESWL should be performed, followed by subsequent ERCP to clear the duct.[10,11] These guidelines were not changed over 7 years, despite advances in technology and technique indicating that ESWL is an established therapy and the standard of care in managing large PC in the MPD.

PATHOGENESIS OF STONE FORMATION AND ITS COMPOSITION

PC consists of a central nidus over which layers of calcium carbonate are deposited. The nidus is amorphous and consists of small quantities of trace elements such as nickel, chromium, and iron. This nidus can be identified and located on scanning electron microscopy and energy dispersive x-ray fluorescence.[12] Over this central nidus, calcium carbonate or calcite is deposited in layers and forms the typical PC.

Precipitation of calcium carbonates in the pancreatic juice is the initial event and dependent on the concentration of the pancreatic stone protein (PSP). Various factors including genetic variants cause reduction in the PSP. This reduction results in supersaturation of calcium carbonate in the pancreatic juice and its eventual deposition in layers

Table 1
Characteristics of patients and extracorporeal shock wave lithotripsy features in 5124 patients

		Number	%
Age	<40 years	3541	69.1
	41–60 years	1035	20.1
	>60 years	548	10.6
Female		*1655*	*32.3*
Etiology	*Alcohol and/or Smoking*	*495*	*9.6*
	Idiopathic	*4629*	*90.4*
Stone characteristics	Single	3851	75.1
	Multiple	1273	24.8
	Radio opaque	4063	79.2
	Radiolucent	820	16.0
	Mixed	241	4.7
Stone location	Head	2824	51.1
	Body	1099	21.4
	Tail	384	7.4
	Head/Body/Tail	817	15.9
Associated stricture		1153	22.5
ESWL sessions	≤4	4920	96
	>5 (maximum 8)	204	4
Fragmentation	Complete	3722	72.6
	Partial	886	17.3
	Unsuccessful	516	10

From Tandan M, Nageshwar Reddy D, Talukdar R, et al. ESWL for large pancreatic calculi: Report of over 5000 patients. Pancreatology. 2019;19(7):916-921.

over the inner nidus.[13] Irrespective of the etiology of CP, the stricture and composition of the PC are similar indicating a common pathway for pancreatolithiasis.[13]

TECHNIQUES OF PANCREATIC DUCTAL STONE EXTRACTION

1. Various endoscopic options exist for the extraction of stones from the MPD. For small calculi, the standard procedure of ERCP and pancreatic sphincterotomy followed by either a balloon trawl or extraction with a basket is recommended. However, the success rate at ERCP and stone extraction are not high in patients with CP. A few studies have revealed clearance rate of 9% in 1041 patients, and 14% in 1834 patients.[14–16] Mechanical lithotripsy for PC is not a procedure of choice because of poor results in extraction and unacceptably high incidence of adverse effects.[17] A retrospective analysis of over 700 patients revealed a complication rate thrice as high as for biliary mechanical lithotripsy.[17] This, as mentioned earlier, is because of the thin diameter of the MPD as well as its tortuosity, as compared to the common bile duct. Manipulation of large accessories in the main MPD is technically challenging and often not very efficient, resulting in many adverse effects.[2] Factors associated with poor results include stones > 10 mm in size, diffuse distribution of calculi, stone impaction in MPD, and a stricture proximal to the calculi.[15,18]

2. Lithotripsy of PC can be performed extracorporeally using ESWL or intraductally using a per oral pancreatoscope with either EHL or LL. These techniques are specifically meant for large and dense calculi which cannot be extracted by the above-mentioned standard ERCP. ESWL has been shown to clear over 80% of PC after an initially failed endotherapy.[14]
3. Chemical dissolution of the stones using an anti-epileptic compound Trimethadione was first reported around four decades ago.[19] The same group has recently published a case series of 13 patients where the compound was used successfully.[20] These results need to be validated by multi-center trials before their acceptance for widespread use. Limitations exist in the form of long duration of therapy required to achieve dissolution. These compounds are seldom used routinely in present-day practice of management of PC.
4. Surgical procedures either in the form of drainage or resection or their combination are well-accepted modes of managing PC. These were the standards of care before the advent of advanced endoscopic procedures. Detailed comparison of pros and cons of ERCP/ESWL and surgery are beyond the scope of this article. Briefly, two earlier studies showed the surgery was superior to endotherapy. In one of these, after a 5-year follow-up, pain was absent in 15% of the endoscopy group versus 34% in the surgery group.[21] This indicated that neither method gave satisfactory results. The other study had only 39 patients and there was selection bias in the two arms of the study that had been highlighted by several experts.[22] A randomized controlled trial revealed that ESWL was effective in providing pain relief in 62% of patients on a 4-year follow-up.[23] Results of ESWL versus surgery were analyzed in a retrospective study of 81 patients with CP. Similar pain relief was reported on follow-up of over 5 years. However, surgery reported more morbidity and higher cost.[24] The issue is not to compare surgery with ESWL but to decide which patient should go for surgery and which for ESWL. ESGE guidelines suggest that early referral for surgery should be advised in case of failure of endotherapy.[11] Both these modalities are complimentary and not competitive.

EXTRACORPOREAL SHOCK WAVE LITHOTRIPSY

ESWL was first introduced in the 1980s for managing urinary tract calculi.[25] However, its indications were quickly expanded to include the gastrointestinal tract and has since been used regularly for fragmenting biliary and pancreatic calculi.[26] Today, it is accepted as the standard of care in the management of large PC in the MPD.[1,2,5,11,27–29]

PRINCIPLES OF EXTRACORPOREAL SHOCK WAVE LITHOTRIPSY

ESWL is based on the principle of shock wave energy. The present-day lithotripters used for fragmenting PC have an electromagnetic device for generating these shock waves. The activated electromagnetic device releases high-energy waves in an enclosed space. These high-energy waves are directed through a cone enclosing water onto the patient's abdominal wall, focusing on the PC. When these waves pass through substances of different acoustic impedance, a compressive stress is produced at the interphase of the two densities. These stresses overcome the inherent tensile strength of the target, which in this case is the PC. Fragmentation of the margin occurs. The shock waves travel through the calculus and are reflected from the posterior surface of the stone resulting in further fragmentation.[30] Presently, at our institute, a third-generation electromagnetic dual-focus lithotripter is used for ESWL. This lithotripter has the facilities for focusing on the calculi either by ultrasound or by fluoroscopy. From our earlier experience, a shock wave rate of 90/minute at a voltage of 16 kv is ideal for fragmenting calculi.[30] Shockwaves at a higher frequency have a tendency to reflect from the calculi and interfere with the efficacy of oncoming shockwaves.[30]

INDICATIONS AND CONTRAINDICATIONS

ESWL is indicated in all patients with painful uncomplicated CP and large radio opaque or radiolucent PC which are not amenable to extraction by the standard procedure of ERCP.[1,2,10,11,27,28,31,32] ESWL should be avoided in patients with extensive calculi involving the head, body, and tail regions. Patients with multiple strictures (chain of lake appearance), as well as suspicious head mass, presence of moderate to severe ascites, should not be taken up for ESWL. Calculi in the pancreatic tail are not targeted at ESWL because of the risk of injury to the spleen.[33] Cholangitis or coagulopathy secondary to biliary obstruction and sepsis should be first controlled and patient subjected to ESWL subsequently.[1,11,32] The aim of ESWL is to achieve fragmentation of the PC to <3 mm in size or demonstrate a decrease in density heterogeneity of the stone mass.[1,11,12,32] Small fragmented calculi either pass off spontaneously or are easily extracted at a subsequent ERCP.

Protocol of Extracorporeal Shock Wave Lithotripsy in Radio Opaque and Radiolucent Pancreatic Calculi

A standard protocol has been devised at our center for performing ESWL (**Fig. 1**).[1,2,32] The presence and size of calculi are confirmed by cross-sectional imaging (MRCP/CT), in those patients who are candidates for ESWL and have large radio opaque PC in the head and body[1,2,32] At our center, fluoroscopic guidance is the preferred method for localizing radio opaque calculi. We carry out the procedure predominantly in a supine position under epidural anesthesia and sedation.[34] Total intravenous analgesia and general anesthesia have occasionally been used for the procedure in a few of our patients as well as at other centers.[2,34]

Between 5000 and 6000 shocks are delivered per session, at a rate of 90/minute and energy level of 16 kv. ESWL is performed on successive days till adequate fragmentation is achieved. An ERCP and pancreatic sphincterotomy is performed subsequently and fragments are cleared. A single pigtail plastic is placed in MPD in those patients who have achieved partial fragmentation as well as in the presence of associated stricture. These stents are removed at a subsequent follow-up between 3 and 6 months after the index procedure, once the MPD is free of any obstructive pathology. A few centers used IV secretin before ESWL as this creates a fluid stone interphase similar to ureteric calculi and results in successful fragmentation.[35] The successful use of a small, mobile, lithotripter has been reported in a small series of patients.[36]

For large radiolucent calculi not extracted at ERCP, a nasopancreatic tube (NPT) is placed in the MPD. This facilitates the use of contrast to localize the PC. The presence of the fluid around the PC also facilitates good fragmentation.[1,2,32] The rest of the protocol is similar to what has been detailed for the radio opaque calculi. An alternative for fragmenting radio lucent calculi would be the use of ultrasound for focusing on the PC, instead of placement of a NPT.

TECHNICAL AND CLINICAL SUCCESS

The following criteria are employed to assess the MPD clearance following ESWL.[1,2,32,37,38]

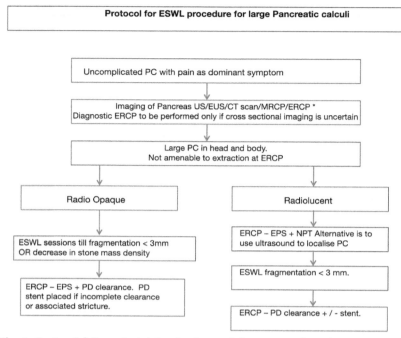

Fig. 1. Protocol followed at Asian Institute of Gastroenterology for extracorporeal shock wave lithotripsy of large PC (* if adequate information is not available with a single imaging technique, then a second imaging procedure was performed). CT, computed tomography; EPS, endoscopic pancreatic sphincterotomy; ERCP, endoscopic retrograde cholangiopancreatography; ESWL, extracorporeal shock wave lithotripsy; EUS, endoscopic ultrasound; MRCP, magnetic resonance cholangiopancreatography; NPT, nasopancreatic tube; PD, pancreatic duct; US, ultrasound. (*Data from* Refs.[1,2])

1. Complete clearance—clearance of >90% of stone volume.
2. Partial clearance—clearance between 50% and 90% of stone volume.
3. Unsuccessful clearance—clearance < 50% of stone volume.

Clinical success is usually assessed based on pain relief, reduction in number of analgesics used, reduction in number and days of hospitalization, and overall improvement in quality of life.

In our experience of over 5000 patients who have undergone ESWL, complete stone clearance was seen in 3722 out of 5124 patients (72.6%), partial clearance in 17.3%, and clearance was unsuccessful in the rest.[2] Significant pain relief was seen in 82.6% on 6 months follow-up (see **Table 1**) (**Figs. 2–4**).

An associated stricture was present in 1153 (22.5%) patients. More than 84% of the patients required three or lesser sessions of ESWL while 3.9% required five sessions or more (maximum of eight sessions) to achieve fragmentation (see **Table 1**).[2] Strictures have been reported approximately in 50% of patients with calculi in the head.[11]

Pain relief was evaluated in a meta-analysis of 27 studies with 3181 patients. ESWL achieved complete clearance in 70% and partial in 22% of patients.[38] On a 2-year follow-up, pain was absent in 52.7% and mild to moderate in 33.4%. Quality of life improved in 88.2% of patients.[38] Other studies have revealed that patients who have no pain relapse at 2 years, rarely have significant pain at a later period. This

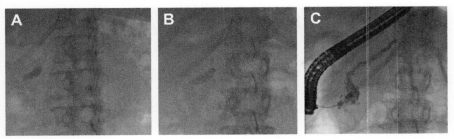

Fig. 2. ESWL procedure for radio opaque PC in the head. (*A*) Pre-ESWL dense radio opaque calculi in the head. (*B*). Post-ESWL reduction in stone density. (*C*) Pancreatic duct calculi fragments cleared during ERCP.

indicates that a good relief from pain in the first 2 years following ESWL is likely to be sustained for a longer period.[23,39] Complete stone clearance was seen in most of these patients with pain relief.

ESWL is established as a standard of care for the management of large PC in centers all over the world.[1,2,27,40–42] ESGE guidelines state that all patients with painful PC > 5 mm especially in the head region should undergo ESWL and subsequent ERCP to clear the MPD.[10,11] An earlier meta-analysis of 17 studies with 489 patients revealed ductal clearance rates between 37% and 100%.[43] A systemic review of over 1000 patients showed successful clearance in 89%.[44]

As CP, especially in our country, is a disease of the young, the long-term effects of ESWL on pain relief following stone clearance are important. Our own experience of 8 years of follow-up has revealed satisfactory pain relief in 60% of patients.[45] This follow-up has now extended to 18 years with similar results. Pain recurrence was present in a few patients even after complete ductal clearance indicating that other mechanisms of pain are also responsible for the pathogenesis.[8,32] Other studies revealed pain relapse between 30% and 50% of patients on follow-up of up to 14 years and 6.9% of these patients required surgery.[11] Similar long-term pain relief and avoidance of surgery have been reported elsewhere.[5,41,46,47] A retrospective long-term follow-up study of 120 patients showed complete pain relief in 50% of patients with avoidance of narcotic use. Partial relief was seen in up to 84% of patients.[48] Higher pain relief has been reported in our patients following treatment as compared to the West because of a higher incidence of alcohol, smoking, and use of opioids in the West.[49,50] It is also a possibility that our patients are more tolerant of pain.[2]

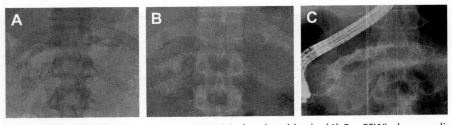

Fig. 3. ESWL procedure for radio opaque PC in head and body. (*A*) Pre-ESWL dense radio opaque calculi in head and proximal body. (*B*) Post-ESWL, majority of stones cleared. (*C*) Pancreatic duct calculi cleared during ERCP.

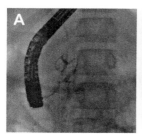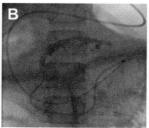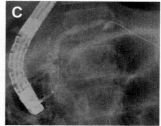

Fig. 4. ESWL procedure for radiolucent pancreatic stones. (*A*) Pre-ESWL multiple large radiolucent calculi in head. (*B*) NPT in situ to localize the calculi. (*C*) Post-ESWL fragmented calculi cleared at ERCP.

A recurrence rate of 22.8% has been reported in patients who had complete MPD clearance, over long-term follow-up.[1,2,47] However, pain recurrence was seen in much lesser numbers. The conclusion is that patients with asymptomatic recurrence of calculi need not undergo repeated endoscopic procedures. A comparison of results of ESWL from different centers is shown in **Table 2**.

COMPLICATIONS OF EXTRACORPOREAL SHOCK WAVE LITHOTRIPSY

ESWL is a safe procedure in large volume centers with very few serious adverse effects or mortality being reported. Our series of over 5000 patients had mild and self-limiting complications in 22% of patients.[2] These included pain at the site of contact of the water cushion in 13.5%, ecchymosis of skin at the site of contact in 19%, and mild pancreatitis in 3.5%.[1,2] Severe post-ESWL and post-ERCP pancreatitis were seen in 0.5% of patients. The incidence of pancreatitis is not higher in ESWL followed by ERCP as compared to ERCP alone. There was no mortality in the study.[2] A meta-analysis of over 1800 patients including 1000 from our center reported a complication rate of 5.8% with a single mortality (0.05%).[10] Another study reported an adverse event rate of 6.7% in over 1470 ESWL procedures.[51] Accurate focusing of the shock-waves on the PC is easier with third-generation lithotripters. This combined with restriction of patient movement with efficient anesthesia help in reducing collateral tissue damage and minimizing complication.[1,31,32,34] A number of rare complications

Table 2
Studies showing efficacy of extracorporeal shock wave lithotripsy for pancreatic calculi

Author	No. of Patients	Complete Clearance (%)	Pain Relief (%)	Follow-up (mo)
Tandan et al,[2] 2019	5124	72.9	82	6
Farnbacher et al,[14] 2002	125	64	48	29
Dumonaceau et al,[23] 2007	29	-	55	51
Delhaye et al,[27] 1992	123	59	85	14
Costamagna et al,[28] 1997	35	74	72	27
Tandan et al,[32] 2010	1006	76	84	6
Kozarek et al,[42] 2002	40	-	80	30
Tandan et al,[45] 2013	272	76	60	96
Adamek et al,[46] 1999	80	-	76	40

have been reported following ESWL. These include hepatic sub-capsular hematoma, biliary obstruction, splenic abscess and rupture, bowel perforation, necrotizing pancreatitis, and liver trauma.[33,52–54] Most of these have been reported in anecdotal case reports. Steinstrasse (street of stones) occurs due to acute stone incarceration at the papilla and may requires early ERCP and pancreatic sphincterotomy to reduce the pain.[11] As technology and techniques improve the incidence of these complications is likely to reduce further.

LIMITATIONS OF EXTRACORPOREAL SHOCK WAVE LITHOTRIPSY

Despite being the standard of care and widely used as the first-line therapy for the large PC, ESWL has limitations too.

1. Failure of fragmentation in approximately 10% of patients has been reported.[1,2] If such patients could be identified before ESWL, they could be subjected to an alternative procedure. Calculi with a density of over 820.5 HU on non-contrast CT (NCCT) have reduced fragmentation rates.[55] Use of NCCT for renal calculi has been reported earlier.[56,57] Another study reported better fragmentation when mean stone density was <375.4 HU on NCCT.[58] A validation of the cut-off value on NCCT could help avoid ESWL in those patients who have high stone density and are poor candidates for this procedure.
2. Recurrence of calculi has been reported in 23% of long-term follow-up.[1,2] Pharmacological agents such as Trimethadone have been successfully used on limited patients in Japan.[19,20] Development of such compounds which can dissolve recurring calculi can minimize repeated endoscopic interventions.
3. Effect of ESWL on the development of exocrine and endocrine insufficiency has not been clarified. Our own study reported improvement in diabetes in a few patients.[32] The numbers are, however, too small to draw any significant conclusion. A few studies reported improvement in both exocrine and endocrine functions, while others have failed to do so.[46,59,60] A recent long-term follow-up study from our center demonstrated that early ductal intervention in CP may delay the onset of diabetes.[61] It is possible that early intervention can alter the course of the disease and its various sequelae.
4. ESWL and its role in preventing the development of pancreatic carcinoma have not yet been evaluated.
5. Limitation in efficacy and success of fragmentation at ESWL has been reported in low-volume centers.[15,16]
6. Special precautions are needed in patients with implanted pacemakers and defibrillators.[62]

A topic of debate has been the use of ERCP after successful and complete fragmentation by ESWL. Two uncontrolled studies revealed that if ESWL is performed adequately, the fragments could spontaneously clear obviating the need for ERCP.[60,63] A randomized trial compared ESWL alone and ESWL followed by ERCP demonstrated equal efficacy between the two arms, but the cost of the procedure is higher in the patient who underwent both procedures.[23] In our experience, the calculi in idiopathic CP, commonly seen at our centers are denser and adherent, and as a practice, we perform ERCP after successful fragmentation.[1,2,32]

COMPARISON WITH OTHER MODALITIES OF TREATMENT OF PANCREATIC CALCULI

Single-operator pancreatoscopy with intraductal lithotripsy (SOPIL), either using EHL or LL is a technique in evolution, and a detailed discussion on comparison with ESWL as well as the pros and cons of surgical removal of PC is beyond the scope of this article. A study comparing 240 patients who underwent ESWL with 19 who underwent SOPIL concluded that both are safe and effective and SOPIL may require lesser sessions for complete fragmentation.[64] SOPIL is emerging as an attractive alternative to ESWL. ESGE guidelines, however, recommend that pancreatoscope guided lithotripsy be used when ESWL is not available or PC are not fragmented after an adequately performed ESWL.[11]

A recent study comparing early surgery versus endoscopy first approach on relief of pain in patients with CP reported that lower pain scores were seen in patients who underwent early surgery. This was a randomized clinical trial with 44 patients in each arm and authors have suggested that further studies are needed to replicate these findings.[65]

SUMMARY

ESWL is a safe and effective procedure for large PC not extracted by the standard technique at ERCP. In properly selected patients, it should be offered as the first line of therapy. Stone clearance as well as short- and long-term pain relief have been well established with this relatively safe procedure. At present, it is considered the standard of care in the management of large PC.

CLINICS CARE POINTS

- ESWL is a very effective technique for large radio opaque or radiolucent PC in uncomplicated painful CP as an alternative to surgery
- ESWL should be avoided in patients with extensive calculi, multiple pancreatic duct strictures, suspected head mass, and isolated pancreatic tail calculi
- ESWL can lead to complete stone clearance in three-fourths of patients.
- Long-term pain relief is achieved in nearly two-thirds of patients after ESWL
- Less than half of the patients require re-intervention after stone clearance with ESWL
- Future prospective studies need to compare this approach with intraductal lithotripsy

DISCLOSURE

None of the authors have any commercial or financial conflicts of interest and any funding sources to disclose.

REFERENCES

1. Tandan M, Talukdar R, Reddy DN. Management of pancreatic calculi: an update. Gut Liver 2016;10(6):873–80.
2. Tandan M, Nageshwar Reddy D, Talukdar R, et al. ESWL for large pancreatic calculi: report of over 5000 patients. Pancreatology 2019;19(7):916–21.
3. Chandak GR, Idris MM, Reddy DN, et al. Absence of PRSS1 mutations and association of SPINK1 trypsin inhibitor mutations in hereditary and non-hereditary chronic pancreatitis. Gut 2004;53(5):723–8.
4. Bhasin DK, Singh G, Rana SS, et al. Clinical profile of idiopathic chronic pancreatitis in North India. Clin Gastroenterol Hepatol 2009;7(5):594–9.

5. Rösch T, Daniel S, Scholz M, et al. Endoscopic treatment of chronic pancreatitis: a multicenter study of 1000 patients with long-term follow-up. Endoscopy 2002; 34(10):765–71.

6. Ammann RW, Akovbiantz A, Largiader F, et al. Course and outcome of chronic pancreatitis. Longitudinal study of a mixed medical-surgical series of 245 patients. Gastroenterology 1984;86(5 Pt 1):820–8.

7. Sharzehi K. Management of pancreatic duct stones. Curr Gastroenterol Rep 2019;21(11):63.

8. Talukdar R, Reddy DN. Pain in chronic pancreatitis: managing beyond the pancreatic duct. World J Gastroenterol 2013;19(38):6319–28.

9. Frulloni L, Gabbrielli A, Pezzilli R, et al. Chronic pancreatitis: report from a multicenter Italian survey (PanCroInfAISP) on 893 patients. Dig Liver Dis 2009;41(4): 311–7.

10. Dumonceau JM, Delhaye M, Tringali A, et al. Endoscopic treatment of chronic pancreatitis: European Society of Gastrointestinal Endoscopy (ESGE) Clinical Guideline. Endoscopy 2012;44(8):784–800.

11. Dumonceau JM, Delhaye M, Tringali A, et al. Endoscopic treatment of chronic pancreatitis: European Society of Gastrointestinal Endoscopy (ESGE) Guideline - Updated August 2018. Endoscopy 2019;51(2):179–93.

12. Pitchumoni CS, Viswanathan KV, Gee Varghese PJ, et al. Ultrastructure and elemental composition of human pancreatic calculi. Pancreas 1987;2(2):152–8.

13. Jin CX, Naruse S, Kitagawa M, et al. Pancreatic stone protein of pancreatic calculi in chronic calcified pancreatitis in man. Jop 2002;3(2):54–61.

14. Farnbacher MJ, Schoen C, Rabenstein T, et al. Pancreatic duct stones in chronic pancreatitis: criteria for treatment intensity and success. Gastrointest Endosc 2002;56(4):501–6.

15. Suzuki Y, Sugiyama M, Inui K, et al. Management for pancreatolithiasis: a Japanese multicenter study. Pancreas 2013;42(4):584–8.

16. Inui K, Masamune A, Igarashi Y, et al. Management of pancreatolithiasis: a nationwide survey in Japan. Pancreas 2018;47(6):708–14.

17. Thomas M, Howell DA, Carr-Locke D, et al. Mechanical lithotripsy of pancreatic and biliary stones: complications and available treatment options collected from expert centers. Am J Gastroenterol 2007;102(9):1896–902.

18. Sherman S, Lehman GA, Hawes RH, et al. Pancreatic ductal stones: frequency of successful endoscopic removal and improvement in symptoms. Gastrointest Endosc 1991;37(5):511–7.

19. Noda A, Hayakawa T, Kondo T, et al. Clinical evaluation of pancreatic excretion test with dimethadione and oral BT-PABA test in chronic pancreatitis. Dig Dis Sci 1983;28(3):230–5.

20. Hamano K, Noda A, Ibuki E, et al. Oral litholysis in patients with chronic calcific pancreatitis unresponsive to or ineligible for extracorporeal shock wave lithotripsy and endoscopic therapy. Digestion 2019;100(1):55–63.

21. Díte P, Ruzicka M, Zboril V, et al. A prospective, randomized trial comparing endoscopic and surgical therapy for chronic pancreatitis. Endoscopy 2003; 35(7):553–8.

22. Cahen DL, Gouma DJ, Nio Y, et al. Endoscopic versus surgical drainage of the pancreatic duct in chronic pancreatitis. N Engl J Med 2007;356(7):676–84.

23. Dumonceau JM, Costamagna G, Tringali A, et al. Treatment for painful calcified chronic pancreatitis: extracorporeal shock wave lithotripsy versus endoscopic treatment: a randomised controlled trial. Gut 2007;56(4):545–52.

24. Jiang L, Ning D, Cheng Q, et al. Endoscopic versus surgical drainage treatment of calcific chronic pancreatitis. Int J Surg 2018;54(Pt A):242–7.

25. Chaussy C, Schmiedt E, Jocham D, et al. First clinical experience with extracorporeally induced destruction of kidney stones by shock waves. J Urol 1982; 127(3):417–20.

26. Sauerbruch T, Stern M. Fragmentation of bile duct stones by extracorporeal shock waves. A new approach to biliary calculi after failure of routine endoscopic measures. Gastroenterology 1989;96(1):146–52.

27. Delhaye M, Vandermeeren A, Baize M, et al. Extracorporeal shock-wave lithotripsy of pancreatic calculi. Gastroenterology 1992;102(2):610–20.

28. Costamagna G, Gabbrielli A, Mutignani M, et al. Extracorporeal shock wave lithotripsy of pancreatic stones in chronic pancreatitis: immediate and medium-term results. Gastrointest Endosc 1997;46(3):231–6.

29. Delhaye M, Arvanitakis M, Bali M, et al. Endoscopic therapy for chronic pancreatitis. Scand J Surg 2005;94(2):143–53.

30. Tandan M, Reddy DN. Extracorporeal shock wave lithotripsy for pancreatic and large common bile duct stones. World J Gastroenterol 2011;17(39):4365–71.

31. Ong WC, Tandan M, Reddy V, et al. Multiple main pancreatic duct stones in tropical pancreatitis: safe clearance with extracorporeal shockwave lithotripsy. J Gastroenterol Hepatol 2006;21(10):1514–8.

32. Tandan M, Reddy DN, Santosh D, et al. Extracorporeal shock wave lithotripsy and endotherapy for pancreatic calculi-a large single center experience. Indian J Gastroenterol 2010;29(4):143–8.

33. Leifsson BG, Borgström A, Ahlgren G. Splenic rupture following ESWL for a pancreatic duct calculus. Dig Surg 2001;18(3):229–30.

34. Darisetty S, Tandan M, Reddy DN, et al. Epidural anesthesia is effective for extracorporeal shock wave lithotripsy of pancreatic and biliary calculi. World J Gastrointest Surg 2010;2(5):165–8.

35. Choi EK, McHenry L, Watkins JL, et al. Use of intravenous secretin during extracorporeal shock wave lithotripsy to facilitate endoscopic clearance of pancreatic duct stones. Pancreatology 2012;12(3):272–5.

36. Milovic V, Wehrmann T, Dietrich CF, et al. Extracorporeal shock wave lithotripsy with a transportable mini-lithotripter and subsequent endoscopic treatment improves clinical outcome in obstructive calcific chronic pancreatitis. Gastrointest Endosc 2011;74(6):1294–9.

37. McHenry L, Watkins JL, Kopecky K, et al. Extracorporeal shock-wave lithoptripsy for pancreatic calculi: a 10-year experience at a single U.S. center. Gastrointest Endosc 2004;59(5):P205.

38. Moole H, Jaeger A, Bechtold ML, et al. Success of extracorporeal shock wave lithotripsy in chronic calcific pancreatitis management: a meta-analysis and systematic review. Pancreas 2016;45(5):651–8.

39. Tadenuma H, Ishihara T, Yamaguchi T, et al. Long-term results of extracorporeal shockwave lithotripsy and endoscopic therapy for pancreatic stones. Clin Gastroenterol Hepatol 2005;3(11):1128–35.

40. Neuhaus H. Fragmentation of pancreatic stones by extracorporeal shock wave lithotripsy. Endoscopy 1991;23(3):161–5.

41. Dumonceau JM, Devière J, Le Moine O, et al. Endoscopic pancreatic drainage in chronic pancreatitis associated with ductal stones: long-term results. Gastrointest Endosc 1996;43(6):547–55.

42. Kozarek RA, Brandabur JJ, Ball TJ, et al. Clinical outcomes in patients who undergo extracorporeal shock wave lithotripsy for chronic calcific pancreatitis. Gastrointest Endosc 2002;56(4):496–500.
43. Guda NM, Partington S, Freeman ML. Extracorporeal shock wave lithotripsy in the management of chronic calcific pancreatitis: a meta-analysis. Jop 2005; 6(1):6–12.
44. Nguyen-Tang T, Dumonceau JM. Endoscopic treatment in chronic pancreatitis, timing, duration and type of intervention. Best Pract Res Clin Gastroenterol 2010;24(3):281–98.
45. Tandan M, Reddy DN, Talukdar R, et al. Long-term clinical outcomes of extracorporeal shockwave lithotripsy in painful chronic calcific pancreatitis. Gastrointest Endosc 2013;78(5):726–33.
46. Adamek HE, Jakobs R, Buttmann A, et al. Long term follow up of patients with chronic pancreatitis and pancreatic stones treated with extracorporeal shock wave lithotripsy. Gut 1999;45(3):402–5.
47. Delhaye M, Arvanitakis M, Verset G, et al. Long-term clinical outcome after endoscopic pancreatic ductal drainage for patients with painful chronic pancreatitis. Clin Gastroenterol Hepatol 2004;2(12):1096–106.
48. Seven G, Schreiner MA, Ross AS, et al. Long-term outcomes associated with pancreatic extracorporeal shock wave lithotripsy for chronic calcific pancreatitis. Gastrointest Endosc 2012;75(5):997–1004.e1.
49. Bhardwaj P, Garg PK, Maulik SK, et al. A randomized controlled trial of antioxidant supplementation for pain relief in patients with chronic pancreatitis. Gastroenterology 2009;136(1):149–59.e2.
50. Siriwardena AK, Mason JM, Sheen AJ, et al. Antioxidant therapy does not reduce pain in patients with chronic pancreatitis: the ANTICIPATE study. Gastroenterology 2012;143(3):655–63.e1.
51. Li BR, Liao Z, Du TT, et al. Risk factors for complications of pancreatic extracorporeal shock wave lithotripsy. Endoscopy 2014;46(12):1092–100.
52. Hirata N, Kushida Y, Ohguri T, et al. Hepatic subcapsular hematoma after extracorporeal shock wave lithotripsy (ESWL) for pancreatic stones. J Gastroenterol 1999;34(6):713–6.
53. Plaisier PW, den Hoed PT. Splenic abscess after lithotripsy of pancreatic duct stones. Dig Surg 2001;18(3):231–2.
54. Karakayali F, Sevmiş S, Ayvaz I, et al. Acute necrotizing pancreatitis as a rare complication of extracorporeal shock wave lithotripsy. Int J Urol 2006;13(5): 613–5.
55. Ohyama H, Mikata R, Ishihara T, et al. Efficacy of stone density on noncontrast computed tomography in predicting the outcome of extracorporeal shock wave lithotripsy for patients with pancreatic stones. Pancreas 2015;44(3):422–8.
56. Pareek G, Hedican SP, Lee FT Jr, et al. Shock wave lithotripsy success determined by skin-to-stone distance on computed tomography. Urology 2005;66(5): 941–4.
57. Lee HY, Yang YH, Lee YL, et al. Noncontrast computed tomography factors that predict the renal stone outcome after shock wave lithotripsy. Clin Imaging 2015; 39(5):845–50.
58. Liu R, Su W, Wang J, et al. Quantitative factors of unenhanced CT for predicting fragmenting efficacy of extracorporeal shock wave lithotripsy on pancreatic duct stones. Clin Radiol 2019;74(5):408, e1-e7.
59. Schneider HT, May A, Benninger J, et al. Piezoelectric shock wave lithotripsy of pancreatic duct stones. Am J Gastroenterol 1994;89(11):2042–8.

60. Inui K, Tazuma S, Yamaguchi T, et al. Treatment of pancreatic stones with extra-corporeal shock wave lithotripsy: results of a multicenter survey. Pancreas 2005; 30(1):26–30.
61. Talukdar R, Reddy DN, Tandan M, et al. Impact of ductal interventions on diabetes in patients with chronic pancreatitis. J Gastroenterol Hepatol 2021;36(5): 1226–34.
62. Crossley GH, Poole JE, Rozner MA, et al. The Heart Rhythm Society (HRS)/American Society of Anesthesiologists (ASA) Expert Consensus Statement on the perioperative management of patients with implantable defibrillators, pacemakers and arrhythmia monitors: facilities and patient management this document was developed as a joint project with the American Society of Anesthesiologists (ASA), and in collaboration with the American Heart Association (AHA), and the Society of Thoracic Surgeons (STS). Heart Rhythm 2011;8(7):1114–54.
63. Ohara H, Hoshino M, Hayakawa T, et al. Single application extracorporeal shock wave lithotripsy is the first choice for patients with pancreatic duct stones. Am J Gastroenterol 1996;91(7):1388–94.
64. Bick BL, Patel F, Easler JJ, et al. A comparative study between single-operator pancreatoscopy with intraductal lithotripsy and extracorporeal shock wave lithotripsy for the management of large main pancreatic duct stones. Surg Endosc 2022;36(5):3217–26.
65. Issa Y, Kempeneers MA, Bruno MJ, et al. Effect of early surgery vs endoscopy-first approach on pain in patients with chronic pancreatitis: the ESCAPE Randomized clinical trial. JAMA 2020;323(3):237–47.

Management of Pancreatic Duct Stones

Nonextracorporeal Approach

Christian Gerges[a],*, Torsten Beyna[b], Horst Neuhaus[c]

KEYWORDS

- Chronic pancreatitis • Pancreatic duct stones • Pancreatoscopy • Pancreatic calculi
- Electrohydraulic lithotripsy

KEY POINTS

- Endoscopic treatment of pancreatic duct stones in patients with chronic pancreatitis is safe and effective and considered as first-line treatment.
- The aim of any endoscopic therapy is to achieve complete duct clearance.
- Pancreatoscopy-guided lithotripsy is a highly effective procedure to achieve complete duct clearance with low adverse event rates in the hands of experts.

INTRODUCTION

Chronic pancreatitis (CP) is a continuous inflammatory condition that impairs pancreatic function by causing fibrotic remodeling of the pancreatic tissue and exocrine and endocrine insufficiency. In a 1761 autopsy report, Jean-Baptista Morgagni made the first mention of CP. Capparelli performed the first successful surgical excision of a pancreatic calculus in 1883. One hundred years later, the first endoscopic pancreatic sphincterotomy was carried out to remove pancreatic duct (PD) stones using a basket. In 1994, Howell and colleagues provided the first description of the removal of main pancreatic duct (MPD) stones while using a 10FR infant endoscope and an electrohydraulic lithotripsy (EHL) probe.

The prevalence of CP is increasing, with a global incidence of 1.6 to 23 per 100.000 people. Pain is the dominant symptom of CP resulting in a reduction of quality of life, unemployment, and major health-care costs.[1] The pathophysiology of pain in CP is multifactorial but is mainly generated by localized pathologic condition, that is, focal PD obstruction leading to ductal hypertension, a localized inflammatory mass,

[a] University Hospital Essen, Essen, North Rhine-Westphalia, Germany; [b] EVLK Duesseldorf, Kirchfeldstr. 40, 40489, Duesseldorf, Germany; [c] RKM 740 Clinic, Pariserstr. 98, 40549, Duesseldorf, Germany
* Corresponding author. Universitätsklinikum Essen, Abteilung Interventionelle gastroenterologische Endoskopie, Hufelandstraße, 55D-45147, Essen
E-mail address: christian.gerges@uk-essen.de

Gastrointest Endoscopy Clin N Am 33 (2023) 821–829
https://doi.org/10.1016/j.giec.2023.04.001
giendo.theclinics.com
1052-5157/23/© 2023 Elsevier Inc. All rights reserved.

elevated interstitial fluid pressure, ischemia, and inflammatory injury to pancreatic neurons are a few of the mechanisms that may contribute to the origin of pain.[2–5] Due to the different causes of pain, it can be challenging to identify the primary cause in a given situation, and there are no established metrics for gauging how well certain therapeutic approaches will work. An increase in ductal and parenchymal pressure that causes discomfort is thought to be indicated by a dilatation of the primary PD of more than 5 mm. Analgesics are the cornerstone of pancreatic pain management.[6] CP with obstruction of the PD is associated with intraductal calculi in 50% of patients, of which 18% is caused by PD stones and 32% due to a combination of PD stricture and PD stones.[7] Invasive treatment with endoscopic PD clearance, either with or without extracorporeal shock wave lithotripsy (ESWL), PD dilatation, and/or PD stenting, is the next course of action in the event that analgesic medication fails.[3,8] According to Guideline recommendations, the first-line treatment of painful, simple CP with an obstruction of the MPD in the head or body of the pancreas should be endoscopic therapy and/or ESWL.[1,8] The justification for invasive procedures is that increasing pancreatic juice flow will relieve pain by lowering ductal pressure.[8] The main limitations of ESWL include limited availability, nonreimbursement, need for (general) anesthesia, variable efficacy (due to operator experience and/or PD stone location and size), adverse events (AEs) and in case of predominant PD strictures, the frequent need for an additional endoscopic retrograde cholangiopancreatography (ERCP).[1,8,9] In addition, calculi with density of greater than 820.5 Hounsfield units seem to respond less effectively to ESWL.[10] Surgery is an additional option in the therapy of CP. The results of the ESCAPE trial have led to an intensive discussion whether early surgery might be the better option for symptomatic patients with CP.[11] However, even in this prospective randomized controlled trial, the difference in Izbicki pain score was statistically not significant during long-term follow-up. Looking into the subgroup analysis of this study, endoscopically treated patients with complete duct clearance perform equally to the surgical arm while patients with partial duct clearance have a significantly worse outcome.

In patients with CP and PD dilatation, digital single-operator pancreatoscopy (DSOP)-guided lithotripsy seems to be an appealing option to ESWL and surgery, especially if the aim is to achieve complete duct clearance.[12,13] DSOP can also be paired with an additional intervention, such as PD stricture dilatation and/or PD stenting, in a single session. Recent meta-analysis of DSOP for tough PD stones revealed a 91% technical success rate and a 14% adverse event rate.[12] DSOP has demonstrated potential in the management of CP. Although former studies have been restricted by a retrospective design, very small patient populations, short follow-up, lack of relevant clinical outcomes, varied patient selection/treatment regimens, and single-center designs, more and more promising prospective data has been published recently.[4,5,14,15]

INDICATIONS

The main indication for endoscopic therapy in chronic calcifying pancreatitis is pain. In case of intraductal stones, endoscopic treatment can help to reduce the intraductal pressure by restoring a sufficient drainage of the MPD. A recent publication showed that achieving a complete duct clearance can lead to a significant size reduction of the MPD and was correlated with pain reduction.[14] This supports the hypothesis that a high intraductal pressure is a main reason for pain in chronic calcifying pancreatitis. However, not every stone case can be managed endoscopically, which makes the selection of the proper candidate crucial for the prevention of AEs and a successful endoscopic treatment. Following the above-mentioned principles, a patient with a

MPD full of stones in head, body, and tail or only in the tail is very unlikely to benefit from an endoscopic approach but has a high risk of complications. The same applies to endoscopic therapy for side branch stones.[16] Patients with 3 or lesser stones in head or body with a dilatated MPD of 5 mm or greater have been shown to be good candidates for an endoscopic approach.[14,17,18] An accurate diagnosis is therefore crucial in order to plan the best treatment strategy for the individual patient. Pre-interventional diagnostic tests should include MRCP or CT and an endoscopic ultrasound. This helps to assess the exact number, position, and size of the stones. It reveals anatomic variances such as pancreas divisum. In this example, it would change the point of access of the PD from major to minor papilla. Ultimately, it clarifies if an endoscopic approach is even possible.

SYSTEMS AND TECHNIQUES

Before attempting to extract pancreatic stones, a sphincterotomy should be performed via a sphincterotome and over a guidewire. This can be done in the major and minor papilla if needed that is, in case of a pancreas divisum. To reduce the risk of post-ERCP pancreatitis through secondary thermal damage, the setting of the electrosurgical device should have less coagulation. Acute pancreatitis (2% to 7%), hemorrhage (0% to 2%), and perforations (1%) are among the early complications of pancreatic sphincterotomy, whereas sphincter stenosis (up to 10%) is a late complication. These risks are similar to those of biliary sphincterotomy.[18–21] In addition, a small balloon sphincteroplasty up to 4 to 6 mm can be performed especially in case of a stricture in the pancreatic head.[14,18] The use of a rat tooth forceps has been described but does not play a major role in standard clinical practice because it is difficult to maneuver the forceps and includes a certain risk of pancreatic trauma and perforation.[22]

Fluoroscopy-Assisted Lithotripsy

After securing a safe and adequate access for stone extraction, baskets or balloons can be used to extract the stones. One of the most common AEs is a trapped or broken basket during stone extraction.[23] Biliary baskets are less likely to break than pancreatic stone baskets and have the option of emergency lithotripsy in case of impaction although they are more difficult to maneuver and less effective in smaller ducts.[24] Another option is to perform mechanical lithotripsy. Due to the higher risk of failure and complications associated with mechanical lithotripsy, it is used less frequently than biliary stone lithotripsy.[25] Stone extraction balloons have shown to be safer because they can be deflated and usually easily extracted if they are trapped.[26] Sharp edges of the pancreatic stones can make this method less effective as they can puncture and destroy the balloon.

Lithotripsy Under Direct Visualization

Visualization systems

In 1976, peroral cholangioscopy and pancreatoscopy were introduced into clinical practice because of technological advancements in fiberoptic duodenoscopy and the development of small caliber flexible fiberoptic instruments.[27–29] For another 23 years, cholangio-pancreaticoscopy could only be used for visualization and had no therapeutic potential. In 1999, Howell used a 10FR fiberoptic "through the scope" endoscope from Olympus Medical Systems Corporation in Tokyo, Japan, to perform therapeutic peroral pancreatoscopy under direct visualization in MPD.[30] In contrast to direct peroral pancreatoscopy, the "mother–baby" procedure is the peroral pancreatoscopy method that is most frequently used. Although the mother–baby technique requires 2 experienced endoscopists, the available reusable scopes are very fragile, have high initial and repair costs, and only offer a small amount of maneuverability and poor irrigation capabilities.[31] As a result, the technique has never gained widespread acceptance in clinical routine. Olympus Medical Systems Corporation, Tokyo, Japan, created a prototype video infant endoscope, which is still being tested in clinical trials.

Single-operator cholangioscopy technology has been developed and introduced in 2007 to address some of the aforementioned constraints (SpyGlass DVS; Boston Scientific, Natick, Mass, US). The old system included a fiberoptic probe with subpar image quality for vision together with a disposable 10F delivery catheter with 4-way deflection capability and specialized irrigation channels. The single-operator digital video cholangioscopy system (SpyGlass DS, Boston Scientific Natick, Massachusetts, US) was introduced in 2015. With a 60% wider field of vision, a larger working channel (1.3 mm), a specialized irrigation channel, and an additional succinate option, the novel technology provides high-resolution imaging. In tertiary referral centers in particular, the SpyGlass technology has increased the use of peroral pancreatoscopy, at least as a third-line option for the treatment of complex pancreatic stones. ERCP requires fragmentation of complicated, difficult-to-extract, and occasionally cast-like stones to allow stone extraction.

Fragmentation systems

EHL and laser lithotripsy (LL) can achieve intraductal lithotripsy despite mechanical lithotripsy and ESWL. EHL-technique comprises a charge generator and a bipolar probe that produces sparks at its tip in an aqueous solution. The sparks produce a vapor plasma and subsequently an oscillating cavitation bubble surrounding the probe's tip. Three different shockwave pulses are generated simultaneously. The first shockwave is generated by the rapid expansion of the vapor plasma, whereas the second and third shockwaves are generated by the cavitation bubble rebounding. Stones nearby absorb the energy of these high-frequency hydraulic pressure waves, resulting in their fragmentation.[32] If the probe is not deployed near to the stone and away from the ductal wall, the shock waves may induce unintended damage or perforation of the bile duct wall. EHL can be conducted using centering balloons or direct cholangioscopic vision under fluoroscopic guidance. The downside of using solely fluoroscopic guidance is the 2-dimensional imaging and inability to validate the probe's precise location. Therefore, direct viewing is typically favored to prevent ductal wall injury. EHL equipment is compact, does not require special electricity, and is reasonably priced.

In LL, laser light of a specific wavelength is concentrated on the stone's surface to produce wave-mediated fragmentation. In 1986, researchers reported the first effective use of a pulsed laser for shock-wave lithotripsy of bile duct stones.[33] Laser technology is often hampered by its lack of portability, its expensive price, and the availability of more affordable alternatives.[34] A neodymium:yttrium-aluminum-garnet (Nd:YAG) laser produces a local shockwave effect, whereas a flash lamp-pulsed laser's mechanism is thermal. The frequency-doubled, double-pulse Nd:YAG system, composed of 532-nm green light (20%) and 1064-nm infrared light (80%), breaks stones by the production of plasma on their surface, which subsequently absorbs the infrared light energy powerfully and generates a strong shockwave. Holmium:YAG lithotripsy fragments stones largely via a photothermal mechanism in which the laser transmits energy directly to the stone.[35] This mechanism is fundamentally distinct from other LL techniques and depends on laser energy absorption of light with a longer wavelength of around 2100 nm on the surface of the stone as well as in the surrounding fluid. At the stone's surface, stone material is melted and ejected. This is then carried away by a vapor bubble produced by the absorption of laser energy by water.[36] Because the holmium laser emits a high amount of effective energy, it is essential to have clear ductal vision to prevent accidental bile duct injury. When performed under cholangioscopic or pancreatoscopic direct vision, the procedure has an excellent safety profile.[36] The first report of Holmium:YAG LL for biliary stones was made in 1998.[35] However, there are limited reports of holmium LL for PD stone removal.[36] There is currently no prospective study comparing the efficacy and safety of these 2 distinct lithotripsy procedures for pancreatic calculi. These 2 main fragmentation techniques can be used individually or combined depending on the success of each system in the target stone. Till date, there is no comparative study evaluating which of these techniques is more effective in pancreatic stone fragmentation.

Technique
To be able to enter the MPD, usually a sphincterotomy and/or a pancreatic sphincteroplasty of 4 mm is necessary. In case of a stricture in front of the stone a step-up dilatation up to 10 FR should be performed before attempting DSOP. The access into the MPD can be simplified by using a guidewire. Stones in the pancreatic head are no contraindication for DSOP.[14] After approaching the stone, lithotripsy can be performed under direct vision. Irrigation should be reduced to a necessary minimum and the patient should receive nonsteroidal anti-inflammatory drugs and saline infusion to reduce the risk of post-ERCP pancreatitis.[14] After DSOP-guided lithotripsy, a large bore stent (8-10 FR) should be placed especially in case of a stricture.[14]

OUTCOMES OF ENDOSCOPIC THERAPY

1. Conventional ERCP: Especially with large symptomatic PD stones, a combination of ERCP and ESWL has the best chance for technical success defined as complete or partial duct clearance and clinical success with complete or partial pain relief.[7,9,37] Therefore, only a small number of studies evaluated the success for ERCP-guided therapy alone. Published clinical success rates are around 65% during long-term follow up.[38,39]

2. DSOP-guided lithotripsy: DSOP-guided lithotripsy is a promising alternative for ESWL in patients with chronic calcifying pancreatitis. From 1999 until 2022, DSOP-guided lithotripsy was mostly reported in small case reports or retrospective trials with mixed population and treatment regimens and, often, a single-center design. Overall success rates in various reviews and meta-analysis are around 91% with adverse event rates around 14%.[4,5,13] In addition, DSOP-guided lithotripsy seems to have a positive effect on quality of life in successfully treated patients up to 95%.[13] A case series of 34 patients reported a complete or partial duct clearance in 70.6% (24/34). Izbicki pain score at 6 months follow-up significantly reduced from 62.3 to 27.5 ($P < .001$). AEs were reported in 40% (10/25) of the cases with 7 cases of post-ERCP pancreatitis. The data of this trial must be interpreted with caution. Previous ERCP with stent therapy was not an exclusion criterion, and in one case, the patient received additional ESWL therapy.[15] In 2022, an international, prospective, multicenter cohort trial was published including only treatment naive patients with a maximum of 3 lumen occluding stones5 mm or greater in head, genu, or body and a dilated MPD.[14] Technical success defined as complete stone clearance was demonstrated in 90% (N = 36/40). Approximately 1.4 procedures were needed to achieve complete stone clearance. MPD diameter was significantly reduced from 8.4 $\pm$ 2.9(35) to 4.9 $\pm$ 1.9(35) (-3.7 ± 2.8(35), $P < .001$). Overall pain relief was reported in 82.4% (N = 28/34)

after 6 months follow-up.[14] The significant change of the MPD after complete stone clearance goes in line with the reduction of pain in this cohort. This underlines the importance of decompression, a key treatment goal in patients with CP. It must be further investigated if the MPD diameter can be another objective parameter for treatment evaluation. However, the results of this study seem to be more realistic taking the structured follow-up and the use of Izbicki pain score (IPS) into account. Hence, only small data are available regarding the clinical success in a long-term follow-up. Reported data suggest a persistent beneficial effect in 80% of the patients on symptom control and quality of life during a long-term follow-up of 36 to 62 months.[40]

DISCUSSION

The treatment of chronic calcifying pancreatitis is very challenging. Patients present mostly with a combination of challenges such as stones, strictures, portal vein thrombosis, and others.[5,10] ESWL mostly in combination with ERCP in the therapy for large intraductal calculi is still the standard therapy in the endoscopic treatment of these patients.[10] For various reasons, ESWL is increasingly limited in access especially in the western world. One reason might be that it lost more of its value in urology, which was often the department in which these devices were used for patients with CP. In addition, most patients need a stenting therapy after successful stone clearance, which makes additional ERCP procedures necessary.[14] It remains unclear if DSOP-guided lithotripsy is cost effective but given the small number of procedures needed to achieve clinical and technical success and the possibility to perform lithotripsy and stricture management in one procedure, it is likely that this therapy has a positive cost–benefit effect. The latest publications especially from the ESCAPE trial suggest an early surgery in the treatment of these patients to not waste precious time in the sufficient treatment and to prevent long-term chronification of the symptoms.[11] CP is an ongoing inflammatory disease. It is therefore still unclear if an invasive intervention such as a surgery can result in a long-term symptom relief, particularly given that surgical data show a high number of patients who experience persistent pain and drug dependence during long-term FU.[10,14] In addition, long-term complications such as anastomotic strictures or significant morbidity must be considered. Real-life data of morbidity and mortality of pancreatic surgery outside of international tertiary referral centers show a significant number of in-hospital mortality rate above 10%.[41] This must be carefully discussed with the patient before referring to surgery and an endoscopic treatment seems to be a safer first-line approach before considering surgery. More data are necessary to compare endoscopic therapy with ESWL and/or DSOP-guided lithotripsy and surgery. As chronic calcifying pancreatitis is a complex disease with various symptoms, it is very likely that it will be hard to define a standard procedure for each patient. Therefore, these therapeutic options should not be considered competitive rather than different approaches in different disease stages in the life of a patient. This makes the discussion of these patients in a multidisciplinary board mandatory because at each stage, all available options should be weighed against each other in a shared decision process.

In conclusion, DSOP-guided lithotripsy for the treatment of large symptomatic PD-stones has been demonstrated to be safe, technically, and clinically effective, and should be regarded as an alternative endoscopic treatment of certain patients. However, the technique is challenging and should be limited to specialized centers for advanced endoscopy. Further randomized controlled trials focusing on total duct clearance are required to determine the function of DSOP in the complex treatment options for patients with CP.

CLINICS CARE POINTS

- When ESWL fails or is not available DSOP-guided lithotripsy is an alternative treatment of certain patients.
- When treating PD stones, always aim to achieve complete duct clearance.
- After endoscopic treatment of PD stones, a consequent stricture therapy for ductal strictures is essential.

DISCLOSURE

The authors have nothing to disclose.

REFERENCES

1. Lohr JM, et al. United European Gastroenterology evidence-based guidelines for the diagnosis and therapy of chronic pancreatitis (HaPanEU). United European Gastroenterol J 2017;5(2):153–99.
2. Anderson MA, et al. Mechanism, assessment and management of pain in chronic pancreatitis: Recommendations of a multidisciplinary study group. Pancreatology 2016;16(1):83–94.
3. Kitano M, et al. International consensus guidelines on interventional endoscopy in chronic pancreatitis. Recommendations from the working group for the international consensus guidelines for chronic pancreatitis in collaboration with the International Association of Pancreatology, the American Pancreatic Association, the Japan Pancreas Society, and European Pancreatic Club. Pancreatology 2020; 20(6):1045–55.
4. Gerges C, et al. Pancreatoscopy in endoscopic treatment of pancreatic duct stones, systematic review. Minerva Chir 2018;74(4):334–47.
5. Beyna T, Neuhaus H, Gerges C. Endoscopic treatment of pancreatic duct stones under direct vision: Revolution or resignation? Systematic review. Dig Endosc 2017;30(1):29–37.
6. Drewes AM, et al. Guidelines for the understanding and management of pain in chronic pancreatitis. Pancreatology 2017;17(5):720–31.
7. Rösch T, et al. Endoscopic treatment of chronic pancreatitis: a multicenter study of 1000 patients with long-term follow-up. Endoscopy 2002;34(10):765–71.
8. Dumonceau JM, et al. Endoscopic treatment of chronic pancreatitis: European Society of Gastrointestinal Endoscopy (ESGE) Guideline - Updated August 2018. Endoscopy 2019;51(2):179–93.
9. Tandan M, Talukdar R, Reddy DN. Management of Pancreatic Calculi: An Update. Gut Liver 2016;10(6):873–80.
10. Dumonceau JM, et al. Endoscopic treatment of chronic pancreatitis: European Society of Gastrointestinal Endoscopy (ESGE) Clinical Guideline. Endoscopy 2012;44(8):784–800.
11. Issa Y, et al. Effect of Early Surgery vs Endoscopy-First Approach on Pain in Patients With Chronic Pancreatitis: The ESCAPE Randomized Clinical Trial. JAMA 2020;323(3):237–47.
12. McCarty TR, Sobani Z, Rustagi T. Per-oral pancreatoscopy with intraductal lithotripsy for difficult pancreatic duct stones: a systematic review and meta-analysis. Endosc Int Open 2020;8(10):E1460–70.

13. Gerges C, et al. SpyGlass DS-guided lithotripsy for pancreatic duct stones in symptomatic treatment-refractory chronic calcifying pancreatitis. Endosc Int Open 2019;7(2):E99–103.

14. Gerges C, et al. Digital single-operator pancreatoscopy for the treatment of symptomatic pancreatic duct stones: a prospective multicenter cohort trial. Endoscopy 2022;55(2):150–7.

15. van der Wiel SE, et al. Pancreatoscopy-guided electrohydraulic lithotripsy for the treatment of obstructive pancreatic duct stones: a prospective consecutive case series. Gastrointest Endosc 2022;95(5):905–914 e2.

16. Tringali A, Boskoski I, Costamagna G. The role of endoscopy in the therapy of chronic pancreatitis. Best Pract Res Clin Gastroenterol 2008;22(1):145–65.

17. Liu BN, et al. Pancreatic duct stones in patients with chronic pancreatitis: surgical outcomes. Hepatobiliary Pancreat Dis Int 2010;9(4):423–7.

18. Kim YH, et al. Endoscopic treatment of pancreatic calculi. Clin Endosc 2014; 47(3):227–35.

19. Cotton PB, et al. Endoscopic sphincterotomy complications and their management: an attempt at consensus. Gastrointest Endosc 1991;37(3):383–93.

20. Freeman ML, et al. Complications of endoscopic biliary sphincterotomy. N Engl J Med 1996;335(13):909–18.

21. Masci E, et al. Complications of diagnostic and therapeutic ERCP: a prospective multicenter study. Am J Gastroenterol 2001;96(2):417–23.

22. Choi EK, Lehman GA. Update on endoscopic management of main pancreatic duct stones in chronic calcific pancreatitis. Korean J Intern Med 2012;27(1):20–9.

23. Thomas M, et al. Mechanical lithotripsy of pancreatic and biliary stones: complications and available treatment options collected from expert centers. Am J Gastroenterol 2007;102(9):1896–902.

24. Payne WG, Norman JG, Pinkas H. Endoscopic basket impaction. Am Surg 1995; 61(5):464–7.

25. Freeman ML. Mechanical lithotripsy of pancreatic duct stones. Gastrointest Endosc 1996;44(3):333–6.

26. Committee AT, et al. Biliary and pancreatic stone extraction devices. Gastrointest Endosc 2009;70(4):603–9.

27. Kawai K, et al. [A new endoscopic method: the peroral choledochopancreatoscopy (author's transl)]. Leber Magen Darm 1976;6(2):121–4.

28. Nakajima M, et al. Peroral cholangiopancreatosocopy (PCPS) under duodenoscopic guidance. Am J Gastroenterol 1976;66(3):241–7.

29. Nakajima M, et al. Direct endoscopic visualization of the bile and pancreatic duct systems by peroral cholangiopancreatoscopy (PCPS). Gastrointest Endosc 1978;24(4):141–5.

30. Howell DA, et al. Endoscopic treatment of pancreatic duct stones using a 10F pancreatoscope and electrohydraulic lithotripsy. Gastrointest Endosc 1999; 50(6):829–33.

31. Chen YK. Preclinical characterization of the Spyglass peroral cholangiopancreatoscopy system for direct access, visualization, and biopsy. Gastrointest Endosc 2007;65(2):303–11.

32. Koch H, Stolte M, Walz V. Endoscopic lithotripsy in the common bile duct. Endoscopy 1977;9(2):95–8.

33. Lux G, et al. The first successful endoscopic retrograde laser lithotripsy of common bile duct stones in man using a pulsed neodymium-YAG laser. Endoscopy 1986;18(4):144–5.

34. Ohara H, et al. Single application extracorporeal shock wave lithotripsy is the first choice for patients with pancreatic duct stones. Am J Gastroenterol 1996;91(7): 1388–94.
35. Vassar GJ, et al. Holmium: YAG lithotripsy: photothermal mechanism. J Endourol 1999;13(3):181–90.
36. Maydeo A, et al. Single-operator cholangioscopy-guided laser lithotripsy in patients with difficult biliary and pancreatic ductal stones (with videos). Gastrointest Endosc 2011;74(6):1308–14.
37. Tandan M, et al. Extracorporeal shock wave lithotripsy and endotherapy for pancreatic calculi-a large single center experience. Indian J Gastroenterol 2010;29(4):143–8.
38. Binmoeller KF, et al. Endoscopic pancreatic stent drainage in chronic pancreatitis and a dominant stricture: long-term results. Endoscopy 1995;27(9):638–44.
39. Farnbacher MJ, et al. Interventional endoscopic therapy in chronic pancreatitis including temporary stenting: a definitive treatment? Scand J Gastroenterol 2006;41(1):111–7.
40. Dertmann TSP, Geenen E-J, et al. Spyglassds-guided lithotripsy for pancreatic duct stones in symptomatic, treatment refractory chronic pancreatitis – long-term (3-5 years) follow-up on clinical success and quality of life. Endoscopy 2022;54(S01):219–20.
41. Nimptsch U, et al. Nationwide In-hospital Mortality Following Pancreatic Surgery in Germany is Higher than Anticipated. Ann Surg 2016;264(6):1082–90.

Management of Benign Biliary Stricture in Chronic Pancreatitis

Mohan Ramchandani, MD, DM[a,b,]*, Partha Pal, MD, DNB, MRCP (UK)[a],
Guido Costamagna, MD[c]

KEYWORDS

- Chronic pancreatitis • Endoscopic retrograde cholangiopancreatography
- Benign biliary stricture • Plastic stent • Self-expandable metal stent • Surgery

KEY POINTS

- Progressive, irreversible fibrosis of pancreatic parenchyma leads to benign biliary strictures (BBSs) in chronic pancreatitis (CP) usually late in the course of the disease.
- Surgical drainage is the definitive therapy for CP-related BBS with high long-term success rates, although surgical morbidity can be substantial.
- First-line therapy for CP-related BBS is endoscopic therapy with multiple plastic stents or fully covered self-expandable metal stents (FCSEMS) in the absence of pancreatic head mass or suspicion of malignancy.
- FCSEMS is non-inferior to multiple plastic stents for BBS due to CP and requires fewer sessions of endoscopic retrograde cholangiopancreatography.
- Failure of stricture resolution after 12 months of endotherapy warrants surgical drainage.

INTRODUCTION

Benign biliary stricture (BBS) due to chronic pancreatitis (CP) is reported to occur in 3% to 46% cases.[1–5] The actual incidence may be higher as many of the cases remain asymptomatic and lack proper follow-up data specially in alcoholic patients who are noncompliant to therapy. BBS complicates the course of CP and it is usually a late phenomenon in the natural history of the disease. Progressive, irreversible fibrosis of the pancreatic parenchyma leads to stricture of the lower, intrapancreatic part of the common bile duct (CBD). Less commonly, BBS can also occur relatively early in the course of CP.

a Department of Medical Gastroenterology, Asian Institute of Gastroenterology, 6-3-661, Somajiguda, Hyderabad, Telangana, India; b Interventional Endoscopy, AIG Hospitals, Plot No 2/3/4/5 Survey, 1, Mindspace Road, Gachibowli, Hyderabad, Telangana 500032, India; c Department of Translational Medicine and Surgery, Catholic University, Rome
* Corresponding author. Interventional Endoscopy, AIG hospitals, Plot No 2/3/4/5 Survey, 1, Mindspace Road, Gachibowli, Hyderabad, Telangana 500032, India.
E-mail address: ramchandanimohan@gmail.com

Gastrointest Endoscopy Clin N Am 33 (2023) 831–844
https://doi.org/10.1016/j.giec.2023.04.002

giendo.theclinics.com

The management of BBS with significant cholestasis requires either endoscopic or surgical biliary drainage. Although there is no prospective study comparing these two approaches, endoscopic therapy is generally the first line of therapy given the high surgical morbidity and mortality as long-term success was better with surgery.[6] However, the response rate of BBS-related CP is lower than what is seen with BBS due to anastomotic strictures and post-liver transplant biliary strictures.[7,8] This could be due to the more fibrotic nature of the biliary strictures in CP. Another drawback of endoscopic therapy compared with surgery is the need for repeated stent exchanges. Poor compliance especially in alcoholic CP could lead to cholangitis if stents are not exchanged in a timely manner. This problem is somewhat circumvented by fully covered self-expanding metal stents (FCSEMS), which requires only two procedures for stent insertion and removal. Surgery should be considered at the first place if there is suspicion of malignancy which can occur in CP-related biliary strictures or in association with an inflammatory pancreatic head mass. However, surgery may not feasible due to poor general condition of the patient and local anatomical issues (eg, portal cavernoma, postoperative adhesions). The authors discuss the pathogenesis, clinical presentation, workup, technical details, and modalities of endoscopic therapy with their drawbacks in this review.

PATHOGENESIS

CP-associated biliary strictures occur in the intrapancreatic portion of the CBD. Such strictures occur in about a third of the patients with CP.[2,5] The variable location of the CBD in relation to the pancreatic tissue can explain its occurrence in few patients. It has been seen that the distal CBD is entirely covered by the pancreatic tissue in 80% cases, whereas it lies in the pancreatic groove and is either not covered or partially covered by pancreatic tissue in 15% and 5% cases, respectively. The variable length of intrapancreatic portion of CBD (1.5–6 cm) can also explain the variable length of strictures encountered in the clinical practice.[9]

There are mainly four different mechanisms contributing to the development of biliary strictures in CP which mechanisms can occur alone or in conjunction.[5] The first one is recurrent bouts of acute and chronic inflammation leading to slow but progressive and irreversible pancreatic parenchymal and periductal fibrosis. The presence of calcifications in pancreatic head leading to fibrosis is usually resistant to therapy.[4,5] These occur late in the course of the disease; however, acute pancreatitis or acute exacerbation of CP can lead to edema in head of pancreas within days of an acute episode (second mechanism). These strictures resolve quickly in a similar way as they appear usually within days to weeks.[5] Third, pancreatic fluid collections (pseudocyst, walled of pancreatic necrosis-walled of pancreatic necrosis [WOPN]) and pancreatic retention cysts can cause extrinsic compression of CBD which usually resolves after drainage of the collections.[10] The presence of clinical or subclinical cholestasis after drainage of collections in this scenario may indicate other underlying mechanisms requiring biliary drainage. Finally, malignancy could result in stricture and should be ruled out in patients whenever biliary stricture is encountered for the first time or in long-standing disease.[5]

CLINICAL PRESENTATION AND WORKUP

BBS in CP can present with asymptomatic elevation of liver function tests, abdominal pain, jaundice, or even rarely cholangitis.[3] Abdominal pain is not specific for biliary stricture as it could be due to pancreatic duct stricture or a bout of acute pancreatitis. Jaundice is present in nearly a third to half of the patients with CP and BBS.[1] Jaudice could be transient if caused by edema due to acute exacerbation of pancreatitis. In these cases, alkaline phosphatase and gamma-glutamyl transferase take more time to normalize after resolution of jaundice. On the other hand, elevated markers of cholestasis usually appear before clinical jaundice. Elevation of alkaline phosphatase two times upper limit of normal for more than a month suggests biliary stricture which needs confirmation by radiologic imaging such as a transabdominal ultrasound (TAS).[5] Apart from TAS, computed tomography (CT) should be the next step of investigation for better understanding the mechanism of biliary stricture (eg, parenchymal and ductal changes, calcifications, fluid collections, or mass lesion) and evaluation for surgical biliary drainage (large pancreatic mass, portal vein thrombosis, metastatic disease in liver and cirrhosis are contraindications). However, CT may not be able to conclusively differentiate inflammatory mass or groove pancreatitis from pancreatic cancer. MRI can help in better delineation of tissue; however, differentiation of benign from malignant stricture may still not be possible.[5] Cholangiographic appearance on magnetic resonance cholangiopancreatography or endoscopic retrograde cholangiopancreatography (ERCP) can be helpful (smooth, regular tapering in benign and tight, abrupt, irregular narrowing in malignant) but not definitive.[1] Marked elevation of carbohydrate antigen 19-9 (CA 19-9) more than 1000 U/mL strongly suggests malignancy but not very common, whereas mild elevation can be due to the leakage of CA 19-9 into serum due to elevated biliary pressure in CP-related BBS.[11,12] Brush cytology and endobiliary biopsy can be helpful but has low sensitivity to diagnose pancreatic malignancy. Endoscopic ultrasound (EUS)-guided tissue acquisition can be particularly helpful in this scenario.[13] If malignancy cannot be ruled out conclusively, surgery is a reasonably good option. If patient is not willing for surgery, close follow-up with repeated histologic sampling is warranted.[5]

INDICATIONS OF BILIARY DRAINAGE

Cholangitis in the settings of CP and BBS is an urgent indication for biliary drainage as with any other indication. Cholangitis is rare with intact papilla but can occur post-biliary sphincterotomy. More commonly, jaundice and subclinical cholestasis (alkaline phosphatase >2–3 times upper limit of normal) are also indications for drainage to prevent the development of secondary biliary cirrhosis.[14] Cirrhosis is reported to occur in 7% of such patients, although alcohol intake could be another plausible explanation of cirrhosis apart from biliary cirrhosis.[4,15] The reversal of fibrosis has been reported on serial liver biopsies after biliary drainage in CP with BBS.[16] It is important to keep in mind that biliary obstruction due to edema after acute exacerbation of CP usually subsides in days to weeks (20%–50% in a month) with normalization of markers of cholestasis. There lies the rationale of biliary drainage in all those with biliary stricture and elevated markers of cholestasis which persisted for more than a month.[4] Usually, most of the biliary strictures in CP are fibrotic and irreversible and hence needs surgical or endoscopic drainage.

Surgical drainage (hepaticojejunostomy or choledochojejunostomy) is the gold standard for biliary drainage and can be performed along with pancreatic duct drainage (pancreaticoduodenectomy/Frey's procedure and duodenum-preserving pancreatic head resection/Berger procedure). However, endoscopic therapy should be considered initially given the substantial morbidity associated with these surgical procedures. Endoscopic therapy should be the initial modality of biliary drainage in the absence of inflammatory head mass.[14] Surgical drainage should be attempted after failure of 1 year or three sessions of endoscopic therapy.[14] If patient compliance is a concern especially in case of alcoholic CP, surgical drainage is a viable initial option.

On the other hand, the presence of comorbidities, portal biliopathy, and postoperative adhesions make surgical therapy (ST) difficult, thus making endoscopic therapy preferable.

ENDOTHERAPY VERSUS SURGERY

A single retrospective study including 39 patients has compared endotherapy (ET) (n = 33, 85%) (35% self-expandable metal stents [SEMS], 65% MPS) with ST (6/39, 15%). The length of hospital stay (ET: 16 days, ST: 24 days, P = .21), success rate at 6 months (75% ET, 74% ST), and 12 months (69% ET, 65% ST) were not significantly different between the two groups. Although morbidity was higher in ST group (ET: 21%, ST: 83%), event-free survival (ET: 5.8 months, ST: 16.9 months) and success at 2 years (ET: 12%, ST: 65%) were significantly higher in ST group.[6] However, the success rate at 2 years was considerably lower compared with other studies including randomized controlled trials (RCTs).[17,18] Nearly half of the patients in ET arm (51.5%, 17/33) were subjected to ST after failure of ET. This is because stricture non-resolution at ERCP was considered as failure of therapy rather than requirement of repeat stenting. Another important finding in the study was that the success rate dropped to 27% at 6 months and 18% at 18 months after more than three sessions of ET.

The study concluded that ST has better long-term outcomes compared with ET. However, given the high rates of surgical morbidity, they also concluded that ET should be used as first-line therapy except in cases of associated pancreatic head mass, when ST should be considered after failure of three sessions or 12 months of ET.[6] This study forms the rationale of current recommendations for the management of BBS due to CP.[14]

TECHNICAL CONSIDERATIONS FOR ENDOSCOPIC THERAPY

Single plastic stent (SPS), multiple plastic stents (MPS) (**Fig. 1**A), and FCSEMS (**Fig. 1**B, C) are the treatment options for endoscopic biliary drainage for BBS due to CP. The technique is relatively simple as these strictures are in the distal CBD which offers a mechanical advantage in putting the stents. After initial cannulation, contrast should be injected to delineate the length of stricture and upstream biliary dilation.

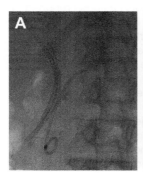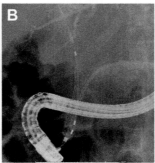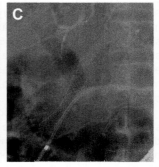

Fig. 1. Multiple plastic stenting (MPS) followed by fully covered self-expanding metal stent (FCSEMS) placement for benign biliary stricture (BBS) due to chronic pancreatitis (CP). (*A*) Two plastic stents with a pancreatic duct stent in a case of chronic calcific pancreatitis which failed to resolve the stricture. (*B*) A 6-cm FCSEMS being placed during endoscopic retrograde cholangiopancreatography for BBS due to CP. (*C*) FCSEMS and pancreatic stent in situ.

Although biliary sphincterotomy may not be required for putting a single 10 Fr stent, it should usually be done before biliary drainage. Single 10 or 11.5 Fr placement can usually be done without any dilation. However, if the stricture is tight, Soehendra dilator (Cook Endoscopy, Winston Salem, NC) can be used to dilate stricture before stent deployment. If MPS placement is planned, prior hydrostatic balloon dilation should be performed. SPS has a patency of 3 to 4 months and hence should be exchanged by that time to avoid stent blockade and cholangitis. If stricture persists, stents should be exchanged. Three to four plastic stents (7 Fr/10 Fr and 5 cm/7 cm) can be placed side by side over a guidewire and catheter loading all plastic stents at once and recannulation with the stent guidewire and catheter after deploying a stent. Alternatively, loading stents one by one alongside each other can also be done. The resolution of stricture is evidenced by disappearance of stricture waist with free flow of injected contrast into the duodenum. The persistence of stricture beyond 1 year indicates the futility of ET and surgical drainage should be offered.[5,19]

Alternatively, FCSEMS can be placed for distal CBD stricture. On cholangiogram, the insertion of cystic duct to common hepatic duct should be delineated to use appropriately sized stent avoiding occlusion of cystic duct orifice by covered SEMS. The insertion of FCSEMS can be done under combined endoscopic and fluoroscopic guidance and is not technically demanding. After the insertion of guidewire and biliary sphincterotomy, stent insertion system is advanced into the bile duct followed by deployment of the stent.[5]

OUTCOMES OF ENDOSCOPIC THERAPY IN BENIGN BILIARY STRICTURE DUE TO CHRONIC PANCREATITIS
Single Plastic Stent

The outcomes of single plastic stenting (**Fig. 2**A) were studied in one prospective and eight retrospective studies (**Table 1**).[20–28] The results were disappointing with long-term success in only up to a third of the patients.[20–28] The presence of calcifications was shown to increase the risk of failure by 17-fold as shown in a prospective study by Kahl and colleagues.[26] In one of the studies by Vitale and colleagues, long-term success was reported in 80% patients. It was explained by the fact that none of the

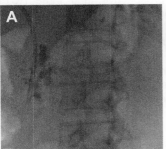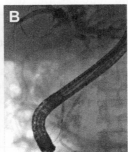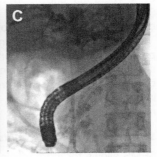

Fig. 2. Single plastic stent followed by fully covered self-expanding metal stent (FCSEMS) with anchoring plastic stent placement for benign biliary stricture (BBS) due to chronic calcific pancreatitis. (*A*) Single plastic stent (10 Fr) placed for a tight distal bile duct stricture in chronic calcific pancreatitis with extensive parenchymal calcification (more in head) which failed to resolve the stricture. (*B*) A 6-cm FCSEMS being placed during endoscopic retrograde cholangiopancreatography for BBS due to CP. The tight stricture can be noted as evidenced by persistence of the waist of FCSEMS. (*C*) FCSEMS was anchored by a plastic stent to prevent migration.

Table 1
Summary of studies on endoscopic placement of single biliary plastic stent for benign biliary strictures related to chronic pancreatitis

Author, Year	Number of Patients	Long-Term Success (%)	Stenting Duration (Months)	Stent Dysfunction of any Cause (%)	Follow-Up Post Stent Removal (Months)	Surgical Drainage (%)
Deviere et al,[52] 1990	25	12	-	72	14	24
Barthet et al,[21] 1994	19	10	10	-	18	21
Smits et al,[22] 1996	58	28	10	64	49	28
Farnbacher et al,[23] 2000	31	32	10	52	28	6
Vitale et al,[24] 2000	25	80	13	20	32	8
Eickoff et al,[25] 2001	39	31	9	42	58	28
Kahl et al,[26] 2003	61	26	12	34	40	49
Catalano et al,[27] 2004	34	24	21	41	50	41
Bartoli et al,[53] 2005	9	44	9	22	16	44
Chaen et al,[54] 2005	58	39	9	48	45	28

patients had calcific pancreatitis.[24] In a comparative study, it was shown that SPS was clearly inferior to MPS with respect to increase in stricture diameter, biochemical normalization of cholestasis markers, need for surgical drainage, and rate of cholangitis.[27] The poor response rate of single stent is due to fibrotic nature of BBS due to CP compared with other etiology. MPS is superior plausibly because it causes gradual remodeling of fibrotic tissue.[5]

Multiple Plastic Stents

MPS (see **Fig. 1**A) is the way to treat BBS due to CP with plastic stents as single plastic stenting has fallen out of favor due to the aforementioned reasons. The long-term success rate of MPS for BBS in CP has ranged from 44% to 92% over maximum follow-up of 4 years as shown in two retrospective, two prospective, and three RCTs (**Table 2**).[17,18,27,29–32] Stent dysfunction and subsequent requirement of surgical drainage was substantially low compared with single plastic stenting.[17,27,30,32]

However, MPS needs re-intervention every 3 months for up to 1 year, and hence, patient compliance is important. Noncompliance is common in alcoholic CP and should warrant surgical drainage. Noncompliance can lead to cholangitis which can be potentially fatal.[33] Stricture recurrence, although less than single plastic stenting, is not uncommon. However, recurrence can be successfully treated with stenting in most of the cases.[5]

Self-Expandable Metal Stents

SEMS allows for more efficient biliary drainage due to its large diameter with longer patency (see **Fig. 1**B, C; **Fig. 2**B, C; **Table 3**). Another advantage is requirement of only two ERCP procedures (one for insertion and one for removal) compared with multiple ERCP sessions with MPS.[5]

An earlier study in 1993 evaluated the role of permanent uncovered SEMS for BBS due to CP. The stent patency was 90% over 33 months in this study of 20 patients. Two patients had stent block due to tissue hyperplasia through the mesh of the SEMS.[34] Later in 2005, Cantu and colleagues evaluated the feasibility of permanent

Table 2
Summary of studies on endoscopic placement of multiple biliary plastic stents for benign biliary strictures related to chronic pancreatitis

Author, Year	Number of Patients	Long-Term Success (%)	Stenting Duration (Months)	Stent Dysfunction of Any Cause (%)	Follow-Up Post-Stent Removal (Months)	Surgical Drainage (%)
Draganov et al,[29] 2002	9	44	14	-	48	-
Pozsarc et al,[30] 2004	29	60	21	-	12	13
Catalan et al,[27] 2004	12	92	14	8	47	8
Happamaki et al,[56] 2015	30	90	6	23	37	-
Ohyama et al,[32] 2017	10	60	12	20	21	-
Ramchandani et al,[18] 2021	84	77.1	12	19	12	-

indwelling partially covered SEMS (PCSEMS) in 14 patients with CP-related BBS. Although all the stents remained patent at a follow-up of 18 months, half of them had stent dysfunction due to tissue hyperplasia or stent migration over mean follow-up of 22 months.[35] The temporary placement of PCSEMS (Wallstent, Boston Sc, Natick, MA, USA) was shown to resolve strictures in 90% after 6 months of SEMS removal, although stent removal was not possible in two patients (10%, 2/20).[36]

To overcome the limitation of tissue ingrowth in uncovered or partially covered SEMS, Kahaleh and colleagues evaluated the feasibility of FCSEMS for BBS due to various causes. Among 22 patients with CP-related BBS, stricture resolution occurred in 77% patients over a period of 1 year. Stent migration was the main drawback of FCSEMS in that study which was higher than described with PCSEMS.[7]

To counteract FCSEMS migration, Park and colleagues studied FCSEMS with anchoring flaps or a proximal flared end. At 6 months, none of them with the anchoring flap and 33% with proximal flared end migrated. All FCSEMS could be removed.[37] Cahen and colleagues described FCSEMS with a distal lasso (Fully covered Hanaro stent, Hanaro; M.I.Tech Co, Ltd, Seoul, South Korea) to pull the SEMS for removal. Stricture resolution at median 5.5 months was only 37% with proximal migration in 2 (33%), which could not be retrieved.[38] A prospective study evaluated FCSEMS with both flared-end SEMS (FE-SEMS, $n = 10$) and un-flared-end SEMS (UE-SEMS, $n = 7$) (Fully covered NITI-S, Taewoong, Seoul, South Korea). The migration rate was 100% for UE-SEMS compared with 40% with FE-SEMS. On 2 years follow-up, stricture resolution rates were 43% and 90% with UE-SEMS and FE-SEMS, respectively.[39] Two more uncontrolled studies showed long-term resolution rates of 70% and 90%, respectively.[8,40] Both the studies used FCSEMS with anchoring fins (Viabil stent, Conmed, Utica, NY, USA).[8,40] The second study also used Fully covered Wallflex (Boston Sc, Natick, MA, USA) stent.[40]

SEMS with anchoring fins (eg, Viabil, Hanaro) were better than SEMS with flared ends (Wallflex) in preventing stent migration. However, they can cause injury to the biliary mucosa and subsequent stricture formation.[8,37,41,42] Secondary stricture after placement of Viabil SEMS was reported in 8% (3/37) as shown in a retrospective study. Out of the three strictures, two were due to distal end of oversized intraductal stent.[43] The short length of fully covered NITI-S (Taewoong, Seoul, South Korea) allows for complete intra-biliary stent placement.[39,42]

In a large ($n = 187$), multicentre, international, prospective, uncontrolled study included all BBS including those due to CP ($n = 127$, stent indwell time for CP

Table 3
Summary of studies on endoscopic placement of fully covered self-expanding metal stents (FCSEMS) for benign biliary strictures related to chronic pancreatitis

Author, Year	Number of Patients	Long-Term Success (%)	Stenting Duration (Months)	Stent Dysfunction of Any Cause (%)	Follow-up Post-Stent Removal (Months)	Surgical Drainage (%)
Cahen et al,[38] 2008	6	50	5	33	28	17
Behm et al,[36] 2009	20	80	5	-	12	13
Mahajan et al,[8] 2009	17	58	3.3	27	3.8	-
Perri et al,[39] 2012	12	92	14	8	47	8
Deviere et al,[55] 2014	127	80	10–12	22	22	-
Happamaki et al,[56] 2015	30	90	6	23	37	-
Saxena et al,[40] 2015	10	60	12	20	21	-
Lakhtakia et al,[45] 2020	118	61.6 (77.4 after complete resolution)	10–12	22.9	58	7.6
Ramchandani et al,[18] 2021	10	75.8	12	23.8	12	-

was 10–12 months). This showed feasibility of FCSEMS (Fully covered Wallflex, Boston Sc, Natick, MA, USA) removal and nearly 75% stricture resolution rates with FCSEMS for BBS.[44]

Long-term follow-up after FCSEMS indwell for 10 to 12 months in BBS related to CP has shown that nearly 60% remain stent free at a median follow-up of 58 months. These results are even better if there is stricture resolution at FCSEMS removal (77.4% remain stent free). Stent-related adverse events can occur in up to a fourth of the patients which is manageable by medical therapy or endoscopy. Severe CP and longer stricture length were the predictors of treatment failure.[45]

Biodegradable Stents

The problem of patient compliance with multiple sessions of ET can be overcome by the use of biodegradable stents (BDBS). Most of the current BDBS stents are made up of polydioxanone and it causes moderate epithelial hyperplasia and stent degradation without stent migration as shown in preclinical study in canine bile ducts. Most of the current existing literature on BDBS for BBS is with percutaneously placed stents.[46] A systematic review of uncontrolled, non-comparative studies have shown that BDBS are non-inferior to MPS in terms of stricture resolution and maintaining long-term bile duct patency.[47] BDBS have been shown to be safe except the fact that it can cause transient cholangitis (24%) and hemobilia (3%).[47] A pilot study showed the feasibility of endoscopically placed BDBS. Out of six patients with BBS, two had BBS related to CP. Overall stricture resolution in BBS was 83% with disappearance of BDBS on MRI at 6 months.[48]

A preclinical porcine study has provided some mechanistic insights into the biocompatibility of BDBS. BDBS normalized galectin-2 levels, the expression of which is lower in BBS compared with intact bile duct. On the other hand, the expression of transgelin, which is low in intact bile duct, increased after FCSEMS placement.[49] However, the current literature is not adequate to recommend this as a treatment option currently. However, this is albeit a promising avenue for treatment of BBS.

Endoscopic Ultrasound-Guided Hepaticoenterostomy

EUS-guided hepaticoenterostomy (HE) can be useful in CP with BBS and inaccessible papilla making ERCP difficult. In a study of 57 patients undergoing EUS-guided HE, two were done for CP-related BBS. EUS-guided hepaticogastrostomy is done by first puncturing with 19G needle and then after passing guidewire and tract dilation followed by specially designed single pigtail plastic stent (total length of 20 cm, effective length 15 cm) (Through and Pass, TYPE-IT, Gadelius Medical Co, Ltd, Tokyo, Japan).[50]

Choice of Endotherapy

A systematic review of non-comparative studies showed that FCSEMS performed better than MPS but a significant proportion of patients (up to a third) in few of the included studies had SPS.[25,42,51]

To compare MPS with FCSEMS, three RCTs have been conducted for BBS that included patients with CP (two had exclusive CP patients, one included other BBS as well).[17,18,31] The study design and stem placement protocols were different. In the first RCT by Haapamaki and colleagues, three plastic stents or FCSEMS were placed initially followed by another three plastic stent after 3 months in the plastic stent group. The 2-year structure free success rates (MPS: 90%, FCSEMS: 92%) were not different between the two arms with comparable migration rates (MPS: 10%, FCSEMS: 7%).[17] The second RCT by Cote and colleagues assessed all BBS including those due to CP. Patients were assessed for stricture resolution 3 months in the MPS group and 6 months in the FCSEMS group and replaced the stents if stricture did not resolve. Stricture resolution at 12 months was not inferior with FCSEMS (92.6%) compared with MPS (85.4%) using a prespecified non-inferiority margin of 15%. However, mean number of ERCPs required with FCSEMS (2.14) was significantly lower than that with MPS (3.24) (P<.001). However, this study was not adequately powered to conduct a subgroup analysis for BBS due to CP.[31] An international multicentre study by Ramchandani and colleagues specifically evaluated patients with CP and BBS. The study used a non-inferiority margin of 20% to calculate sample size which was 164. In the MPS group, at least two to four plastic stents were placed (8.5 Fr or 10 Fr) and exchanged every 4 months over 1 year. In the FCSEMS group, the indwell period was 12 months; 12 months after the treatment completion, stricture resolution rates were non-inferior with FCSEMS (75.8%) compared with MPS (77.1%) (P = .008, non-inferiority analysis). The mean number of ERCPs in FCSEMS (2.6) was lower compared with that in MPS group (3.9). Any serious adverse event or stent migration rates were not different between the two arms.[18]

Based on these evidences, FCSEMS is non-inferior to MPS for BBS due to CP with lower requirement of ERCP sessions. Hence, FCSEMS can be used as one of the first-line therapies in BBS due to CP obviating multiple stent exchanges and improvement in treatment compliance.[14,42,45]

SUMMARY

BBS due to CP is difficult to treat endoscopically compared with other causes due to its fibrotic nature especially in calcific, severe pancreatitis with longer strictures.

Even asymptomatic, persistent cholestasis warrants biliary drainage to prevent the development of secondary biliary cirrhosis. Malignancy should be ruled out.

Surgical biliary drainage provides higher long-term stricture resolution rates at the cost of high surgical morbidity. Hence, endoscopic therapy is the preferred initial option except in case of associated pancreatic head mass, and ST should be considered after failure of 12 months of endoscopic therapy.

SPSs have poor long-term outcomes. MPS exchanged over time can give good long-term results, and restenosis can be successfully retreated endoscopically. FCSEMS placement for up to 12 months provides similar results with fewer sessions. Novel BDBS are promising and can obviate stent removal altogether thus addressing non-compliance.

CLINICS CARE POINTS

- Endoscopic therapy should be considered the first line of therapy for chronic pancreatitis (CP)-related benign biliary stricture.
- Surgical therapy is preferred initially if there is pancreatic head mass or suspicion of malignancy.
- Multiple plastic stents and fully covered self-expanding metal stents are preferred modalities of endotherapy and have comparable efficacy, although the later requires fewer endoscopic retrograde cholangiopancreatography sessions.
- Head calcifications, severe CP, and long stricture length are predictors of treatment failure.
- The failure of endotherapy at 1 year should be considered for surgery which has high long-term efficacy but substantial morbidity.

DISCLOSURE

None of the authors have any commercial or financial conflicts of interest and any funding sources to disclose. *The figures are the authors' original work and have not been used elsewhere.*

REFERENCES

1. Sarles H, Sahel J. Cholestasis and lesions of the biliary tract in chronic pancreatitis. Gut 1978;19(9):851–7.
2. Eckhauser FE, Knol JA, Strodel WE, et al. Common bile duct strictures associated with chronic pancreatitis. Am Surg 1983;49(7):350–8.
3. Kalvaria I, Bornman PC, Marks IN, et al. The spectrum and natural history of common bile duct stenosis in chronic alcohol-induced pancreatitis. Ann Surg 1989; 210(5):608–13.
4. Abdallah AA, Krige JE, Bornman PC. Biliary tract obstruction in chronic pancreatitis. HPB (Oxford) 2007;9(6):421–8.
5. Familiari P, Boškoski I, Bove V, et al. ERCP for biliary strictures associated with chronic pancreatitis. Gastrointest Endosc Clin N Am 2013;23(4):833–45.
6. Regimbeau JM, Fuks D, Bartoli E, et al. A comparative study of surgery and endoscopy for the treatment of bile duct stricture in patients with chronic pancreatitis. Surg Endosc 2012;26(10):2902–8.
7. Kahaleh M, Behm B, Clarke BW, et al. Temporary placement of covered self-expandable metal stents in benign biliary strictures: a new paradigm? (with video). Gastrointest Endosc 2008;67(3):446–54.
8. Mahajan A, Ho H, Sauer B, et al. Temporary placement of fully covered self-expandable metal stents in benign biliary strictures: midterm evaluation (with video). Gastrointest Endosc 2009;70(2):303–9.
9. Hollinshead WH. The lower part of the common bile duct: a review. Surg Clin North Am 1957;37(4):939–52.
10. Delhaye M, Arvanitakis M, Bali M, et al. Endoscopic therapy for chronic pancreatitis. Scand J Surg 2005;94(2):143–53.
11. Steinberg W. The clinical utility of the CA 19-9 tumor-associated antigen. Am J Gastroenterol 1990;85(4):350–5.
12. Minghini A, Weireter LJ Jr, Perry RR. Specificity of elevated CA 19-9 levels in chronic pancreatitis. Surgery 1998;124(1):103–5.
13. Lewis JJ, Kowalski TE. Endoscopic ultrasound and fine needle aspiration in pancreatic cancer. Cancer J 2012;18(6):523–9.
14. Dumonceau JM, Delhaye M, Tringali A, et al. Endoscopic treatment of chronic pancreatitis: European Society of Gastrointestinal Endoscopy (ESGE) Guideline - Updated August 2018. Endoscopy 2019;51(2):179–93.
15. Frey CF, Suzuki M, Isaji S. Treatment of chronic pancreatitis complicated by obstruction of the common bile duct or duodenum. World J Surg 1990;14(1): 59–69.
16. Hammel P, Couvelard A, O'Toole D, et al. Regression of liver fibrosis after biliary drainage in patients with chronic pancreatitis and stenosis of the common bile duct. N Engl J Med 2001;344(6):418–23.
17. Haapamäki C, Kylänpää L, Udd M, et al. Randomized multicenter study of multiple plastic stents vs. covered self-expandable metallic stent in the treatment of biliary stricture in chronic pancreatitis. Endoscopy 2015;47(7):605–10.
18. Ramchandani M, Lakhtakia S, Costamagna G, et al. Fully Covered Self-Expanding Metal Stent vs Multiple Plastic Stents to Treat Benign Biliary Strictures

Secondary to Chronic Pancreatitis: A Multicenter Randomized Trial. Gastroenterology 2021;161(1):185–95.

19. Law R, Baron TH. 22 - Plastic Pancreaticobiliary Stents and Nasopancreaticobiliary Tubes: Concepts and Insertion Techniques. In: Baron TH, Kozarek RA, Carr-Locke DL, editors. Ercp. 3rd edition. Philadelphia: Elsevier; 2019. p. 196–205.e1.

20. Devière J, Devaere S, Baize M, et al. Endoscopic biliary drainage in chronic pancreatitis. Gastrointest Endosc 1990;36(2):96–100.

21. Barthet M, Bernard JP, Duval JL, et al. Biliary stenting in benign biliary stenosis complicating chronic calcifying pancreatitis. Endoscopy 1994;26(7):569–72.

22. Smits ME, Rauws EA, van Gulik TM, et al. Long-term results of endoscopic stenting and surgical drainage for biliary stricture due to chronic pancreatitis. Br J Surg 1996;83(6):764–8.

23. Farnbacher MJ, Rabenstein T, Ell C, et al. Is endoscopic drainage of common bile duct stenoses in chronic pancreatitis up-to-date? Am J Gastroenterol 2000;95(6):1466–71.

24. Vitale GC, Reed DN Jr, Nguyen CT, et al. Endoscopic treatment of distal bile duct stricture from chronic pancreatitis. Surg Endosc 2000;14(3):227–31.

25. Eickhoff A, Jakobs R, Leonhardt A, et al. Endoscopic stenting for common bile duct stenoses in chronic pancreatitis: results and impact on long-term outcome. Eur J Gastroenterol Hepatol 2001;13(10):1161–7.

26. Kahl S, Zimmermann S, Genz I, et al. Risk factors for failure of endoscopic stenting of biliary strictures in chronic pancreatitis: a prospective follow-up study. Am J Gastroenterol 2003;98(11):2448–53.

27. Catalano MF, Linder JD, George S, et al. Treatment of symptomatic distal common bile duct stenosis secondary to chronic pancreatitis: comparison of single vs. multiple simultaneous stents. Gastrointest Endosc 2004;60(6):945–52.

28. Cahen DL, van Berkel AM, Oskam D, et al. Long-term results of endoscopic drainage of common bile duct strictures in chronic pancreatitis. Eur J Gastroenterol Hepatol 2005;17(1):103–8.

29. Draganov P, Hoffman B, Marsh W, et al. Long-term outcome in patients with benign biliary strictures treated endoscopically with multiple stents. Gastrointest Endosc 2002;55(6):680–6.

30. Pozsár J, Sahin P, László F, et al. Medium-term results of endoscopic treatment of common bile duct strictures in chronic calcifying pancreatitis with increasing numbers of stents. J Clin Gastroenterol 2004;38(2):118–23.

31. Coté GA, Slivka A, Tarnasky P, et al. Effect of Covered Metallic Stents Compared With Plastic Stents on Benign Biliary Stricture Resolution: A Randomized Clinical Trial. JAMA 2016;315(12):1250–7.

32. Ohyama H, Mikata R, Ishihara T, et al. Efficacy of multiple biliary stenting for refractory benign biliary strictures due to chronic calcifying pancreatitis. World J Gastrointest Endosc 2017;9(1):12–8.

33. Kiehne K, Fölsch UR, Nitsche R. High complication rate of bile duct stents in patients with chronic alcoholic pancreatitis due to noncompliance. Endoscopy 2000;32(5):377–80.

34. Deviere J, Cremer M, Baize M, et al. Management of common bile duct stricture caused by chronic pancreatitis with metal mesh self-expandable stents. Gut 1994;35(1):122–6.

35. Cantù P, Hookey LC, Morales A, et al. The treatment of patients with symptomatic common bile duct stenosis secondary to chronic pancreatitis using partially covered metal stents: a pilot study. Endoscopy 2005;37(8):735–9.

36. Behm B, Brock A, Clarke BW, et al. Partially covered self-expandable metallic stents for benign biliary strictures due to chronic pancreatitis. Endoscopy 2009;41(6):547–51.
37. Park DH, Lee SS, Lee TH, et al. Anchoring flap versus flared end, fully covered self-expandable metal stents to prevent migration in patients with benign biliary strictures: a multicenter, prospective, comparative pilot study (with videos). Gastrointest Endosc 2011;73(1):64–70.
38. Cahen DL, Rauws EA, Gouma DJ, et al. Removable fully covered self-expandable metal stents in the treatment of common bile duct strictures due to chronic pancreatitis: a case series. Endoscopy 2008;40(8):697–700.
39. Perri V, Boškoski I, Tringali A, et al. Fully covered self-expandable metal stents in biliary strictures caused by chronic pancreatitis not responding to plastic stenting: a prospective study with 2 years of follow-up. Gastrointest Endosc 2012; 75(6):1271–7.
40. Saxena P, Diehl DL, Kumbhari V, et al. A US Multicenter Study of Safety and Efficacy of Fully Covered Self-Expandable Metallic Stents in Benign Extrahepatic Biliary Strictures. Dig Dis Sci 2015;60(11):3442–8.
41. Blero D, Huberty V, Devière J. Novel biliary self-expanding metal stents: indications and applications. Expert Rev Gastroenterol Hepatol 2015;9(3):359–67.
42. Dumonceau JM, Tringali A, Papanikolaou IS, et al. Endoscopic biliary stenting: indications, choice of stents, and results: European Society of Gastrointestinal Endoscopy (ESGE) Clinical Guideline - Updated October 2017. Endoscopy 2018;50(9):910–30.
43. Kasher JA, Corasanti JG, Tarnasky PR, et al. A multicenter analysis of safety and outcome of removal of a fully covered self-expandable metal stent during ERCP. Gastrointest Endosc 2011;73(6):1292–7.
44. Devière J, Nageshwar Reddy D, Püspök A, et al. Successful management of benign biliary strictures with fully covered self-expanding metal stents. Gastroenterology 2014;147(2):385–95 [quiz: e15].
45. Lakhtakia S, Reddy N, Dolak W, et al. Long-term outcomes after temporary placement of a self-expanding fully covered metal stent for benign biliary strictures secondary to chronic pancreatitis. Gastrointest Endosc 2020;91(2):361–9.e3.
46. Fan Z, Zhao X, Ji R, et al. Endoscopic treatment of benign biliary stricture using different stents: a systematic review and meta-analysis. Wideochir Inne Tech Maloinwazyjne 2022;17(1):35–60.
47. Almeida GG, Donato P. Biodegradable versus multiple plastic stent implantation in benign biliary strictures: A systematic review and meta-analysis. Eur J Radiol 2020;125:108899.
48. Siiki A, Rinta-Kiikka I, Sand J, et al. A pilot study of endoscopically inserted biodegradable biliary stents in the treatment of benign biliary strictures and cystic duct leaks. Gastrointest Endosc 2018;87(4):1132–7.
49. Siiki A, Jesenofsky R, Löhr M, et al. Biodegradable biliary stents have a different effect than covered metal stents on the expression of proteins associated with tissue healing in benign biliary strictures. Scand J Gastroenterol 2016;51(7):880–5.
50. Matsunami Y, Itoi T, Sofuni A, et al. EUS-guided hepaticoenterostomy with using a dedicated plastic stent for the benign pancreaticobiliary diseases: A single-center study of a large case series. Endosc Ultrasound 2021;10(4):294–304.
51. Siiki A, Helminen M, Sand J, et al. Covered self-expanding metal stents may be preferable to plastic stents in the treatment of chronic pancreatitis-related biliary strictures: a systematic review comparing 2 methods of stent therapy in benign biliary strictures. J Clin Gastroenterol 2014;48(7):635–43.

52. Deviere J, Devaere S, Baize M, et al. Endoscopic biliary drainage in chronic pancreatitis. Gastrointest Endosc 1990;36:96–100.
53. Bartoli E, Delcenserie R, Yzet T, et al. Endoscopic treatment of chronic pancreatitis. Gastroenterol Clin Biol 2005;29:515–21.
54. Cahen DL, van Berkel AM, Oskam D, et al. Long-term results of endoscopic drainage of common bile duct strictures in chronic pancreatitis. Eur J Gastroenterol Hepatol 2005;17(1):103–8.
55. Devière J, Nageshwar Reddy D, Püspök A, et al. Successful management of benign biliary strictures with fully covered self-expanding metal stents. Gastroenterology 2014;147(2):385–95.
56. Haapamäki C, Kylänpää L, Udd M, et al. Randomized multicenter study of multiple plastic stents vs. covered self-expandable metallic stent in the treatment of biliary stricture in chronic pancreatitis. Endoscopy 2015;47(7):605–10.

Endoscopic Ultrasound-Guided Pancreatic Duct Interventions

Jacques Devière, MD, PhD

KEYWORDS

- EUS-guided pancreatic duct drainage • Surgically altered anatomy
- Transmural drainage • Chronic pancreatitis • Disconnected pancreatic duct
- Pancreatic leak

KEY POINTS

- Endoscopic ultrasound (EUS)-guided pancreatic duct drainage is a technically challenging therapeutic procedure, which should be performed in tertiary centers by highly qualified endoscopists in a multidisciplinary environment.
- The major clinical indication is pain associated with segmental dilatation of the pancreatic duct after Whipple resection, secondary to a disconnection of the duct after severe pancreatitis.
- Pain in patients with advanced chronic pancreatitis and no access to the duct by endoscopic retrograde approach is another potential indication.
- It may be indicated in pancreatic leaks but alternative routes of pancreatic fluid diversion (drainage of a communicating collection or EUS-guided internalization of an external fistula) should be considered first.

INTRODUCTION

Symptomatic obstruction of the pancreatic duct (PD) is usually managed with a step-up approach including, after failure of medical therapy, endoscopy (possibly combined with percutaneous access) and surgery.[1] Although the endoscopic transpapillary approach to the PD is obviously the preferred approach, there are clinical and anatomic situations where direct endoscopic access is difficult or impossible through endoscopic retrograde pancreatography (ERCP).[2,3] These include (1) patients with pain and stenosis of a pancreatico-jejunal or pancreatico-gastric anastomosis after duodenopancreatectomy, (2) patients with pain and/or acute relapsing pancreatitis (ARP) after severe acute pancreatitis complicated by disconnected pancreatic tail syndrome (DPTS), and (3) patients with painful chronic pancreatitis in whom drainage

Department of Gastroenterology, Hepatopancreatology and Digestive Oncology, Erasme Hospital, Université Libre de Bruxelles, 808 Route de Lennik, Brussels B1070, Belgium
E-mail address: Jacques.deviere@hubruxelles.be

Gastrointest Endoscopy Clin N Am 33 (2023) 845–854
https://doi.org/10.1016/j.giec.2023.04.005
1052-5157/23/© 2023 Elsevier Inc. All rights reserved.

giendo.theclinics.com

of a dilated duct is not possible due to stones or nonpassable strictures. Postoperative leaks or collections communicating with a functional distal pancreas represent a fourth clinical indication where drainage of the PD can be obtained indirectly either by drainage of the collection or internalization of the leak.[3–6] Although some of these conditions can be treated with either enteroscopy-guided pancreatography (with a very-low success rate) or using combined percutaneous and endoscopic access. The advent of therapeutic endoscopic ultrasound (EUS) has dramatically broadened the indications that can be addressed and have improved clinical outcomes.[7–9]

EUS-guided PD drainage includes the EUS rendezvous technique, in which a guide wire is passed into the PD, in cases of failed retrograde access, to facilitate transpapillary or transanastomotic cannulation,[10] and EUS anterograde drainage (pancreatico-gastro-stomy, pancreatico-duodenostomy, pancreatico-enterostomy), which consists of the EUS-guided transmural placement of a stent into the main pancreatic duct (MPD), with or without additional EUS-guided access to the jejunum through the anastomosis.[11] This latter procedure has become the preferred technique for most indications.

Although it offers new therapeutic opportunities, EUS-guided PD drainage is recognized as a very challenging, advanced technique that should only be performed in tertiary referral centers. Even in these cases, retrospective series have shown that the indications for the technique are rare (ranging from 2 to 5 patients/y)[12–14] while the number of cases to reach competency may be greater than 20.[15] Reported technical success is less than 90% and overall clinical success is 75% to 80%, at the cost of around 20% immediate complications including pancreatitis, bleeding, and leakage.[2,3,16,17]

INDICATIONS AND CONTRAINDICATIONS FOR ENDOSCOPIC ULTRASOUND-GUIDED PANCREATIC DUCT DRAINAGE

The main clinical indications for endoscopic ultrasound-guided pancreatic duct drainage (EUS-PDD) are pain and/or ARP associated with an anastomotic stricture after duodenopancreatectomy (pancreatico-jejunal or pancreatico-gastric anastomosis) or with an unpassable stricture (or inaccessible papilla due to stricture or duodenal pancreatitis) in the setting of chronic pancreatitis. The purpose of treatment is to reduce proximal ductal hypertension and to restore drainage of the pancreatic fluid to the stomach, duodenum, and/or jejunum. Indications for malignant obstruction are extremely rare because this is rarely associated with obstructive pain. Steatorrhea, anecdotally reported in retrospective series, is not an indication for EUS-PDD. Given the complexity of the technique, every indication should be discussed in a multidisciplinary environment and balanced with the risk/benefit ratio.[2,3,16]

Pancreatic fistula is another indication where the need for direct EUS-PDD is less frequent[18] because the duct feeding the leak is rarely dilated and other routes for diverting the pancreatic fluid to the gastrointestinal (GI) tract exist, including drainage of associated collections[19,20] or a combined percutaneous and EUS-guided approach to internalize the pancreatic leak.[4,6]

Contraindications for EUS-PDD include the lack of clinical indication (pain or ARP), or the presence of severe coagulopathy, thrombocytopenia, or hemodynamic instability. From a technical point of view, nondilated ducts, multiple strictures, or the inability to clearly locate the PD are the most frequent contraindications. The minimal diameter of the MPD for these procedures has not been determined but is probably 4 to 6 mm, as quoted in many studies.[12,13,21,22] Failure of cannulation of the PD in a patient with Sphincter of Oddi dysfunction or pancreas divisum without PD dilation is, in our opinion, not an indication for EUS-PDD, not only because of the difficulty of reaching the PD but also because of the risk of pancreatitis associated with the puncture, dilation and/or cautery, and passage of the stent through an almost normal parenchyma.

TECHNIQUES

EUS-PDD is performed by highly trained physicians and nurse assistants under general anesthesia with intubation. A high-quality fluoroscopy is needed and the patient is either in prone or in supine position (left lateral does not allow adequate visualization of the PDs). Prophylactic antibiotic therapy is given. In addition, even if not proven in this specific indication, we now give the patient prophylaxis for post-ERCP pancreatitis, including non-steroid antiinflammatory drug (NSAIDs) and hyperhydration. Anticoagulation and antithrombotic agents should be stopped according to guidelines.

A therapeutic linear EUS scope is used for the procedure and access to the pancreas can be obtained from the stomach to perform a EUS-guided pancreatico-gastrostomy or, in a long scope position from the duodenum to perform a EUS-guided pancreatico-duodenostomy. The latter offers a more stable position but can only be performed when the dilated duct is visible (and present) up to the genu of the pancreas, excluding postsurgical anastomotic strictures and most PD dilations after DPTS (**Figs. 1** and **2**).

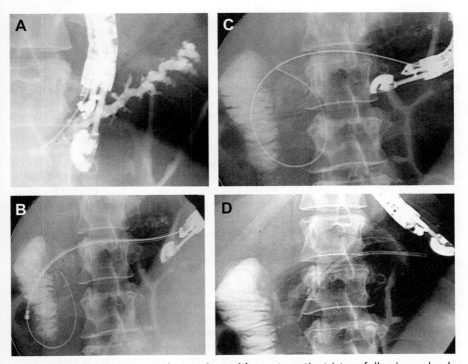

Fig. 1. Pancreatico-gastrostomy in a patient with anastomotic stricture following a duodenopancreatectomy. The PD is punctured with a 19G FNA needle (*A*), over a guide wire passed through the duct and the anastomosis, a cystotome is used to enlarge the transgastric tract and provide an easier access to the duct (*B*). Over this GW (*C*) a 7 French stent is inserted with its distal end in the jejunal loop, distal to the anastomosis and its proximal end into the stomach (*D*).

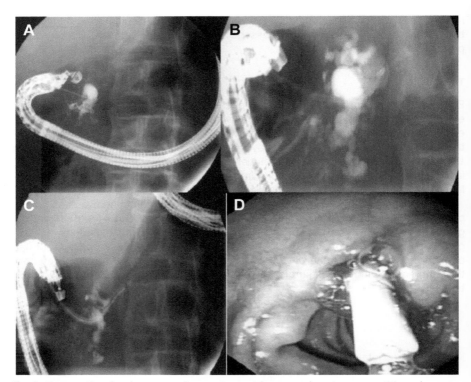

Fig. 2. Pancreatico-duodenostomy in a patient with severe chronic pancreatitis and unpassable stricture at ERP. Puncture of the duct is obtained in a long scope position (*A*), at the level of the genu of the MPD, and after dilation with a 6 French cystotome (*B*), a 7 French stent is inserted (*C,D*).

Access to the PD is obtained most often by using a 19G needle inserted under EUS guidance, followed by minimal contrast and saline injection and insertion of a hydrophilic 0.035-inch guidewire (GW).[3,23] The axis of puncture should be toward the anastomosis or the papilla to have a chance to reach it with the wire. Alternatively, especially in patients with advanced chronic pancreatitis, with a dilated duct and fibrotic parenchyma that is difficult to traverse, a diathermy needle (Zimmon, Cook Endoscopy, Winston Salem, NC) can be used but requires precise targeting, using pure cutting current delivered immediately before starting the advancement of the needle to avoid the risk of kinking.[12]

Once the GW is guided into the PD, either it passes the stenosis or the strictured anastomosis and reaches the papilla and the duodenum or the jejunum distal to the anastomosis, or it curves into the PD. In the first case, a rendezvous technique may be attempted when the papilla is still anatomically accessible, and the wire has looped into the duodenum. The wire is left in place and the scope exchanged for a standard duodenoscope, allowing the performance of standard transpapillary endotherapy.[23] One must be aware about the risk of GW dislodgement during stent exchange as well as the risk associated with manipulation of the GW once it has been grasped with a snare to perform the rendezvous procedure if too much traction is applied (butter-cutter wire effect). We currently almost never perform a rendezvous and prefer, if the duodenum has been reached, to leave a stent in place which allows, in a second session, the endoscopist to choose between transpapillary and transgastric access to the PD.[12,13]

In all the other cases (which means the vast majority), pancreatic access should be followed by dilation of the tract and placement of a plastic stent. Dilation of the tract can be performed with either a balloon (Hurricane Rx, Boston Scientific, Marlborough, MA) or a 6Fr Cystotome (Endoflex, Voerde, Germany). The passage of a balloon, especially when puncture has been obtained with a standard (noncautery) needle, can be extremely difficult due to the lack of stability into the stomach and the hardness of the pancreatic parenchyma. Some authors[24] have recommended the use of a thinner angioplasty balloon in this indication (Sterling, Boston Scientific, Marlborough, MA). The 6Fr cystotome[12] is, in our hands, the preferred technique, which allows for the creation of a safe and easy tract toward the PD. In addition, when in place in the PD, it allows further manipulation of the GW without the risk of peeling it, which often occurs when a wire is manipulated into a 19G needle. This has been associated with a possible higher risk of bleeding,[24] which is, in our opinion, possibly associated with the type of electrocautery used. This device provides easier access and less current diffusion when used with pure cutting current applied only during the passage through the GI wall[25] and the pancreatic parenchyma. Blended or Endocut currents are less effective and favor uncontrolled current diffusion with a higher risk of damaging an adjacent vessel.

Transmural stenting is performed using a 7Fr or 5Fr plastic stent after 4-mm balloon dilation of the tract and, if passable, of the distal/anastomotic stricture. In case of retrograde (toward the pancreatic tail) or antegrade (toward the pancreatic head) stenting and when the stricture cannot or has not been passed through the stricture, straight stents are preferred. When the GW has passed the stricture, we prefer to use double pigtail stents to reduce the risk of migration. It is our policy, when EUS is performed for a benign indication, to follow-up with the patient after 2 to 3 months when the tract to the PD has matured and to replace the single stent with 2 7Fr (Or 5 Fr) stents placed side-by-side to ensure the longevity of the tract without the need for further interventions. In such cases, similarly to when transmural stenting is performed to drain a collection associated with a DPTS,[26,27] the stents act as a wick to maintain the open communication even if they become occluded. No systematic exchange is needed at this point.

Uncovered self-expandable metal stents (SEMS) and lumen-apposing metal stents have no indication in EUS-PDD for obvious reasons. Fully covered SEMS, recommended by some[28] are associated with specific adverse events (side branch occlusion, migration, ductal injuries) and have no advantage over plastic stents for PD drainage. Once a tract has been created and matured, it can possibly be used for additional interventions, including dilation or stent revision but also to perform direct pancreatoscopy, if indicated. The major potential indication[29] is the performance of electrohydraulic lithotripsy of pancreatic stones using a cholangioscope (Spyscope DS, Boston Sc, Marlborough, MA, USA). However, this indication must be evaluated with the risk balance in comparison with other stone fragmentation techniques such as extracorporeal shock wave lithotripsy.

Alternative routes to divert the pancreatic fluid to the GI tract, especially in cases of DPTS with or without external leak include the following:

1. The drainage of associated collections using plastic stents, which can be left in place for years,[26] the technique for which is described elsewhere in this issue.
2. When an external postoperative leak is present after pancreatic surgery or severe pancreatitis with DPTS, with or without an external drain in place, an

internalization[4,30] of the leak is probably the easiest and least invasive technique. In this case, an EUS-guided transmural puncture of the fistula tract is facilitated by injection of saline or contrast through the drain or a catheter placed in the fistula. This transiently recreates a collection, which can be punctured and stented (usually with a 7 Fr pigtail stent), diverting the pancreatic fluid back to the GI tract.

OUTCOMES

Most of the studies published so far have been retrospective studies or multicentric retrospective analyses of prospectively acquired data, and this field is currently still waiting for a multicentric prospective evaluation of the technique with standardization of indications and techniques to provide unbiased data on success, adverse events, and outcomes.

That being said, a recent meta-analysis[16] of 16 studies[9,12,15,21,28,31–38] including 503 patients treated by EUS-PDD for PD decompression reported a technical success rate of 81.4% (95% confidence interval [CI]: 72–88), and that the method of dilation (diathermy vs balloon) was a significant covariate affecting technical success. Ten studies reported clinical outcomes of pain resolution after EUS-PDD with an overall clinical success rate of 84.6% (95%CI: 75–91). The overall pooled adverse event rate was 21.3% (95%CI:17–27), most commonly postprocedural abdominal pain. Bleeding (usually self-resolving) after stent placement and collection formation (possibly associated with stent dislodgement) were other possible complications. There was no procedure-related mortality. The overall pooled incidence of post-EUS-PDD pancreatitis was 5% (95%CI: 3–8) with no covariate significantly affecting this. These results confirm that the technique is challenging, with a technical success rate less than other EUS-guided therapies but which can offer improved clinical outcomes in more than 80% of the cases at the cost of a still reasonable (although high in such a group of patients) rate of complications, especially postprocedural pancreatitis.

In a recent dual center retrospective study (28 patients during 3 years), Krafft and colleagues[13] reported similar rates for technical (81%) and clinical (75%) success, and 15% complications at index pancreato-gastrostomy while reinforcing the concept described above of a second procedure, performed 1 to 3 months after the first procedure, to achieve definitive therapy (ie, transpapillary/anastomotic drainage combined with transmural drainage). Another study evaluated the impact of EUS-PDD availability on the outcomes of patients undergoing PD drainage due to stricture/obstruction of the MPD due to chronic pancreatitis.[39] Endoscopic transpapillary drainage, the preferred approach, was successful in 35 out of 45 cases and EUS-PDD allowed the achievement of technical success in 8 out of 10 of the remaining cases, providing an overall clinical success rate of more than 95%, with a cumulative 3-year relapse rate of 27%. Rates of postprocedural pancreatitis were, however, higher in the EUS-PDD group. This suggests that, in the group of patients with pain associated with chronic pancreatitis and ductal hypertension, EUS-PDD is a useful add-on for achieving technical success which should, however, be performed with caution in case of failure of the safer transpapillary therapy.

As far as pancreatic anastomotic leakage after duodenopancreatectomy, a recent retrospective analysis[40] reported on 110 patients who experienced a pancreatic leakage after pancreatic resection with pancreatico-gastric anastomosis. Of these, 32 were treated by EUS-guided, perianastomotic, pigtail stent placement while 50 received a percutaneous drainage as first interventional therapy. The authors observed better primary (78% vs 54%) and secondary (86% vs 68%) success rates of the therapy as well as much earlier primary resolution (11 vs 37 days) in patients who received endoscopic versus percutaneous management. This also suggests a paradigm change in the management of postoperative leaks in which an endoscopic approach should be performed as a first interventional therapy, avoiding, when expertise is available, primary external drainage.

PERSPECTIVES

Twenty-one years after its first description, EUS-PDD drainage has started to become part of the armamentarium for treating selected difficult cases of pancreatic disease. Its development has been slower than that of other EUS-guided therapeutic approaches, such as drainage of pseudocysts or biliary drainage, for various reasons including the paucity of real clinical indications, the difficulty of the technique (small therapeutic target, lack of stability in the stomach, fibrotic tissue to be traversed), and the potential risk of complications associated with injury to the pancreatic parenchyma. The contrast between the estimated 27 cases that should be performed in order to reach mastery of the technique, as reported recently,[15] and the low mean number of cases treated per year and per center, most often between 2 and 5 in tertiary centers, suggests that, in most cases, gaining full expertise in this technique is an impossible mission.

Despite this limitation, it appears that this technique has a role in the clinic. This is even more true for alternative drainage techniques proposed for patients with external postsurgical or postsevere pancreatitis leaks where endoscopic approaches have surpassed other techniques. Dedicated devices should be developed to facilitate EUS-PDD, among which diathermic and safe access devices will likely be most prominent. Standardization of the approach and of the indication, including clear definitions of the pretherapeutic imaging required (MRI and/or computed tomography), will allow clinicians to reach consensus and avoid nonindicated, risky procedures such as puncture of a normal duct or treatment proposed without a clear and clinically relevant indication. Training remains an important issue and should be offered to senior endoscopists who are highly qualified in both ERCP and therapeutic EUS. These can be limited in number because patient numbers will never be sufficient to require multiple operators in a single center. Trainees should probably already have training in the technique of hepatico-gastrostomy, a very similar but easier technique in terms of access and passage of the parenchyma. This challenging technique has, in every case, to be discussed and performed in a multidisciplinary environment where all other therapeutic alternatives are available.

CLINICS CARE POINTS

- Do not perform EUS-guided drainage in patients with nondilated ducts and normal pancreatic parenchyma.
- Be sure about clinical indication, pain associated with ductal hypertension and dilation is the major one. Steatorrhea or failed cannulation (without dilation) is not an indication for EUS PDD.
- Once the puncture has been obtained, the procedure is done under almost exclusive fluoroscopic guidance. Do not try to have an endoscopic view up to the time of stent release.
- EUS-PDD should be performed by the most experienced endoscopist and GI assistants under general anesthesia.

- Place only one stent at the first procedure and consider a second one, few weeks later when the tract between the MPD and the GI tract has matured.

DISCLOSURES

Institutional research support from Boston Sc (USA) and Olympus (Japan) for IRB approved studies. Consultancy from Olympus (Japan).

REFERENCES

1. Dumonceau J-M, Delhaye M, Tringali A, et al. Endoscopic treatment of chronic pancreatitis : ESGE guideline-updated 2018. Endoscopy 2019;51:179–92.
2. van der Merwe SW, van Wanrooij RLJ, Bronswijk M, et al. Therapeutic endoscopic ultrasound: European Society of Gastrointestinal Endoscopy (ESGE) Guideline. Endoscopy 2022;54:185–205.
3. Teh JL, Teoh AYB. Techniques and outcomes of endoscopic ultrasound guided pancreatic duct drainage-EUS-PDD. J Clin Med 2023;12:1626.
4. Arvanitakis M, Delhaye M, Bali MA, et al. Endoscopic treatment of external pancreatic fistulas: When draining the main pancreatic duct is not enough. Am J Gastroenterol 2007;102:516–24.
5. Bang JY, Wilcox CM, Navaneethan U, et al. Impact of disconnected pancreatic duct syndrome on the endoscopic management of pancreatic fluid collections. Ann Surg 2018. https://doi.org/10.1097/SLA.0000000000002082.
6. Deviere J, Bueso H, Baize M, et al. Complete disruption of the main pancreatic duct: endoscopic management. Gastrointest Endosc 1995;42:445–51.
7. Farrell J, Carr-Locke D, Garrido T, et al. Endoscopic retrograde cholangiopancreatography after pancreaticoduodenectomy for benign and malignant disease: indications and technical outcomes. Endoscopy 2006;38:1246–9.
8. Chahal P, Baron TH, Topazian MD, et al. Endoscopic retrograde cholangiopancreatography in post-Whipple patients. Endoscopy 2006;38:1241–5.
9. Chen YI, Levy MJ, Moreels TG, et al. An international multicenter study comparing EUS-guided pancreatic duct drainage with enteroscopy-assisted endoscopic retrograde pancreatography after Whipple surgery. Gastrointest Endosc 2017;85:170–7.
10. Bataille L, Deprez P. A new application for therapeutic EUS: Main pancreatic duct drainage with a "pancreatic rendezvous technique". Gastrointest Endosc 2002; 55:740–3.
11. François E, Kahaleh M, Giovannini M, et al. EUS-guided pancreaticogastrostomy. Gastrointest Endosc 2002;56:128–33.
12. Tessier G, Bories E, Arvanitakis M, et al. EUS -guided pancreatogastrostomy and pancreatobulbostomy for the treatment of pain in patients with pancreatic ductal dilatation inaccessible for transpapillary endoscopic therapy. Gastrointest Endosc 2007;65:233–41.
13. Krafft MR, Croglio MP, James TW, et al. Endoscopic endgame for obstructive pancreatopathy: Outcomes of anterograde EUS-guided pancreatic duct drainage. A dual-center study. Gastrointest Endosc 2020;92:1055–66.
14. Tyberg A, Sharaiha RZ, Kedia P, et al. EUS-guided pancreatic drainage for pancreatic strictures after failed ERCP: a multicenter international collaborative study. Gastrointest Endosc 2017;85:164–9.

15. Tyberg A, Bodiwala V, Kedia P, et al. EUS-guided pancreatic drainage: A steep learning curve. Endosc. Ultrasound 2020;9:175–9.
16. Devière J. EUS-guided pancreatic duct drainage: A rare indication in need of prospective evidence. Gastrointest Endosc 2017;85:178–80.
17. Bhurwal A, Tawadros A, Mutneja H, et al. EUS guided pancreatic duct decompression in surgically altered anatomy or failed ERCP—A systematic review, meta-analysis and meta-regression. Pancreatology 2021;21:990–1000.
18. Toshima T, Fujimori N, Yoshizumi T, et al. A Novel Strategy of Endoscopic Ultrasonography-Guided Pancreatic Duct Drainage for Pancreatic Fistula After Pancreaticoduodenectomy. Pancreas 2021;50:e21–2.
19. Gupta T, Lemmers A, Tan D, et al. EUS-guided transmural drainage of postoperative collections. Gastrointest Endosc 2012;76:1259–65.
20. Ghandour B, Akshintala VS, Bejjani M, et al. A modified approach for endoscopic ultrasound-guided management of disconnected pancreatic duct syndrome via drainage of a communicating collection. Endoscopy 2022;54:917–9.
21. Fujii LL, Topazian MD, Abu Dayyeh BK, et al. EUS-guided pancreatic duct intervention: Outcomes of a single tertiary-care referral center experience. Gastrointest Endosc 2013;78:854–64.e1.
22. Chen YI, Saxena P, Ngamruengphong S, et al. Endoscopic ultrasound-guided pancreatic duct drainage: Technical approaches to a challenging procedure. Endoscopy 2016;48(Suppl. 1):E192–3.
23. Itoi T, Kasuya K, Sofuni A, et al. Endoscopic ultrasonography-guided pancreatic duct access: Techniques and literature review of pancreatography, transmural drainage and rendezvous techniques. Dig Endosc 2013;25:241–52.
24. Hayat U, Freeman ML, Trikudanathan G, et al. Endoscopic ultrasound-guided pancreatic duct intervention and pancreaticogastrostomy using a novel cross-platform technique with small-caliber devices. Endosc Int Open 2020;8: E196–202.
25. Cremer M, Devière J, Baize M, et al. New device for endoscopic cystoenterostomy. Endoscopy 1990 Mar;22(2):76–7.
26. Gkolfakis P, Bourguignon A, Arvanitakis M, et al. Indwelling double-pigtail plastic stents for treating disconnected pancreatic duct syndrome-associated peripancreatic fluid collections: long-term safety and efficacy. Endoscopy 2021; 53(11):1141–9.
27. Téllez-Aviña FI, Casasola-Sánchez LE, Ramírez-Luna M, et al. Permanent Indwelling Transmural Stents for Endoscopic Treatment of Patients with Disconnected Pancreatic Duct Syndrome: Long-term Results. J Clin Gastroenterol 2018;52:85–90.
28. Oh D, Park DH, Cho MK, et al. Feasibility and safety of a fully covered self-expandable metal stent with antimigration properties for EUS-guided pancreatic duct drainage: Early and midterm outcomes (with video). Gastrointest Endosc 2016;83:366–73.e2.
29. Suzuki A, Ishii S, Fujisawa T, et al. Efficacy and Safety of Peroral Pancreatoscopy Through the Fistula Created by Endoscopic Ultrasound-Guided Pancreaticogastrostomy. Pancreas 2022;51:228–33.
30. Jürgensen C, Distler M, Arlt A, et al. EUS guided drainage in the management of postoperative pancreatic leaks and fistulas (with video). Gastrointest Endosc 2019;89:311–9.
31. Barkay O, Sherman S, McHenry L, et al. Therapeutic EUS-assisted endoscopic retrograde pancreatography after failed pancreatic duct cannulation at ERCP. Gastrointest Endosc 2010;71:1166–73.

32. Ergun M, Aouattah T, Gillain C, et al. Endoscopic ultrasound-guided transluminal drainage of pancreatic duct obstruction: Long-term outcome. Endoscopy 2011; 43:518–25.

33. Kahaleh M, Hernandez AJ, Tokar J, et al. EUS-guided pancreaticogastrostomy: analysis of its efficacy to drain inaccessible pancreatic ducts. Gastrointest Endosc 2007;65:224–30.

34. Vila JJ, Pérez-Miranda M, Vazquez-Sequeiros E, et al. Initial experience with EUS-guided cholangiopancreatography for biliary and pancreatic duct drainage: A Spanish national survey. Gastrointest Endosc 2012;76:1133–41.

35. Shah JN, Marson F, Weilert F, et al. Single-operator, single-session EUS-guided anterograde cholangiopancreatography in failed ERCP or inaccessible papilla. Gastrointest Endosc 2012;75:56–64.

36. Will U, Reichel A, Fueldner F, et al. Endoscopic ultrasonography-guided drainage for patients with symptomatic obstruction and enlargement of the pancreatic duct. World J Gastroenterol 2015;21:13140–51.

37. Matsunami Y, Itoi T, Sofuni A, et al. Evaluation of a new stent for EUS-guided pancreatic duct drainage: Long-term follow-up outcome. Endosc Int Open 2018;6:E505–12.

38. Uchida D, Kato H, Saragai Y, et al. Indications for Endoscopic Ultrasound-Guided Pancreatic Drainage: For Benign or Malignant Cases? Can J Gastroenterol Hepatol 2018;8216109.

39. Sakai T, Koshita S, Kanno Y, et al. Early and long-term clinical outcomes of endoscopic interventions for benign pancreatic duct stricture/obstruction-the possibility of additional clinical effects of endoscopic ultrasonography-guided pancreatic drainage. Pancreatology 2022;22:58–66.

40. Felsenstein M, Amini A-C, Dorfer S, et al. Internal drainage for interdisciplinary management of anastomotic leakage after pancreaticogastrostomy. Surg Endosc 2023. epub march 6th.

Radiofrequency Ablation of Pancreatic Solid Tumors

Marc Giovannini[a,*], Mariola Marx[b]

KEYWORDS

- Radiofrequency ablation • Pancreatic tumors • Neoplastic lesions

KEY POINTS

- Endoscopic ultrasound-guided radiofrequency ablation (EUS-RFA) has become increasingly accepted for the treatment of different precancerous and neoplastic lesions of the pancreas, particularly in patients who are unfit for surgery.
- EUS-RFA seems to be a promising treatment strategy for the management of small pancreatic neuroendocrine tumors (pNETs) with excellent efficacy.

INTRODUCTION

Today, endoscopic ultrasound-guided radiofrequency ablation (EUS-RFA) has become increasingly accepted for the treatment of different precancerous and neoplastic lesions of the pancreas, particularly in patients who are unfit for surgery. However, thermal ablation has long been suspected to induce pancreatitis or to injure adjacent structures, such as the bile duct, large vessels, or gastrointestinal wall.[1] Published case reports and case series on this topic are of limited size and are often based on a heterogeneous study population, reporting on functional and nonfunctional (NF) pancreatic neuroendocrine tumors (pNETs), as well as cystic lesions such as cystic neoplasms or intraductal papillary mucinous neoplasms (IPMNs). Nevertheless, the overall results are promising, with high technical success and low complication rates.[2–5]

In this chapter, we will discuss

1. Technique and device of EUS-guided RFA
2. Place of EUS-RFA for the pancreatic insulinoma
3. Place of EUS-RFA in NF pNETs
4. Place of EUS-RFA for pancreatic adenocarcinoma
5. Place of EUS-RFA for pancreatic metastasis from renal cancer

[a] Paoli-Calmettes Institute, 232 Boulevard St-Marguerite, Marseille Cedex 9 13273, France;
[b] Unit of Hepato-Gastroenterology, CHUV, Rue Du Bugnon 46 Street, Lausanne 1011, Switzerland
* Corresponding author.
E-mail address: UEMCO@IPC.UNICANCER.FR

Gastrointest Endoscopy Clin N Am 33 (2023) 855–865
https://doi.org/10.1016/j.giec.2023.04.013
1052-5157/23/© 2023 Elsevier Inc. All rights reserved.

TECHNIQUE AND DEVICE FOR ENDOSCOPIC ULTRASOUND-GUIDED RADIOFREQUENCY ABLATION

EUS-RFA was performed with a therapeutic linear array echoendoscope under CO_2 insufflation using a EUSRA EUS-RFA system from Taewoong Medical (STARmed/ TaeWoong Medical, Gimpo, South Korea). All procedures should be performed under general anesthesia or propofol sedation. The EUSRA device is composed of a 19 G radiofrequency monopolar electrode (**Fig. 1**) that is cooled by a chilled saline solution to decrease the risk of tissue damage. We accepted a maximum of 3 passes to correctly position the needle within the target lesion. A dedicated radiofrequency current generator allows the control of power and impedance (VIVA combo from STARmed, Goyang, South Korea). Radiofrequency current is applied under EUS control at a power setting of 30 to 50 W in 1 to 5 cycles, each with a maximum duration of 10 to 12 s or until the appearance of hyperechoic bubbles (**Fig. 2**). We start from the most difficult-to-reach area of the lesion, as treatment-induced artifacts may appear and thus obscure the EUS view. The procedure is stopped whenever the impedance exceeds 1000 Ω.

Barret and colleagues[6] analyzed tissue ablation of the EUSRA probe in a porcine model, suggesting that the cooling system probably accounts for the absence of a plateau in the ablation depth when increasing the power settings. A higher electrode temperature, however, induces tissue charring, increasing tissue impedance and thus reducing the coagulative necrosis of surrounding healthy tissue. This means that the charred tissue acts as an insulator, protecting the pancreatic tissue surrounding the ablation site. Kim and colleagues[7] performed EUS-RFA in 10 pigs using the EUSRA probe (power 50 W, time 5 min): the mean diameter of the ablated lesions was 23.0 ± 6.9 mm, and necropsy findings revealed normal pancreatic parenchyma around the ablated lesion, devoid of any evidence of parenchymal necrosis or pancreatic duct injury.

EUS-RFA uses high-frequency alternating current to induce coagulation necrosis in neoplastic cells. In addition, EUS-RFA also induces immunomodulation with the secretion of cytokines and killer lymphocytes, which have a delayed antitumoral effect.

When the tumor and the main pancreatic duct (MPD) are in close proximity, we place a prophylactic pancreatic stent (5 F/5 or 7 cm). A strict threshold distance

A   **B**

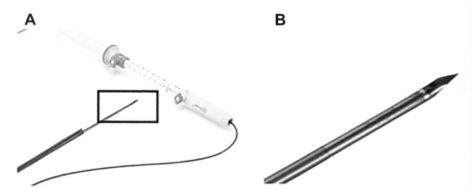

Fig. 1. (*A*) EUSRA endoscopic ultrasound-guided radiofrequency ablation (EUS-RFA) system (ST ARmed, Taewoong Medical) using a 19G-needle. (*B*) The active tip lacks insulation and measures 10 mm. (With permission from STARmed Co., Ltd.)

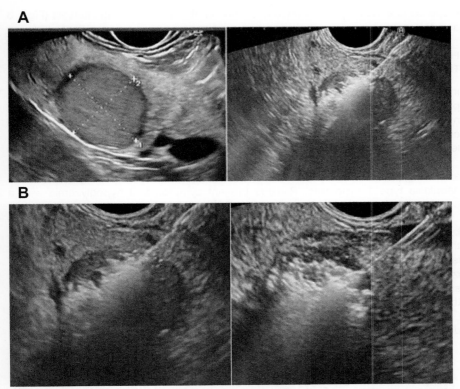

Fig. 2. (*A* and *B*) RF energy (50 W) is applied under endoscopic ultrasound (EUS) view, starting from the most difficult-to-reach area of the lesion. Maximum duration of 10 to 12 s or until the appearance of hyperechoic bubbles. (*From* Marx M, Godat S, Caillol F, et al. Management of non-functional pancreatic neuroendocrine tumors by endoscopic ultrasound-guided radiofrequency ablation: Retrospective study in two tertiary centers. Dig Endosc. 2022;34(6):1207-1213.)

between the target lesion and the main pancreas has not been defined, and the need for preventive pancreatic stent placement is at the endoscopist's discretion. However, stent placement is always performed when the lesion is in direct contact with the MPD. Rectal or intravenous diclofenac or indomethacin, respectively, is given at the beginning of each procedure to prevent post-ERCP pancreatitis. Periprocedural antibiotic prophylaxis is administered.

All patients are hospitalized for the surveillance of early complications and discharged the following day after clinical evaluation. Perioperative adverse events occurring during the 30 days after treatment are described according to the Clavien–Dindo classification of surgical complications.[8]

Abdominal cross-sectional imaging control by computed tomography (CT) or MRI is performed between 1 and 3 months after EUS-RFA. Images are interpreted by an experienced radiologist specializing in gastrointestinal tumor disease and by a gastroenterologist. Treatment response is defined as the diminution or absence of enhancing residual tissue on the tumor site and is classified as partial or complete, respectively. In case of doubt, an independent reinterpretation is asked. If a residual tumor is suspected, a new session of EUS-RFA is performed. Once a complete radiological response is achieved, surveillance is continued at 6 and 12 month intervals (**Figs. 3 and 4**).

PLACE OF ENDOSCOPIC ULTRASOUND-GUIDED RADIOFREQUENCY ABLATION FOR THE PANCREATIC INSULINOMA

Insulinoma is the most frequent functional neuroendocrine tumor of the pancreas, and preserving surgery is the treatment of choice. EUS-guided radiofrequency ablation is a novel and promising technique that induces tissue necrosis in localized lesions. This chapter presents a preliminary clinical experience in treating pancreatic insulinomas less than 2 cm by EUS-RFA, focusing on safety and efficacy.

The incidence of insulinomas is 1 to 3 per 1 million persons per year. More than 90% are benign, and in 5% to 10%, there is an association with multiple endocrine neoplasia type 1 syndrome. Patients present symptoms of hypoglycemia with a considerable impact on their quality of life.[9–11]

Insulinomas are generally small NETs (82%, <2 cm; 47%, <1 cm) and may be localized throughout the pancreas gland (30% in the head, 30% in the body, and 30% in the tail).[9–11] Visualization by cross-sectional imaging remains challenging, and EUS is the diagnostic procedure of choice if noninvasive strategies fail. EUS is characterized by a sensitivity of 70% to 95%, allowing tissue sampling by fine-needle biopsy sampling for histologic classification, and may evaluate the exact distance between the lesion and the MPD and major vessels.[12,13]

Management of insulinomas was defined in 2012 as part of the European Neuroendocrine Tumor Society (ENETS) Consensus Guidelines[2] for functional pancreatic

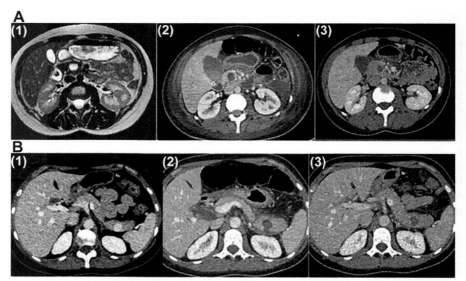

Fig. 3. CT scan evaluation of RFA for (*A*) insulinoma of the head of the pancreas: (1) before the RFA, (2) 1 week after RFA: necrotic area without enhancement after contrast injection, (3) 6 months after RFA residual hypodense area as complete ablation. (*B*) Pancreatic neuroendocrine tumor grade 1 of the tail of the pancreas: (1) before RFA, (2) 1 week after RFA: necrotic area without enhancement after contrast injection and pancreatic edema due to mild acute pancreatitis post ablation, and (3) 6 months after RFA residual hypodense area as complete ablation.

Before EUS-RFA   2-months later, first evaluation   Complete necrosis

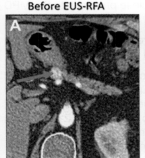 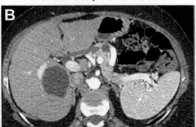 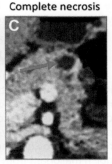

Fig. 4. RF ablation of a small pancreatic metastasis from renal cancer. (*From* Chanez B, Caillol F, Ratone JP, et al. Endoscopic Ultrasound-Guided Radiofrequency Ablation as an Future Alternative to Pancreatectomy for Pancreatic Metastases from Renal Cell Carcinoma: A Prospective Study. Cancers (Basel). 2021;13(21):5267. Published 2021 Oct 20.)

endocrine tumor syndromes and was revised in 2017. Accordingly, surgery is the standard treatment for nonmetastatic, sporadic, or multiple endocrine neoplasia type 1-associated disease, and laparoscopy should be the preferred approach in preoperatively imaged tumors. In most cases, enucleation or limited resection is possible, and lymphadenectomy is not needed.[14] However, with regard to the benign nature (>90%) and solitary occurrence (>90%) of insulinomas, it is worth discussing whether surgery-associated morbidity and mortality and a potential impairment of pancreatic function are justified in all patients.

Results in the literature reported technical and clinical success rates of almost 100% without significant treatment-associated morbidity. Presently, 8 case reports, series, or retrospective studies report the outcomes of 29 insulinoma patients (outlined in **Table 1**).[2,15–20] Two patients in the series by Oleinikov and colleagues 13 with nonfunctional pancreatic NETS measuring 25 and 10 mm developed mild pancreatitis 10 days after ablation, which resolved with conservative measures after 2 to 3 days. It

Table 1
Literature on EUS-guided RFA for pancreatic neuroendocrine tumors

First Author, Year	No. of Patients	Mean Size	Multiple Endocrine Neoplasia Type 1	Efficacy (%)	Adverse Events	Mean Follow-up (mo)
Lakhtakia et al,[15] 2016	3	16.7	No	100	No	11.7
Waung et al,[16] 2016	1	18	No	100	No	10
Bas-Cutrina et al,[17] 2017	1	10	No	100	No	10
Choi et al,[2] 2018	1	12	No	100	No	13
Oleinikov et al,[18] 2019	7	14.8	1/7	100	No	9.7
De Nucci et al,[19] 2020	5	12.8	No	100	No	12
Furnica et al,[20] 2020	4	12	No	100	No	22
Marx et al,[28] 2022	7	13.3	No	85.7	2/7*	21

is worth mentioning that the 25 mm lesion was ablated in close proximity to the MPD without preventive stent placement.

- 1 patient had abdominal pain and fever who recovered in 7 days with medical treatment, and 1 patient developed a pancreatic fluid collection.

Currently, the long-term outcome in terms of disease recurrence or progression of insulinomas treated by EUS-RFA is still unknown. Thus, surgery remains the recommended treatment. As more than 90% of insulinomas are benign, systematic lymphadenectomy is not recommended. According to a systematic review of 6222 insulinoma patients, the surgery-associated morbidity rate is approximately 35%.[21–24] Surgical resection provides more definitive pathologic analysis; nevertheless, criteria to distinguish malignant from benign insulinomas are lacking, and the definition of malignancy is mainly based on lymph node involvement and typically found with larger lesions.[25–27]

The study of Marx and colleagues[28] refers to EUS-RFA in small insulinomas (range, 8–20 mm), histologically classified as grade 1 in 4 of 5 patients. None of these patients showed disease recurrence, and 4 patients had a long follow-up time of 18, 24, 34, and 38 months, respectively, as confirmed by high-resolution imaging. In 1 patient, the first radiologic evaluation showed partial treatment success (70% of the lesion), but complete necrosis was confirmed by 2 consecutive abdominal CTs after 12 and 18 months of follow-up. This delayed response might be explained by radiofrequency-induced immunomodulation.[24] The decision for treatment by EUS-RFA was based on the algorithm shown in **Fig. 3**. Larger prospective studies with longer-term follow-up as well as clarification of the role of pancreatic stents are needed.

PLACE OF ENDOSCOPIC ULTRASOUND-GUIDED RADIOFREQUENCY ABLATION IN NONFUNCTIONAL PANCREATIC NEUROENDOCRINE TUMORS

Current ENETS guidelines state that close follow-up is a reasonable management strategy for patients with small, low-grade NF pNETs. In cases of tumor progression, pancreatic surgery is the standard of care, with a nonnegligible morbidity rate. However, successful surveillance depends on patient compliance, requires iterative imaging controls, and might cause a psychological burden for the patient. With the development of endoscopic ultrasound techniques, EUS-RFA has become an alternative to surgical resection and might reduce the need for the life-long surveillance of patients.[9,10,12–14]

The study of Marx and colleagues[29] is one of the largest case series to date, reporting on the outcome of 27 patients treated by EUS-RFA for NF pNETs. Complete treatment responses were observed in 25/27 (93%) patients, as confirmed by radiological follow-up (15.7 ± 12.2 months; range 2–41 months). Two patients required 2 treatment sessions to achieve necrosis in the lesion, and re-treatment is pending for one patient. These results are consistent with previous studies.

There have been 4 prospective studies on EUS-RFA in solid and cystic precancerous lesions of the pancreas, as well as some retrospective case series.[2–5,30] A recently published review on interventional EUS showed treatment success in 42/51 (82.4%) pNETs treated by EUS-RFA. In contrast, the efficacy of EUS-guided ethanol ablation was lower (36/58 lesions, 62.1%).[31] The largest studies have been conducted by Barthet and colleagues, reporting on 12 patients with 14 NF pNETs treated by EUS-RFA; after 1 year of follow-up, 12/14 lesions had completely disappeared.[4] In a retrospective study by Oleinikov and colleagues[3], a complete treatment response was confirmed in 8/11 patients treated for NF pNETs (8 G1 lesions and 2 G3 lesions), whereas one patient had a partial response, and 2 patients could not be assessed. Two patients presented with metastatic disease at the time of diagnosis.[3]

Regarding complication rate, acute periprocedural pancreatitis occurred in 4/27 patients in the study of Marx and colleagues,[29] 3 of them underwent endoscopic cystogastrostomy for drainage of peripancreatic collections (3/27; 11.1%).

A similar morbidity rate has been shown in a recent review of EUS-RFA (13.7%).[32] However, complications described in the mentioned review seem less severe than in our case series. The authors included studies about functional and NF lesions, and patients with advanced disease. This might have an impact on the adverse event rate because complete ablation of NF pNETs with treatment of the tumor borders may increase the risk of acute pancreatitis. In contrast, for functional tumors, the treatment goal is to alleviate symptoms, and an "oncological" ablation may not always be mandatory. Furthermore, two-thirds of the included studies were case reports or small series with 2 to 3 patients. Thus, selection bias is not excluded. Currently, how to select patients for EUS-RFA remains controversial. Treatment decisions should take into account tumor features, patient comorbidities, and life expectancy, as well as surgery-associated morbidity and mortality rates. The results of larger cohort studies that evaluate long-term treatment responses and prognostic factors are needed. EUS-RFA is a promising treatment strategy for the management of small NF pNETs with excellent efficacy. Adverse events can often be managed by endoscopic or medical treatment. As tumor-free margins cannot be evaluated, further evidence focusing on long-term survival, follow-up modalities, and recurrence is needed.

PLACE OF ENDOSCOPIC ULTRASOUND-GUIDED RADIOFREQUENCY ABLATION FOR PANCREATIC ADENOCARCINOMA

Local radiofrequency ablation (RFA) technology is being developed as a supplementary therapy in the multimodal therapy strategy for unresectable nonmetastatic tumors.[33] However, the clinical application of intraoperative or percutaneous RFA for pancreatic ductal adenocarcinoma (PDAC) is limited because of the higher mortality and incidence of adverse events.

The first feasibility study was performed by Crinio and colleagues.[34] They evaluated the feasibility, safety, and technical success of pancreatic EUS-RFA.[9] Consecutive patients (8 with pancreatic adenocarcinoma and 1 with renal cancer metastasis) were referred for EUS-RFA. EUS-RFA was performed using an 18 gauge internally cooled electrode with a 5 or 10 mm exposed tip. Feasibility, technical success, or early and late adverse events were assessed.

One patient was excluded because of a large necrotic area. EUS-RFA was feasible in all the other 8 (100%) cases. An ablated area inside the tumor was achieved in all treated patients. No early or late major adverse event was observed after a mean follow-up of 6 months. Three patients experienced mild post-procedural abdominal pain. EUS-RFA seems a feasible and safe procedure for pancreatic neoplasms.

More recently, Jiang and colleagues[35] reported their experience in 8 patients with locally advanced pancreatic adenocarcinomas. The mean tumor sizes measured by EUS 1 month post-procedure were significantly reduced than those at pre-procedure (46.9 mm × 38.1 mm vs 39.5 mm × 29.5 mm); the pancreatic cancer mass was reduced by 34.3% 1 month after RFA treatment. The mean survival of the patients after EUS-RFA was 10.7 months and 16.1 months from the diagnosis. All patients did not have serious early adverse events. Only mild abdominal pain and mild pancreatitis occurred, suggesting that the power of 5 W and the time of 90 to 120 s were safe. The limitation of this study is that there is no control group, and it is a single-center study with a small sample size.

Another recent study has evaluated the association between EUS-RFA and chemotherapy.[36] A total of 22 patients with unresectable pancreatic cancer (n = 14, locally advanced unresectable; n = 8, metastatic) underwent EUS-RFA. The median CA19 to 9 levels before RFA were 200.8 U/mL. Among these patients, CA19 to 9 levels were greater than 200 U/mL in 11 patients (50%). Pancreatic cancer was located in the head of the pancreas in 14 patients (63.6%), in the pancreas body in 4 patients (18.2%), in the tail of the pancreas in 3 patients (13.6%), and in the resection margin in 1 patient (4.5%). The median size of the primary tumor was 38 mm. Sixteen patients (72.7%) had nodal involvement. All patients underwent gemcitabine-based chemotherapy before (n = 19) and after (n = 3) EUS-RFA. Among these patients, 18 (81.8%) received induction chemotherapy.

EUS-RFA was performed successfully in all patients. The median number of RFA sessions was 5. Over a median follow-up period of 21.23 months, 17 patients (77.3%) died because of disease progression. Twenty patients (95.5%) experienced treatment failure. Among these patients, treatment failure was first associated with local progression in 13 patients (59.1%), distant metastasis in 7 patients (31.8%), and both in one patient (4.5%). Early procedure-related adverse events occurred in 4 out of 107 sessions (3.74%), including peritonitis (n = 1) and abdominal pain (n = 3). There were no severe adverse events, and the patients improved completely after conservative treatment. Subsequent systemic chemotherapy was performed within 2 days. Randomized, large-sample, multicenter studies are needed to shed light on the efficacy of EUS-RFA, optimize RFA parameters (such as ablation time, power, and interval time), and explore whether the survival time of patients can be further improved by RFA and combined chemotherapy.

PLACE OF ENDOSCOPIC ULTRASOUND-GUIDED RADIOFREQUENCY ABLATION FOR PANCREATIC METASTASIS FROM RENAL CANCER

Glandular metastases, and more precisely, pancreatic metastases (PMs) from renal cell carcinoma (mRCC), are associated with long survival. Focal treatment to control oligo-metastatic disease and avoid systemic therapy is standard in RCC. However, pancreatic RFA remains a marginal and under-evaluated technique. Standard treatment remains pancreatectomy, with hazardous outcomes. Endoscopic ultrasound-guided radiofrequency ablation is an innovative approach to treating focal deep metastases and could be a relevant technique to control PM from RCC.

Chanez and colleagues[37] reported the largest series in the literature. They performed 26 EUS-RFA sessions to treat a total of 21 PMs in 12 patients. Nine patients underwent $\geq$2 EUS-RFA due to an incomplete necrosis of PM at first evaluation.

A second and third session for the same patient could be motivated by the presence of untreated metastases in the first session and uncomplete PM necrosis evaluated by CT scan defined by contrast-enhanced remnant tissue. All procedures achieved technical success with no immediate complications and all patients spent 2 days at the hospital for each session.

Two patients experienced complications requiring hospitalization and intervention (grade IIIb Clavien-Dindo). In the first patient, treated by a tyrosine kinase inhibitor at the time of EUS-RFA, a duodenal abscess occurred 2 months after the 2nd EUS-RFA. In the second patient, the only one with a biliary stent, a symptomatic hepatic abscess occurred 1 week after the EUS-RFA. At the time of analysis, all adverse effects had been resolved, and no further complications were detected in any patient. Median follow-up as the first EUS-RFA was 27.7 months (range 6.4–57.1).

Among the 21 PMs treated, 40% had a complete response at 12 months. The 6 month and 12 month focal control rates were 84.2% and 73.3%, respectively, among evaluable PMs. Progressive disease was observed in only 15.8% and 26.7% of evaluable PMs at 6 and 12 months, respectively. All patients were alive at the time of analysis and median progression-free survival for PM was 25.38 months. Comparing PM > 20 mm to those less than 20 mm, the 6 month focal control rate was lower (92% vs 71%) and the time to progression was shorter, although the difference was not statistically significant ($P = .06$). Tumor size was not significantly associated with a better response (OR 0.37, $P = .43$) in logistic regression analysis.

SUMMARY

EUS-RFA seems to be a promising treatment strategy for the management of small NF pNETs with excellent efficacy. Further evidence focusing on long-term survival, safety profile, and recurrence is needed.

Regarding pancreatic adenocarcinoma, EUS-RFA is technically feasible and safe for the management of unresectable tumors. EUS-RFA combined with systemic chemotherapy may be associated with favorable survival outcomes. A further larger-scale prospective comparative study is required to confirm these findings.

CLINICS CARE POINTS

- RFA for pancreatic net should be applied only to patients with a lesion of less than 2 cm and grade 1 on histology.
- RFA for pancreatic metastasis of renal cancer should be performed only for lesions of less than 2 cm.
- RFA of pancreatic adenocarcinoma should be performed only in the case of research protocols.

DISCLOSURE

The authors have nothing to disclose.

REFERENCES

1. Zhang L, Tan S, Huang S, et al. The safety and efficacy of endoscopic ultrasound-guided ablation therapy for solid pancreatic tumors: A systematic review. Scand J Gastroenterol 2020;55:1121–31.
2. Choi J-H, Seo D-W, Song TJ, et al. Endoscopic ultrasound-guided radiofrequency ablation for management of benign solid pancreatic tumors. Endoscopy 2018;50:1099–104.
3. Oleinikov K, Dancour A, Epshtein J, et al. Endoscopic ultrasound-guided radiofrequency ablation: A new therapeutic approach for pancreatic neuroendocrine tumors. J Clin Endocrinol Metab 2019;104:2637–47.
4. Barthet M, Giovannini M, Lesavre N, et al. Endoscopic ultrasound-guided radiofrequency ablation for pancreatic neuroendocrine tumors and pancreatic cystic neoplasms: A prospective multicenter study. Endoscopy 2019;51:836–42.

5. de Nucci G, Imperatore N, Mandelli ED, et al. Endoscopic ultrasound-guided radiofrequency ablation of pancreatic neuroendocrine tumors: A case series. Endosc Int Open 2020;8:E1754–8.
6. Barret M, Leblanc S, Rouquette A, et al. EUS-guided pancreatic radiofrequency ablation: Preclinical comparison of two currently available devices in a pig model. Endosc Int Open 2019;7:E138–43.
7. Kim HJ, Seo D-W, Hassanuddin A, et al. EUS-guided radiofrequency ablation of the porcine pancreas. Gastrointest Endosc 2012;76:1039–43.
8. Dindo D, Demartines N, Clavien P-A. Classification of surgical complications: A new proposal with evaluation in a cohort of 6336 patients and results of a survey. Ann Surg 2004;240:205–13.
9. Service FJ, McMahon MM, O'Brien PC, et al. Functioning insulinoma—incidence, recurrence, and long-term survival of patients: a 60-year study Mayo. Clin Proc 1991;66:711–9.
10. Jensen RT, Cadiot G, Brandi ML, et al. ENETS consensus guidelines for the management of patients with digestive neuroendocrine neoplasms: functional pancreatic endocrine tumor syndromes. Neuroendocrinology 2012;95:98–119.
11. Guettier J-M, Gorden P. Insulin secretion and insulin-producing tumors Expert. Rev Endocrinol Metab 2010;5:217–27.
12. Kitano M, Kudo M, Yamao K, et al. Characterization of small solid tumors in the pancreas: the value of contrast-enhanced harmonic endoscopic ultrasonography. Am J Gastroenterol 2012;107:303–10.
13. Patel KK, Kim MK. Neuroendocrine tumors of the pancreas: endoscopic diagnosis. Curr Opin Gastroenterol 2008;24:638–42.
14. Falconi M, Eriksson B, Kaltsas G, et al. ENETS consensus guidelines update for the management of patients with functional pancreatic neuroendocrine tumors and non-functional pancreatic neuroendocrine tumors. Neuroendocrinology 2016;103:153–71.
15. Lakhtakia S, Ramchandani M, Galasso D, et al. EUS-guided radiofrequency ablation for management of pancreatic insulinoma by using a novel needle electrode (with videos). Gastrointest Endosc 2016;83:234–9.
16. Waung JA, Todd JF, Keane MG, et al. Successful management of a sporadic pancreatic insulinoma by endoscopic ultrasound-guided radiofrequency ablation. Endoscopy 2016;48(Suppl 1):E144–5.
17. Bas-Cutrina F, Bargalló D, Gornals JB. Small pancreatic insulinoma: successful endoscopic ultrasound-guided radiofrequency ablation in a single session using a 22-G fine needle Dig. Endosc 2017;29:636–8.
18. Oleinikov K, Dancour A, Epshtein J, et al. Endoscopic ultrasound-guided radiofrequency ablation: a new therapeutic approach for pancreatic neuroendocrine tumors. J Clin Endocrinol Metab 2019;104:2637–47.
19. de Nucci G, Imperatore N, Mandelli ED, et al. Endoscopic ultrasound-guided radiofrequency ablation of pancreatic neuroendocrine tumors: a case seriesEndosc. Int Open 2020;8:E1754–8.
20. Furnica RM, Deprez P, Maiter D, et al. Endoscopic ultrasound-guided radiofrequency ablation: an effective and safe alternative for the treatment of benign insulinoma. Ann Endocrinol 2020;81:567–71.
21. Mehrabi A, Fischer L, Hafezi M, et al. A systematic review of localization, surgical treatment options, and outcome of insulinoma. Pancreas 2014;43:675–86.
22. Han SH, Han IW, Heo JS, et al. Laparoscopic versus open distal pancreatectomy for nonfunctioning pancreatic neuroendocrine tumors: a large single-center study. Surg Endosc 2018;32:443–9.

23. Jilesen APJ, van Eijck CHJ, in't Hof KH, et al. Postoperative complications, in-hospital mortality and 5-year survival after surgical resection for patients with a pancreatic neuroendocrine tumor: a systematic review World. J Surg 2016;40: 729–48.

24. Jeune F, Taibi A, Gaujoux S. Update on the surgical treatment of pancreatic neuroendocrine tumors. Scand J Surg 2020;109:42–52.

25. Sada A, Yamashita TS, Glasgow AE, et al. Comparison of benign and malignant insulinoma. Am J Surg 2021;221:437–47.

26. Câmara-de-Souza AB, Toyoshima MTK, Giannella ML, et al. Insulinoma: a retro-spective study analyzing the differences between benign and malignant tumors. Pancreatology 2018;18:298–303.

27. Andreassen M, Ilett E, Wiese D, et al. Surgical management, preoperative tumor localization, and histopathology of 80 patients operated on for insulinoma. J Clin Endocrinol Metab 2019;104:6129–38.

28. Marx M, Trosic-Ivanisevic T, Caillol F, et al. EUS-guided radiofrequency ablation for pancreatic insulinoma: experience in 2 tertiary centers. Gastrointest Endosc 2022;95(Issue 6):1256–63.

29. Marx M, Godat S, Caillol F, et al. Management of non-functional pancreatic neuro-endocrine tumors by endoscopic ultrasound-guided radiofrequency ablation: Retrospective study in two tertiary centers. Dig Endosc 2022;34(6):1207–13.

30. Pai M, Habib N, Senturk H, et al. Endoscopic ultrasound guided radiofrequency ablation, for pancreatic cystic neoplasms and neuroendocrine tumors. World J Gastrointest Surg 2015;7:52–9.

31. Rimbaş M, Horumbă M, Rizzatti G, et al. Interventional endoscopic ultrasound for pancreatic neuroendocrine neoplasms. Dig Endosc 2020;32:1031–41.

32. Imperatore N, de Nucci G, Mandelli ED, et al. Endoscopic ultrasound-guided ra-diofrequency ablation of pancreatic neuroendocrine tumors: A systematic review of the literature. Endosc Int Open 2020;8:E1759–64.

33. Siegel RL, Miller KD, Jemal A. Cancer statistics, 2020. CA Cancer J Clin 2020; 70:7–30.

34. Crinò SF, D'Onofrio M, Bernardoni L, et al. EUS-guided radiofrequency ablation (EUS-RFA) of solid pancreatic neoplasm using an 18-gauge needle electrode: Feasibility, safety, and technical success. J Gastrointestin Liver Dis 2018;27: 67–72.

35. Jiang J, Lou Q, Yang J, et al. Feasibility and safety of EUS-guided radiofrequency ablation in treatment of locally advanced, unresectable pancreatic cancer. En-dosc Ultrasound 2021 Sep-Oct;10(5):398–9.

36. Oh D, Seo D-W, Jun Song T, Park D-H, Koo Lee S, 1, Kim M-H. Clinical outcomes of EUS-guided radiofrequency ablation for unresectable pancreatic cancer: A prospective observational study. Endosc Ultrasound 2022;11(1):68–74.

37. Chanez B, Caillol F, Ratone J-P, et al. Endoscopic Ultrasound-Guided Radiofre-quency Ablation as an Future Alternative to Pancreatectomy for Pancreatic Me-tastases from Renal Cell Carcinoma: A Prospective Study. Cancers 2021; 13(21):5267.

Endoscopic Interventions in Pancreatic Cystic Neoplasms

Sung Hyun Cho, MD, Dong-Wan Seo, MD, PhD*

KEYWORDS

- Endosonography • Interventional • Pancreatic cyst • Pancreatic neoplasms
- Ethanol • Injection • Radiofreuqency ablation

KEY POINTS

- Endoscopic ultrasound (EUS)-guided through-the-needle biopsy provides histologic diagnoses that conventional modalities, such as cross-sectional imaging, EUS-morphology, and cystic fluid analysis cannot provide. This procedure helps avoid unnecessary lifelong surveillance.
- In patients who refuse surgery or have high surgical risk, EUS-guided pancreatic cystic ablation, including EUS-guided fine needle injection (FNI) using ethanol and/or paclitaxel and EUS-guided radiofrequency ablation (RFA) can be an optional therapeutic modality as an alternative to surgical resection.
- In unilocular or oligolocular pancreatic cystic neoplasms (PCNs) (>2 cm), EUS-FNI can be performed safely.
- In multilocular PCNs, such as microcystic serous cyst neoplasm, EUS-RFA can be performed by ablating multiple septations.

BACKGROUND

The incidence of pancreatic cystic neoplasms (PCNs) increased due to increases in incidental detection of the lesions on high-quality cross-sectional imaging.[1,2] The surveillance and therapeutic strategy for PCNs vary depending on their types because each type of cyst has different malignant potentials.[3,4] Among the various PCN types, mucinous cysts, such as intraductal papillary mucinous neoplasms (IPMNs) and mucinous cystic neoplasms (MCNs), have the potential for malignant transformation. The malignancy risk stratification should be evaluated in those cysts to establish therapeutic strategies such as life-long surveillance or surgical resection.[3,4] For nonmucinous cysts, such as serous cystic neoplasm (SCN), follow-up is recommended. Surgical resection, however, can be considered when symptomatic or in cases of continuous growth during follow-up.

Department of Gastroenterology, Asan Medical Center, University of Ulsan College of Medicine, 88, Olympic-ro 43-gil, Songpa-gu, Seoul 05505, South Korea
* Corresponding author. .
E-mail address: dwseoamc@amc.seoul.kr

Gastrointest Endoscopy Clin N Am 33 (2023) 867–877
https://doi.org/10.1016/j.giec.2023.04.007
1052-5157/23/© 2023 Elsevier Inc. All rights reserved.

An accurate diagnosis of the specific PCN type is important to avoid unnecessary life-long surveillance or surgical resection. However, an accurate diagnosis of PCN type is challenging in real-world clinical practice because cross-sectional imaging and endoscopic ultrasound (EUS) have limitations for accurate differential diagnosis of PCN types.[4] The presumptive diagnosis of PCNs is not always concordant with the histologic diagnosis of surgical specimens.[5,6] The presumptive diagnosis is traditionally based on the combination of diagnostic modalities, including cross-sectional imaging (computed tomography [CT], or MRI), EUS morphology, and EUS-guided fine needle aspiration (FNA) for cystic fluid analysis and cytology. However, these conventional modalities do not provide a definitive diagnosis of specific types of PCN; thus, tissue is still the issue. Considering the high morbidity of surgical resection, the therapeutic strategy should be established based on an accurate categorization of PCN types. With this background, EUS-guided through-the-needle biopsy (EUS-TTNB) using microforceps was introduced for tissue confirmation.[7] Tissues obtained from the cystic wall or mural nodule using EUS-TTNB can provide a histologic diagnosis. This procedure showed encouraging results in the efficacy and safety profile in categorizing types of PCNs.[8]

Surgical resection is the standard treatment in the management of mucinous cysts with concerning features or symptomatic non-mucinous cysts.[3,4] However, pancreatectomy entails high morbidity (20%–40%) and mortality (2%) rates.[9,10] EUS-guided pancreatic cystic ablation (EUS-PCA) is the alternative to surgical resection as a minimally invasive therapeutic modality, especially in high surgical risk patients. EUS-PCA can be performed safely with fewer major adverse events in patients who refuse surgery or have high surgical risks. EUS-PCA can be categorized into EUS-guided fine needle injection (FNI) using ethanol and/or other ablative agent and EUS-guided radiofrequency ablation (EUS-RFA). The type of EUS-PCA (EUS-FNI or EUS-RFA) can be chosen according to the characteristics of the PCNs.

ENDOSCOPIC ULTRASOUND FOR EVALUATION OF PANCREATIC CYSTIC NEOPLASM

Before the interventional EUS, PCNs should be fully evaluated by EUS, including EUS morphology and EUS-FNA for cystic fluid analysis. EUS morphology includes the evaluation of locularity, size, location, and presence of mural nodule, septation, and thickened wall. EUS morphology alone has limitations in accurately differentiating the type of PCNs because of interobserver variation. Therefore, EUS-FNA for cystic fluid analysis, including carcinoembryonic agent (CEA), amylase/lipase, and cytology, is generally performed for the differential diagnosis of PCN types. An elevated level of cystic fluid CEA (>192 ng/mL) can differentiate mucinous cysts from non-mucinous cysts with a sensitivity of 63% and a specificity of 93%.[11,12] The cytology of cystic fluid can identify mucinous cysts; however, it is not very useful because of the low cellularity of samples and low sensitivity.[13] The combination of EUS morphology and cystic fluid analysis showed better diagnostic results in the differential diagnosis between mucinous cysts and non-mucinous cysts.[12,14] However, cystic fluid CEA analysis and/or cytology cannot differentiate between IPMN and MCN and cannot identify cysts with high-grade dysplasia. Molecular markers of cystic fluid, such as DNA, RNA, and protein, have been introduced for the identification of mucinous cysts.[15,16]

ENDOSCOPIC ULTRASOUND-GUIDED THROUGH-THE-NEEDLE BIOPSY
Preprocedural Preparation

The potential indications for EUS-TTNB are as follows: (1) unilocular or oligolocular cysts (largest locule >2 cm); (2) indeterminate PCN in which conventional diagnostic modalities cannot provide a diagnosis of specific PCN type, thus, the result of EUS-TTNB is expected to change the strategy of surveillance and management of PCNs; and (3) before EUS-PCA to exclude high-grade dysplasia of mucinous cysts. The relative contraindication is cysts highly suspicious of malignancy because these PCNs require upfront surgical resection. The absolute contraindication for the EUS-TTNB is the same as that of other endoscopic procedures, including irreversible coagulopathy, active inflammation in the cyst such as abscess and infected necrosis, and short life expectancy.

Before the procedure, PCNs should be fully evaluated by cross-sectional imaging and EUS evaluation, including cyst size, thickened wall, and mural nodules. During the procedure, the patients are placed under conscious sedation or general anesthesia and are administered prophylactic antibiotics intravenously.

Techniques

EUS is initially performed using a conventional linear array echoendoscope to evaluate and record the characteristics of the cyst. The transgastric or transduodenal needle puncture by a 19-gauge needle is performed while avoiding any intervening vessels using Doppler imaging. To increase the accuracy of diagnosis of PCN type, FNA to obtain cystic fluid for analysis, including CEA, amylase/lipase, and cytology, should be performed during the same session of EUS-TTNB, which is recommended to be performed before TTNB to avoid contamination of cystic fluid to be analyzed. Although the cystic fluid is aspirated through a 19-gauge needle for cystic fluid analysis, a sufficient amount of cystic fluid should remain to secure enough space for the advancement of the microforceps. If the cyst collapses after cystic fluid aspiration, the same volume of normal saline injection can be instilled through a 19-gauge needle. After EUS-FNA, a microforceps is passed through the 19-gauge needle and advanced into the cyst (**Fig. 1**A). The targeted lesions can be cystic walls, septations, solid components, or mural nodules; mural nodules and thickened walls are preferentially targeted if possible. The microforceps in the pancreatic cyst is opened and gently pushed against the target lesion, then closed and pulled back to see the "tent sign" on the EUS image (**Fig. 1**B–C). Confirmation of the tent sign under EUS imaging is an important step to obtain a sufficient amount of specimen. The microforceps showing the tent sign is pulled back to obtain the specimen and retrieved from the 19-gauge needle, maintaining the needle tip inside the cysts. If the tissue grasped by the microforceps is too large to be retrieved through the 19-gauge needle, the microforceps and 19-gauge needle can be retrieved from the cyst simultaneously. This method has advantages in obtaining large tissues grasped by forceps and avoiding the squeezing artifact developed while retrieving through the 19-gauge needle. The microforceps passes through the 19-gauge needle or needle passes are performed multiple times until sufficient specimens (three to four visible tissue fragments) are obtained. After confirmation of visible tissues on the jaw of the microforceps, the specimens are deposited in a formalin jar and processed as routine histologic samples for histologic diagnosis (**Fig. 1**D). After completion of TTNB, residual cystic fluid is fully aspirated.

Postprocedural Consideration

Monitoring for at least 2 days after the procedures is recommended while maintaining the administration of intravenous antibiotics to observe possible postprocedural adverse events. A laboratory test and simple abdominal radiograph are carried out the next day. Diet can be resumed 24 hour after the procedure.

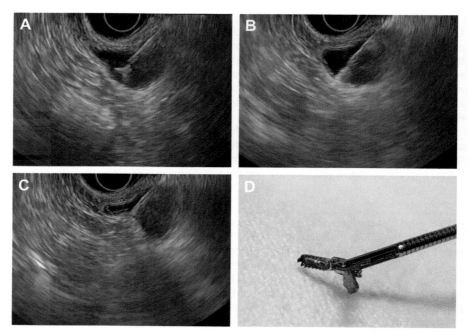

Fig. 1. EUS-TTNB. (*A*) After the cyst was punctured by a 19-gauge needle, the microforceps was introduced into the cyst through the 19-gauge needle. (*B*) The cystic wall was captured by closing the microforceps. (*C*) When pulling back the closed microforceps, the tent sign was noted on EUS image. (*D*) The specimen on the jaw of the microforceps was grossly confirmed. EUS-TTNB, endoscopic ultrasound-guided through-the-needle biopsies; IPMN, intraductal papillary mucinous neoplasm.

In a recent study, EUS-TTNB showed high rates of technical (100%) and diagnostic yield (82%) and a low rate of procedure-related adverse events (7%).[8] The most common adverse events were mild acute pancreatitis, followed by intracystic bleeding. All those adverse events were treated with conservative management without any interventions. In the subgroup analysis, a smaller number of visible biopsy specimens (<4 fragments) per session were associated with diagnostic failure.

ENDOSCOPIC ULTRASOUND-GUIDED FINE NEEDLE INJECTION
Preprocedural Preparation

The aim of EUS-FNI is to prevent the malignant transformation of mucinous cysts or treat PCN-related symptoms of non-mucinous cysts by ablating the lining epithelium of the cystic wall. The potential indications for the EUS-FNI are as follows: (1) unilocular cysts or oligolocular cysts (2–6 locules) with presumed or histologically confirmed mucinous cyst or symptomatic non-mucinous cyst and (2) a diameter of the largest locule greater than 2 cm. The relative contraindications are concerning features suggestive of malignant transformation or high malignant potential, including enhancing mural nodules, significant solid portion, and main pancreatic duct dilatation greater than 5 mm. The absolute contraindications include irreversible coagulopathy, high suspicion of pancreatic malignancy, acute pancreatitis, pancreatic abscess or necrosis, or short life expectancy.[17]

The candidates for the EUS-FNI should be carefully selected by a full evaluation of cysts based on cross-sectional imaging and EUS evaluation. EUS evaluation includes EUS morphology (cyst size, septation, wall thickness, mural nodule, solid portion, and communication with the pancreatic duct), cystic fluid analysis, and TTNB, if possible. The additional contrast-enhanced-EUS (CE-EUS) may be helpful for differentiation between mural nodules and mucin plugs in mucinous cysts. EUS-FNI is recommended to be performed after confirmation of the results of FNA and/or TTNB rather than at the same session of FNA and/or TTNB because diagnosing the PCN type is mandatory to select the candidates for the procedure. In the case of branch-duct IPMN, which is communicated with the pancreatic duct on EUS image, prophylactic plastic pancreatic stenting via endoscopic retrograde cholangiopancreatography (ERCP) is recommended before EUS-FNI to prevent acute pancreatitis. Before the procedure, the patients are administered prophylactic antibiotics intravenously.

Techniques

After delineation of the targeted PCN, the PCN is punctured by a 22-gauge needle under EUS guidance. In the case of a PCN with high viscosity of the cystic fluid, confirmed in the session of EUS-FNA, a 19-gauge needle with high suction pressure is preferred to a 22-gauge needle to aspirate cystic fluid smoothly during EUS-FNI. After insertion of the needle, the maximum possible volume of cystic fluid is aspirated while maintaining the tip of the needle in the cyst. The exact amount of aspirated cystic fluid should be recorded to prepare the same volume of ethanol or other ablative agents. Ninety-nine percent ethanol is injected into the cyst through the needle with equal volume to that of the aspirated cystic fluid and re-aspirated immediately. This procedure is referred to as lavage. The lavage is repeated carefully three to four times. After the lavage, injected ethanol and residual cystic fluid are fully aspirated, and the needle is retrieved from the cyst. In the case of PCN with a thickened wall and multiple septations, paclitaxel can be injected after full aspiration of ethanol and left in the cyst. The ethanol contacts the epithelium, causing protein denaturation, membrane lysis, and vascular occlusion of the epithelium.[18] Paclitaxel is a chemotherapeutic agent that arrests cellular microtubule assembly and interferes with cell replication, which induces a synergic ablative effect when remaining in the closed cystic cavity following ethanol lavage.[19]

Postprocedural Consideration

After the procedure, monitoring for at least 2 days is recommended while maintaining intravenous prophylactic antibiotics to observe possible postprocedural adverse events, including fever, abdominal pain, acute pancreatitis, and infection. A simple abdominal radiograph and laboratory test, including complete blood count, liver function tests, and amylase and/or lipase, is carried out the next day. Diet can be resumed 24 hour after the procedure. EUS-FNI shows a low rate of adverse events.[19,20] Potential procedural adverse events include abdominal pain, acute pancreatitis, and rarely thromboembolism, most of which show mild severity and can be treated with conservative management.

The treatment responses are evaluated by comparing the treated cyst volume with the original cyst volume, which can be calculated by measuring the diameter of the cyst on cross-sectional imaging (**Fig. 2**A–D). The responses are categorized into complete radiologic resolution, partial resolution, or persistence, corresponding to less than 5%, 5% to 25%, and greater than 25% of the original cyst volume, respectively.[17] Six-month interval follow-up CT scans are carried out until cyst resolution and yearly after that. The unilocularity and smaller cyst diameter may be the factors associated

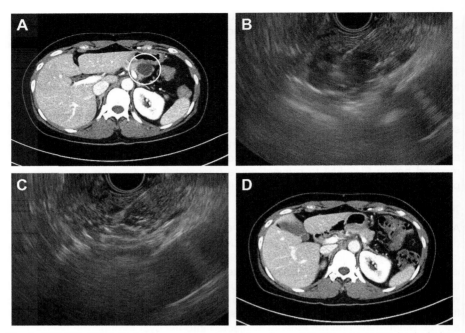

Fig. 2. EUS-FNI. (*A*). Initial CT scan showed a unilocular cyst in the pancreatic body (*white circle*). (*B*) After aspiration of the cystic fluid, the ethanol was injected into the cyst through the 19-gauge needle. (*C*) After completion of ethanol lavage, the injected ethanol and residual cystic fluid were fully aspirated. (*D*) One-year follow-up CT after the procedure showed complete resolution of the PCN. CT, computed tomography; EUS-FNI, EUS-guided fine needle injection; PCN, pancreatic cystic neoplasm.

with complete resolution.[20] Long-term follow-up after a complete resolution is recommended considering the possibility of relapse. In the long-term follow-up, the relapse rate after a complete resolution was reported to be 1.7%.[20]

ENDOSCOPIC ULTRASOUND-GUIDED RADIOFREQUENCY ABLATION
Preprocedural Preparation

EUS-FNI is not feasible in the management of multilocular PCNs, such as microcystic SCN, because it is challenging to inject the ablative agent into hundreds of small locules. In such cases, EUS-RFA can be an optional therapeutic modality. Microcystic SCNs showing a honeycomb appearance can be good candidates for EUS-RFA, which aims to ablate the septations within the cysts (**Fig. 3**A–F). Although SCNs are generally slow-growing PCNs and have a low risk of malignancy, they should only be treated when they are continuously growing or become symptomatic. Before the procedure, the patients are administered prophylactic antibiotics intravenously.

Techniques

In microcystic SCNs with lots of locules and a large amount of fluid, the duration of ablation time is lengthened due to water heating, and the delivery of uniform power of the radiofrequency current to the cystic wall is challenging. Therefore, the cystic fluid should be aspirated until a thin layer of fluid enough to maintain the needle tip

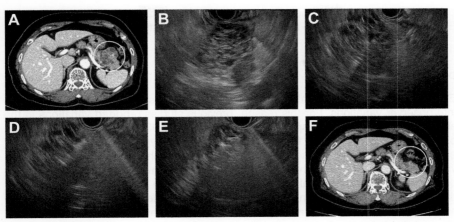

Fig. 3. EUS-RFA. (*A*) Initial CT scan showed microcystic SCN in the pancreatic tail (*white circle*). (*B*) EUS image showed microcystic SCN with honeycomb appearance. (*C*) The dedicated RFA needle punctured the PCN. (*D*) The white bubble sign on real-time EUS was visualized around the RFA needle tip during the ablation. (*E*) Additional needle puncture followed by ablation was performed to ablate other areas in the same cyst. (*F*) Six-month follow-up CT scan showed a reduction in the size of PCN (*white circle*). CT, computed tomography; EUS-RFA, EUS-guided radiofrequency ablation; PCN, pancreatic cystic neoplasm; SCN, serous cystic neoplasm.

remains. The dedicated 19-gauge RFA needle is inserted into the SCN under EUS guidance. After placing the tip of the needle at the septum of SCNs, the dedicated RF generator is activated with 50 W of power. The ablation is continued until the hyperechoic zone, referred to as the "white bubble" is visualized around the needle tip on a real-time EUS image. Additional needle passes can be performed to target different non-ablated zone within the same lesion for sufficient ablation of SCN. To avoid pancreatic duct injury, it is important to maintain a minimum safety margin of 5 mm between the needle tip and the main pancreatic duct.

Postprocedural Consideration

A laboratory test and a simple abdominal radiograph are performed the next day. Diet can be resumed 24 hour after the procedure. After the procedure, monitoring for at least 2 days is recommended while maintaining intravenous antibiotics to observe possible postprocedural adverse events.

Follow-up CE-EUS is performed to evaluate the initial treatment responses within 1 week after the first EUS-RFA. When CE-EUS shows viable lesions, a second session of EUS-RFA is performed to ablate residual lesions. After completion of EUS-RFA sessions, the follow-up strategy is similar to that of EUS-FNI (6 months follow-up CT until resolution and yearly after that). A pilot study reported a reduction in all cases of SCN, including 62% partial response, 38% stable disease, and 0% complete response.[21] Considering the ablative zone and concerns about adverse events, EUS-RFA should only target the septations within the cysts rather than margin of the cyst (cystic wall) to be ablated. Therefore, it is challenging to ablate SCNs completely (complete response) using EUS-RFA. However, EUS-RFA can reduce the volume of microcystic SCN and alleviate cyst-related symptoms. Possible adverse events include abdominal pain, acute pancreatitis, and pancreatic duct stricture. When the targeted ablative zone is close to the main pancreatic duct, prophylactic plastic pancreatic stenting via ERCP may be considered to prevent pancreatic ductal stricture.

DISCUSSION

EUS morphology alone for categorizing the types of PCNs has limitations arising from interobserver variations. For this reason, previous studies reported variations in the sensitivity (36%–91%) and specificity (48%–94%) of EUS in differentiating the type of PCNs.[12,14,22,23] However, the categorization of cyst type often depends on EUS-based diagnoses made by the combination of EUS morphology and cystic fluid analysis. EUS-TTNB provides a histologic diagnosis that conventional modalities cannot provide. With the histological diagnosis of the PCN type by EUS-TTNB, malignancy risk stratification of PCNs can be established; hence, patients can avoid unnecessary surgical resection, which entails high morbidities. In a previous study, 10 of 37 cases showed discrepancies between the diagnosis of EUS-TTNB and presumptive diagnosis based on conventional modalities, such as cross-sectional imaging and EUS-based evaluation for categorizing the types of PCNs.[8] Of these, EUS-TTNB changed the therapeutic strategies in four patients.[8] This suggests that EUS-TTNB helps avoid unnecessary life-long surveillance or surgical resection.

Crinò and colleagues[24] reported that two visible specimens obtained from EUS-TTNB reached 100% histologic adequacy and specific diagnosis in 74%. Cho and colleagues[8] reported that a higher number of biopsies increased the diagnostic yield (≥ 4 biopsies, 93% vs <4 biopsies, 67%; $P = .045$). Yet, considering that repeated punctures and biopsies can lead to the leakage of PCNs, repeated needle punctures are considered only when the cyst volume is large enough to be punctured. Further well-designed prospective studies are needed to establish standardized protocols, including the cutoff number of needle passages and biopsies in EUS-TTNB.

The recent clinical guidelines did not describe the role of EUS-PCA in detail as a therapeutic modality.[3,4] However, as EUS-PCA has gained popularity, it has been performed more widely in patients who refuse or cannot undergo surgery. A position statement on EUS-PCA was also published recently.[17]

Ethanol and paclitaxel were first introduced as ablative agents in EUS-FNI. Other agents, such as the combination of paclitaxel and gemcitabine without ethanol, and lauromacrogol were introduced as effective ablative agents in previous clinical trials.[25,26] Owing to the absence of unified protocols of procedure and case selection, it is difficult to compare ablative agents, and varying results of efficacy and safety have been reported. One of the major challenges of EUS-PCA is selecting an appropriate candidate for the procedure because PCNs with a high risk of malignancy should be excluded in candidates for the procedure considering the complete resolution rate (62%–72%).[19,20] EUS-TTNB may help select the appropriate candidate by histologic diagnosis.

Another concern regarding EUS-PCA is whether PCA can complete ablation histologically and consequently change its biological behavior. The treatment response was evaluated by measuring the treated cystic volume compared with the original cystic volume in EUS-FNI-related studies because the biological response cannot be easily evaluated in real-world clinical practice.[17,19,20,25] Previous studies reported genetic change after EUS-FNI by measuring the cystic fluid DNA, with loss of mutations, such as KRAS, found in some cases.[27] Oh and colleagues[19] reported cases of PCNs subjected to surgery after EUS-FNI, wherein histology showed the histologic degree of epithelial ablation ranging from 0% to 100%. Therefore, a surrogate marker of biologic response rather than radiologic response is needed to evaluate the efficacy of EUS-FNI.

Despite the low malignant potential, SCN can be a candidate for EUS-PCA when symptomatic. EUS-RFA has shown promising results in terms of treating pancreatic tumors.[28,29] This procedure can also be performed in microcystic SCN by ablating multiple septations. In a retrospective study, although a complete resolution was not observed in the study population during follow-up, all patients achieved a reduction in cyst volume.[21] Considering that SCN has benign biologic behavior and the aim of the procedure is to alleviate symptoms, EUS-RFA is clinically efficacious in treating symptomatic microcystic SCN.

SUMMARY

EUS-guided diagnostic and therapeutic interventions in PCNs have been considered alternatives to conventional modalities. EUS-TTNB has advantages over the conventional modalities for diagnosing PCNs in providing histologic diagnosis, including the degree of dysplasia. Considering the possibility of diagnostic failure in EUS-TTNB, a combination with other diagnostic modalities, including cystic fluid analysis, cytology, and imaging modalities, is recommended for evaluating PCNs.

EUS-PCA can be performed to treat PCNs in patients who refuse surgery or have high surgical risk. Unlike surgical resection, complete resolution cannot be achieved in all cases. Therefore, before the procedure, a thorough evaluation of PCNs, including cross-sectional imaging and EUS, should be conducted to select appropriate candidates for EUS-PCA. EUS-TTNB can help select a candidate for EUS-PCA by excluding the high risk of malignancy. Generally, EUS-FNI is performed as EUS-PCA. In the case of microcystic SCN, in which EUS-FNI is not feasible, EUS-RFA can be performed. Considering its good safety profile, EUS-PCA is a good optional modality for selected patients.

CLINICS CARE POINTS

- Endoscopic ultrasound (EUS)-guided through-the-needle biopsy can help patients avoid unnecessary surgery or life-long surveillance when the type of cyst is indeterminate by conventional modalities.

- Before endoscopic ultrasound-guided pancreatic cystic ablation (EUS-PCA), evaluation of malignancy risk stratification of pancreatic cystic neoplasms (PCNs) for excluding PCNs with high malignancy potential is necessary to select the appropriate candidate for the procedure.

- The type of EUS-PCA (EUS-guided radiofrequency ablate [EUS-FNI] or EUS-guided radiofrequency ablation [EUS-RFA]) and additional ablative agent in EUS-FNI is decided based on the characteristics of PCNs. Unilocular or oligolocular cysts (>2 cm) are appropriate for EUS-FNI, and microcystic SCN is appropriate for EUS-RFA. EUS-FNI is generally performed using ethanol. In cases with a thickened cystic wall or complicated septation, additional retention of paclitaxel following ethanol lavage can be considered.

- Even in cases of complete resolution after EUS-RFA, cross-sectional imaging follow-up with regular intervals should be continued, considering the possibility of relapse and incomplete epithelial ablation.

CONFLICT OF INTEREST DISCLOSURE

The authors declare no conflicts of interest or financial relationships relevant to this publication.

REFERENCES

1. Lee KS, Sekhar A, Rofsky NM, et al. Prevalence of incidental pancreatic cysts in the adult population on MR imaging. Am J Gastroenterol 2010;105(9):2079–84.
2. Laffan TA, Horton KM, Klein AP, et al. Prevalence of unsuspected pancreatic cysts on MDCT. AJR Am J Roentgenol 2008;191(3):802–7.
3. Elta GH, Enestvedt BK, Sauer BG, et al. ACG clinical guideline: diagnosis and management of pancreatic cysts. Am J Gastroenterol 2018;113(4):464–79.
4. European evidence-based guidelines on pancreatic cystic neoplasms. Gut 2018; 67(5):789–804.
5. Gaujoux S, Brennan MF, Gonen M, et al. Cystic lesions of the pancreas: changes in the presentation and management of 1,424 patients at a single institution over a 15-year time period. J Am Coll Surg 2011;212(4):590–600 [discussion: 600-3].
6. Valsangkar NP, Morales-Oyarvide V, Thayer SP, et al. 851 resected cystic tumors of the pancreas: a 33-year experience at the Massachusetts General Hospital. Surgery 2012;152(3 Suppl 1):S4–12.
7. Aparicio JR, Martínez J, Niveiro M, et al. Direct intracystic biopsy and pancreatic cystoscopy through a 19-gauge needle EUS (with videos). Gastrointest Endosc 2010;72(6):1285–8.
8. Cho SH, Song TJ, Seo DW, et al. Efficacy and safety of EUS-guided through-the-needle microforceps biopsy sampling in categorizing the type of pancreatic cystic lesions. Gastrointest Endosc 2022;95(2):299–309.
9. Brugge WR, Lauwers GY, Sahani D, et al. Cystic neoplasms of the pancreas. N Engl J Med 2004;351(12):1218–26.
10. Allen PJ, D'Angelica M, Gonen M, et al. A selective approach to the resection of cystic lesions of the pancreas: results from 539 consecutive patients. Ann Surg 2006;244(4):572–82.
11. Thornton GD, McPhail MJ, Nayagam S, et al. Endoscopic ultrasound guided fine needle aspiration for the diagnosis of pancreatic cystic neoplasms: a meta-analysis. Pancreatology 2013;13(1):48–57.
12. Brugge WR, Lewandrowski K, Lee-Lewandrowski E, et al. Diagnosis of pancreatic cystic neoplasms: a report of the cooperative pancreatic cyst study. Gastroenterology 2004;126(5):1330–6.
13. de Jong K, Poley JW, van Hooft JE, et al. Endoscopic ultrasound-guided fine-needle aspiration of pancreatic cystic lesions provides inadequate material for cytology and laboratory analysis: initial results from a prospective study. Endoscopy 2011;43(7):585–90.
14. Cizginer S, Turner BG, Bilge AR, et al. Cyst fluid carcinoembryonic antigen is an accurate diagnostic marker of pancreatic mucinous cysts. Pancreas 2011;40(7): 1024–8.
15. Springer S, Wang Y, Dal Molin M, et al. A combination of molecular markers and clinical features improve the classification of pancreatic cysts. Gastroenterology 2015;149(6):1501–10.
16. Singhi AD, Zeh HJ, Brand RE, et al. American Gastroenterological Association guidelines are inaccurate in detecting pancreatic cysts with advanced neoplasia: a clinicopathologic study of 225 patients with supporting molecular data. Gastrointest Endosc 2016;83(6):1107–17.e2.

17. Teoh AY, Seo DW, Brugge W, et al. Position statement on EUS-guided ablation of pancreatic cystic neoplasms from an international expert panel. Endosc Int Open 2019;7(9):E1064–77.
18. Gelczer RK, Charboneau JW, Hussain S, et al. Complications of percutaneous ethanol ablation. J Ultrasound Med 1998;17(8):531–3.
19. Oh HC, Seo DW, Song TJ, et al. Endoscopic ultrasonography-guided ethanol lavage with paclitaxel injection treats patients with pancreatic cysts. Gastroenterology 2011;140(1):172–9.
20. Choi JH, Seo DW, Song TJ, et al. Long-term outcomes after endoscopic ultrasound-guided ablation of pancreatic cysts. Endoscopy 2017;49(9):866–73.
21. Oh D, Ko SW, Seo DW, et al. Endoscopic ultrasound-guided radiofrequency ablation of pancreatic microcystic serous cystic neoplasms: a retrospective study. Endoscopy 2021;53(7):739–43.
22. de Jong K, van Hooft JE, Nio CY, et al. Accuracy of preoperative workup in a prospective series of surgically resected cystic pancreatic lesions. Scand J Gastroenterol 2012;47(8–9):1056–63.
23. Sedlack R, Affi A, Vazquez-Sequeiros E, et al. Utility of EUS in the evaluation of cystic pancreatic lesions. Gastrointest Endosc 2002;56(4):543–7.
24. Crinò SF, Bernardoni L, Brozzi L, et al. Association between macroscopically visible tissue samples and diagnostic accuracy of EUS-guided through-the-needle microforceps biopsy sampling of pancreatic cystic lesions. Gastrointest Endosc 2019;90(6):933–43.
25. Moyer MT, Sharzehi S, Mathew A, et al. The safety and efficacy of an alcohol-free pancreatic cyst ablation protocol. Gastroenterology 2017;153(5):1295–303.
26. Linghu E, Du C, Chai N, et al. A prospective study on the safety and effectiveness of using lauromacrogol for ablation of pancreatic cystic neoplasms with the aid of EUS. Gastrointest Endosc 2017;86(5):872–80.
27. DeWitt JM, Al-Haddad M, Sherman S, et al. Alterations in cyst fluid genetics following endoscopic ultrasound-guided pancreatic cyst ablation with ethanol and paclitaxel. Endoscopy 2014;46(6):457–64.
28. Song TJ, Seo DW, Lakhtakia S, et al. Initial experience of EUS-guided radiofrequency ablation of unresectable pancreatic cancer. Gastrointest Endosc 2016;83(2):440–3.
29. Choi JH, Seo DW, Song TJ, et al. Endoscopic ultrasound-guided radiofrequency ablation for management of benign solid pancreatic tumors. Endoscopy 2018;50(11):1099–104.

Statement of Ownership, Management, and Circulation
(All Periodicals Publications Except Requester Publications)

1. Publication Title	2. Publication Number	3. Filing Date
GASTROINTESTINAL ENDOSCOPY CLINICS OF NORTH AMERICA	012 – 603	9/18/2023

4. Issue Frequency	5. Number of Issues Published Annually	6. Annual Subscription Price
JAN, APR, JUL, OCT	4	$381.00

7. Complete Mailing Address of Known Office of Publication (Not printer) (Street, city, county, state, and ZIP+4®)

ELSEVIER INC.
230 Park Avenue, Suite 800
New York, NY 10169

Contact Person
Malathi Samayan

Telephone (Include area code)
91-44-4299-4507

8. Complete Mailing Address of Headquarters or General Business Office of Publisher (Not printer)

ELSEVIER INC.
230 Park Avenue, Suite 800
New York, NY 10169

9. Full Names and Complete Mailing Addresses of Publisher, Editor, and Managing Editor (Do not leave blank)

Publisher (Name and complete mailing address)

Dolores Meloni, ELSEVIER INC.
1600 JOHN F KENNEDY BLVD. SUITE 1600
PHILADELPHIA, PA 19103-2899

Editor (Name and complete mailing address)

KERRY HOLLAND, ELSEVIER INC.
1600 JOHN F KENNEDY BLVD. SUITE 1600
PHILADELPHIA, PA 19103-2899

Managing Editor (Name and complete mailing address)

PATRICK MANLEY, ELSEVIER INC.
1600 JOHN F KENNEDY BLVD. SUITE 1600
PHILADELPHIA, PA 19103-2899

10. Owner (Do not leave blank. If the publication is owned by a corporation, give the name and address of the corporation immediately followed by the names and addresses of all stockholders owning or holding 1 percent or more of the total amount of stock. If not owned by a corporation, give the names and addresses of the individual owners. If owned by a partnership or other unincorporated firm, give its name and address as well as those of each individual owner. If the publication is published by a nonprofit organization, give its name and address.)

Full Name	Complete Mailing Address
WHOLLY OWNED SUBSIDIARY OF REED/ELSEVIER US HOLDINGS	1600 JOHN F KENNEDY BLVD. SUITE 1600 PHILADELPHIA, PA 19103-2899

11. Known Bondholders, Mortgagees, and Other Security Holders Owning or Holding 1 Percent or More of Total Amount of Bonds, Mortgages, or Other Securities. If none, check box ▶ ☐ None

Full Name	Complete Mailing Address
N/A	

12. Tax Status (For completion by nonprofit organizations authorized to mail at nonprofit rates) (Check one)
The purpose, function, and nonprofit status of this organization and the exempt status for federal income tax purposes:
☒ Has Not Changed During Preceding 12 Months
☐ Has Changed During Preceding 12 Months (Publisher must submit explanation of change with this statement)

PS Form 3526, July 2014 [Page 1 of 4 (see instructions page 4)] PSN: 7530-01-000-9931   PRIVACY NOTICE: See our privacy policy on www.usps.com.

---

13. Publication Title	14. Issue Date for Circulation Data Below
GASTROINTESTINAL ENDOSCOPY CLINICS OF NORTH AMERICA	JULY 2023

15. Extent and Nature of Circulation			Average No. Copies Each Issue During Preceding 12 Months	No. Copies of Single Issue Published Nearest to Filing Date
a. Total Number of Copies (Net press run)			115	113
b. Paid Circulation (By Mail and Outside the Mail)	(1)	Mailed Outside-County Paid Subscriptions Stated on PS Form 3541 (Include paid distribution above nominal rate, advertiser's proof copies, and exchange copies)	57	59
	(2)	Mailed In-County Paid Subscriptions Stated on PS Form 3541 (Include paid distribution above nominal rate, advertiser's proof copies, and exchange copies)	0	0
	(3)	Paid Distribution Outside the Mails Including Sales Through Dealers and Carriers, Street Vendors, Counter Sales, and Other Paid Distribution Outside USPS®	33	26
	(4)	Paid Distribution by Other Classes of Mail Through the USPS (e.g. First-Class Mail®)	6	8
c. Total Paid Distribution [Sum of 15b (1), (2), (3), and (4)]		▶	96	95
d. Free or Nominal Rate Distribution (By Mail and Outside the Mail)	(1)	Free or Nominal Rate Outside-County Copies Included on PS Form 3541	18	17
	(2)	Free or Nominal Rate In-County Copies Included on PS Form 3541	0	0
	(3)	Free or Nominal Rate Copies Mailed at Other Classes Through the USPS (e.g. First-Class Mail)	0	0
	(4)	Free or Nominal Rate Distribution Outside the Mail (Carriers or other means)	1	1
e. Total Free or Nominal Rate Distribution (Sum of 15d (1), (2), (3) and (4))		▶	19	18
f. Total Distribution (Sum of 15c and 15e)		▶	115	113
g. Copies not Distributed (See Instructions to Publishers #4 (page 83))		▶	0	0
h. Total (Sum of 15f and g)		▶	115	113
i. Percent Paid (15c divided by 15f times 100)		▶	83.84%	84.07%

* If you are claiming electronic copies, go to line 16 on page 3. If you are not claiming electronic copies, skip to line 17 on page 3.

16. Electronic Copy Circulation		Average No. Copies Each Issue During Preceding 12 Months	No. Copies of Single Issue Published Nearest to Filing Date
a. Paid Electronic Copies	▶		
b. Total Paid Print Copies (Line 15c) + Paid Electronic Copies (Line 16a)	▶		
c. Total Print Distribution (Line 15f) + Paid Electronic Copies (Line 16a)	▶		
d. Percent Paid (Both Print & Electronic Copies) (16b divided by 16c × 100)	▶		

☒ I certify that 50% of all my distributed copies (electronic and print) are paid above a nominal price.

17. Publication of Statement of Ownership

☒ If the publication is a general publication, publication of this statement is required. Will be printed   ☐ Publication not required.
in the OCTOBER 2023 issue of this publication.

18. Signature and Title of Editor, Publisher, Business Manager, or Owner

Malathi Samayan

Malathi Samayan - Distribution Controller   Date 9/18/2023

I certify that all information furnished on this form is true and complete. I understand that anyone who furnishes false or misleading information on this form or who omits material or information requested on the form may be subject to criminal sanctions (including fines and imprisonment) and/or civil sanctions (including civil penalties).

PS Form 3526, July 2014 (Page 3 of 4)   PRIVACY NOTICE: See our privacy policy on www.usps.com

Moving?

Make sure your subscription moves with you!

To notify us of your new address, find your **Clinics Account Number** (located on your mailing label above your name), and contact customer service at:

Email: journalscustomerservice-usa@elsevier.com

800-654-2452 (subscribers in the U.S. & Canada)
314-447-8871 (subscribers outside of the U.S. & Canada)

Fax number: 314-447-8029

Elsevier Health Sciences Division
Subscription Customer Service
3251 Riverport Lane
Maryland Heights, MO 63043

Printed and bound by CPI Group (UK) Ltd, Croydon, CR0 4YY

08/05/2025

01864749-0004